D0936268

# SOME CLINICAL APPROACHES TO PSYCHIATRIC NURSING

# SOME CLINICAL APPROACHES TO PSYCHIATRIC NURSING

*Edited by*

### SHIRLEY F. BURD, B.S., M.S., R.N.

Assistant Professor, Nursing, Graduate Program in Advanced Psychiatric Nursing, College of Nursing and Graduate School, Rutgers, The State University of New Jersey, Newark, New Jersey

### MARGARET A. MARSHALL, B.S., M.S., R.N.

Instructor, Nursing, Graduate Program in Advanced Psychiatric Nursing, College of Nursing and Graduate School, Rutgers, The State University of New Jersey, Newark, New Jersey

The Macmillan Company, New York
Collier-Macmillan Limited, London

*First Printing,* April, 1963

Library of Congress catalog card number: 63–11787

The Macmillan Company, New York
*Collier-Macmillan Canada, Ltd., Toronto, Ontario*
DIVISIONS OF THE CROWELL-COLLIER PUBLISHING COMPANY

*Printed in the United States of America*


DESIGNED BY RONALD FARBER

*To the Renaissance of
Clinical Practice
of Nursing*

# FOREWORD

This work is another indication of a groundswell of interest in clinical problems in nursing situations. Nurses have always said their interest lay with clinical problems in nursing care of patients, but since the turn of the century there have been many counterpulls. Nurses have been distracted by many new demands upon their time—to administer hospital units, to teach nonprofessional personnel, to prepare work situations for other disciplines not previously concerned in the direct care of patients, to orient lay volunteers who assist in hospitals, and in general to complete any chore not claimed by other hospital personnel. But more nurses are awakening to the fact that what they really want is direct care of patients, and a chorus of grass-roots voices is petitioning for this return to the bedside. This book will help nurses to see and seize the opportunities before them.

In psychiatric work the possibility of nurses working psychotherapeutically in the direct care of patients is also being realized. In psychiatric settings the problem is compounded by a shortage of professional personnel, particularly professional nurses are in short supply. There are many reasons for this shortage: too few positions for nurses are budgeted, public mental hospitals are often located in remote places, salaries are unattractive, supervision of the novice nurse is inept or absent, the size of the patient load is often staggering, auxiliary personnel to assist the professional nurse are too often adapted to custodial ways, and the possibility of reduction in their power and change in their behavior is too often remote, professional stimulation by way of the library and professional colleague relationships is often meager at best. But these reasons are not the main ones. Nurses are "doers"; they are energetic, active people who, through their basic nursing education, have come to expect rather dramatic recoveries, usually in a short hospital stay, in most of their patients. This expectation in the psychiatric setting is not realistic. Yet, even the "psychiatric affiliation"—that portion of the basic nursing curriculum which is supposed to prepare all nurse students for staff nurse positions in psychiatric settings—has the same expectation hidden in it. In most schools

—vii

a period of 8 to 16 weeks (of a total of 120 to 144 weeks of basic nursing education) is devoted to the "psychiatric affiliation." In other words about one-fifteenth of the curriculum is devoted to preparing nurses to do staff nursing with the mentally ill, who comprise over 50 per cent of the hospitalized patient population. The main reason more nurses do not seek work in psychiatric facilities upon graduation from basic schools of nursing is that their preparation has not really fitted them for the work of a staff nurse in such units. At least six months for the psychiatric affiliation are necessary.

It is possible that directors of diploma schools of nursing and deans of collegiate schools of nursing need help in grasping the nature of clinical problems faced by nurses in the psychiatric setting. These problems are not completely different from interpersonal problems seen in a general hospital setting, except in their intensity and their scope as an interference to effective personal living. In the general hospital the nurse can gain satisfactions from her work and assume the "wellness" of the patient once an invading organism or dysfunctioning body part has been dealt with and the patient has been discharged. If the nurse does not notice interpersonal difficulties of patients, she will not be concerned about them. While it is desirable for the nurse to make such observations and to consider suitable assistance to the general hospital patient, it is likely that her failure to notice generally will not lead to chronicity for the patient, as it does in the psychiatric setting. The general hospital patient has at least one foot in the community and can seek other sources of help if he recognizes his need. In the psychiatric hospital the patient is trapped by his illness; if professional personnel do not realize the patient's "trap adaptation" and find the ways to work with patients so that their problems can be solved, the patient is trapped forever. And so public mental hospitals have this huge backlog of chronic patients—a way out must be found for them and the backlog must be released!

In order for professional workers, including nurses, to be fully useful to patients, the clinical problems the patients present must be seen and understood. Painstaking study of such clinical problems and reporting results so that all psychiatric workers can benefit from the experience of nurses are tasks of nurses working in the psychiatric setting. Learning from the experiences of other nurses is a beginning step for nurses who have not yet begun such studies as a part of their work. Learning how to study a clinical problem in the psychiatric setting is an aspect of the psychiatric affiliation. And stimulating this trend, as an aspect of the groundswell of interest in clinical problems in nursing situations, is a responsibility of graduates of master's and doctoral programs in psychiatric nursing, for these nurses are initiating new insights and new practices of nursing in the psychiatric setting.

In this work are samples of the many interpersonal problems of psychiatric patients. Nurses in psychiatric facilities can check the problems reported in this book against their own everyday observations of psychiatric patients and report through some media any new understanding of the nature of the problem or any approaches not discussed in this volume that work better. Every nurse who works in a psychiatric unit can decide today to study one small problem that interests her. This work provides several different models for reporting results of study of such problems. The practicing nurse has a gold mine of opportunity to collect data, every day, from many patients. This can be done through her own observations and those of students and psychiatric attendants of one clinical problem. Such data can be recorded verbatim in some form for simple and easy study. Then reporting the results, not only to nurse colleagues but, through publication, to other professional colleagues as well, enables the nurse practitioner to contribute insights deriving from clinical practice.

The nursing profession is on the way to becoming a profession in the full sense of this word. This forward movement will be speeded when nurses the country over take it as their responsibility to observe, study, and report findings on a clinical problem of interest and concern to each nurse. There is no limit to the contribution that the profession of nursing can make in an understanding of problems of human relatedness; the failures to achieve human relationships are everywhere apparent in the behavior of the mentally ill. Nursing as a social force must help undo these failures, and it must cite the preventive interventions that will obviate them in time. Nursing must also share its insights with other disciplines concerned in the field of mental health and psychiatric work; it cannot continue only to borrow theories from other professions but must offer also viable theories for its own use and for consideration by other disciplines. This work is a step in these directions, it is written by the "next generation" of nurse leaders, and in turn it should spur more widespread interest and the development of still other contributors to nursing literature on clinical problems in nursing in psychiatric facilities.

HILDEGARD E. PEPLAU, R.N., ED.D.
Professor in Nursing,
Director, Graduate Program in
   Advanced Psychiatric Nursing
Rutgers, The State University of
   New Jersey

# PREFACE

*Some Clinical Approaches to Psychiatric Nursing* is a compilation of clinical papers, research reports, and conceptual frameworks. These papers have been available to students, faculty, and others as they have become available to the editors over the course of six years. Interest in such endeavors has been increasing recently, as evidenced by more frequent requests to make the papers available to other nurses and other schools. Similarly, the number of such papers has increased with the passing of each year. These facts assisted us in determining that this volume should be made available to the general reading public of nursing.

All contributors have been graduate fellows enrolled in the Program in Advanced Psychiatric Nursing at the Graduate School, Rutgers, The State University of New Jersey. Generally, contributions were written during the authors' appointments as graduate fellows in the master's program. These chapters, therefore, represent the authors' competencies and views at various times during their program of study, and in varying years of the initial six years of our graduate program.

For ease in reading, this book has been sectioned as follows: Section I deals with problems in communication. While the emphasis is on verbal communication, or spoken language, nonverbal communication is of recognizable importance as well. That unspoken communication is of vital concern in interpersonal relationships can be noted by the many books and articles that have been published of late on the subjects of nonverbal communication, the language of gestures, body language, dreams, and the like. While these systems of communication are valuable for those who work with people—be they peers, friends, or the general public—the first section of this text is concerned primarily with spoken or written language.

Section II is concerned with a diversity of topics. These problems are some of those encountered by all nurses whether they work in nonpsychiatric or psychiatric facilities. Generally, the authors have attempted to communicate the essential elements of professional nursing care—clinical observations, explanatory theory of those observations, and methods of applying this theory to clinical practice of nursing. Chapters 24, 26, and

29 are exceptions to this section in that they were written during the educative process of the program.

Section III includes reports of clinical research endeavors of the fellows, with the exception of Chapter 39. The initial four chapters are portions of clinical research or papers based on the research. The final three reports are presented in their entirety since they are not available through interuniversity library loan.

Section IV is comprised of conceptual frameworks. Throughout the compilation of this volume, we noted recurringly the stated or apparent employment of conceptual frameworks by the various authors. These frameworks were used either in the intellectual process that "bridges the gap" between theory and clinical practice of nursing, or to place the elements of theory and their relationships in logical and rational order. Since these conceptual frameworks have been used by many of the contributors to this text, they are included as a separate section. The initial five chapters of this section were developed by the authors following completion of their last educative program of study rather than while they were on student status.

The glossary includes definitions developed and used by the various contributors in their papers. Many of these definitions are operational in form and have been excerpted from the papers by the editors and presented in simple form. All are labeled with the name of the contributors.

Finally, we wish to acknowledge that this compilation has been prepared with the assistance of many people. We are indebted to all those who contributed chapters. Further, we would like to thank all of those many people who encouraged us and who made valuable suggestions during the months this text was in preparation. Specifically, we wish to thank several persons for their roles in bringing the volume to fruition. Dr. Peplau encouraged and held high expectations of the contributors and the editors, in addition to which she prepared the Foreword. We wish to thank Mrs. Jacqueline Gettings and Mrs. Mary Griffin for their efforts in preparing the manuscript in its final form.

Newark, New Jersey

SHIRLEY F. BURD
MARGARET A. MARSHALL

# CONTRIBUTORS

ARMSTRONG, SHIRLEY W., R.N., M.S., Instructor, Psychiatric Nursing, College of Nursing, Rutgers, The State University of New Jersey, Newark, New Jersey

BAKER, JOAN BACHAND, R.N., M.S., Acting Instructor, School of Nursing, University of Washington, Seattle, Washington

BURD, SHIRLEY FARLEY, R.N., M.S., Assistant Professor, Nursing, Graduate Program in Advanced Psychiatric Nursing, College of Nursing and Graduate School, Rutgers, The State University of New Jersey

CARTER, ELIZABETH WACKERMAN, R.N., M.S., Assistant in Nursing, Executive Division of Psychiatry, Montefiore Hospital, The Bronx, New York

CLACK, JANICE, R.N., M.S., Clinical Specialist, Psychiatric Nursing, Plymouth State Home and Training School, Northville, Michigan

DAVIS, SHIRLEY EBERLEIN, R.N., M.S., Assistant Director of Nursing, Clinical Specialist, New Jersey State Hospital, Greystone Park, New Jersey

DE AUGUSTINIS, JANE, R.N., B.S., Graduate Fellow, Graduate Program in Advanced Psychiatric Nursing, College of Nursing and Graduate School, Rutgers, The State University of New Jersey

FRANCEL, CLAIRE GRIFFIN, R.N., M.S. Formerly, Clinical Specialist, Psychiatric Nursing, Franklin D. Roosevelt Hospital, Veterans Administration, Montrose, New York

GRAVENKEMPER, KATHERINE HEPP, R.N., M.S. Formerly, Clinical Instructor, Psychiatric Nursing, De Pauw University, Greencastle, Indiana

HADLEY, ALICE A. H., R.N., B.S., Assistant Educational Director, Psychiatric Nursing, Langley Porter Neuropsychiatric Institute, San Francisco, California

HAYS, DOROTHEA RICHTER, R.N., M.S., Public Health Nurse, Knox County Health Department, Barbourville, Kentucky

HURTEAU, M. PHYLLIS, R.N., B.S., Associate Director of Nurses, Inservice Education, Hillside Hospital, Glen Oaks, New York

ISANI, REBECCA S., R.N., B.S., Graduate Fellow, Graduate Program in Advanced Psychiatric Nursing, College of Nursing and Graduate School, Rutgers, The State University of New Jersey

KUMLER, FERN R., R.N., B.S., Graduate Fellow, Graduate Program in Advanced Psychiatric Nursing, College of Nursing and Graduate School, Rutgers, The State University of New Jersey

LAZAROFF, URA ANN LANTZ, R.N., M.S., Assistant Director of Nursing, Essex County Overbrook Hospital, Cedar Grove, New Jersey

MARSHALL, MARGARET A., R.N., M.S., Instructor, Nursing, Graduate Program in Advanced Psychiatric Nursing, College of Nursing and Graduate School, Rutgers, The State University of New Jersey

NEWSOM, BETTY HARMUTH, R.N., M.S. Formerly, Graduate Fellow, Graduate Program in Advanced Program of Psychiatric Nursing, College of Nursing and Graduate School, Rutgers, The State University of New Jersey

ODEN, GLORIA, R.N., M.S., Instructor, Graduate Program in Psychiatric Nursing, Catholic University of America, Washington, D.C.

PEPLAU, HILDEGARD E., R.N., ED.D., Professor of Nursing and Director of Graduate Program in Advanced Psychiatric Nursing, College of Nursing and Graduate School, Rutgers, The State University of New Jersey

RICHTER, BETTIJEAN, R.N., M.S., Director, Mental Health Program, Harris College of Nursing, Texas Christian University, Fort Worth, Texas

ROSENBLUM, ELIZABETH PARKER, R.N., B.S. Formerly, Instructor in Psychiatric Nursing, University of Virginia School of Nursing, Charlottesville, Virginia

ROUSLIN, SHEILA, R.N., M.S., Instructor, Psychiatric Nursing, Graduate Program in Advanced Psychiatric Nursing, College of Nursing and Graduate School, Rutgers, The State University of New Jersey

SMOYAK, SHIRLEY A., R.N., M.S., Instructor, Nursing, Graduate Program in Advanced Psychiatric Nursing, College of Nursing and Graduate School, Rutgers, The State University of New Jersey

STUEKS, ALICE, R.N., M.S., Mental Health Consultant, South Shore Child Guidance Clinic, Quincy, Massachusetts

UMLAND, THEO J., R.N., M.S., Assistant Professor, Psychiatric Nursing, College of Nursing, University of Wyoming, Laramie, Wyoming

WERNER, ANITA M., R.N., M.S., Clinical Specialist, Psychiatric Nursing, Essex County Overbrook Hospital, Cedar Grove, New Jersey

# CONTENTS

III. CLINICAL RESEARCH

# SECTION

# I

COMMUNICATION PROBLEMS
MANIFESTED IN INTERPERSONAL
RELATIONSHIPS IN NURSING

# 1 AN OUTLINE OF THE NORMAL THOUGHT PROCESS

*Gloria Oden*

The thought process in the human organism is a highly complex integrated physiological and psychological operation. This operation is an inherent potential in man. However, the development of this intrinsic ability depends on extrinsic factors.

Diagramatically, the initial considerations in the development of man's thought process follow:

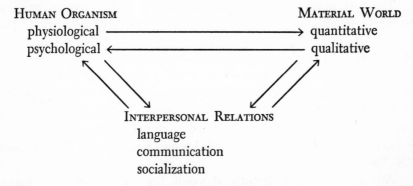

| HUMAN ORGANISM | | MATERIAL WORLD |
| physiological ⟶ | | quantitative |
| psychological ⟵ | | qualitative |

INTERPERSONAL RELATIONS
language
communication
socialization

The interdependence of man and his environment extends to all his activities, including higher mental functioning. This paper is limited, however, to the progressive evolvement of man's capacity to think rationally, from early undifferentiated perception to the ability to think in abstract logical constructs. The physiological, interpersonal, and material aspects of the thought process are considered only to the extent that they bring the human organism into contact with his environment. Piaget's conceptualization of the major stages in the development of the thought process is used to catalogue its emergent operations.

## STAGE 1

### SENSORIMOTOR PHASE—0 TO 2 YEARS

During the early sensorimotor stage, the environment is represented as a motile observable universe, a series of representations centered around activity and devoid of any intrinsic stability. There is no differentiation between self and environment, with the notion of self omnipotent. This merging of self and environment in activity is dependent solely on the action of self.

At approximately the fourth month, there is an increased perceptual capacity, indicated by prolonged inspection of objects placed in the field of vision. By the fifth or sixth month, generalization, recognition, and reproduction begin by assimilation. Concurrently, the reality of objects ceases without perception of the object. This mode of perception persists until the ninth or tenth month, when a notion of real exterior permanence begins. This notion is not based upon spatial construction or external displacement in space, rather it is predicated upon former self-action on a sensorimotor level which is successful.

The first indication of immediate memory ability appears at nine to twelve months, evidenced by imitation of perceived actions. At this point in development, there are significant tokens of discriminative and elaborative behavior. The organism evidences a primitive, ambiguous analytic ability in segregating a single detail for attention and in reacting successively to two details or objects. A dim sense of twoness emerges. Repeatable noises are made which are the first type of speech representative of the syntaxic mode which will occur when speech acquires meaning that is consensually validated. Response to his own name and to the command "No" occurs.

At twelve months differentiated sounds begin with the use of nouns. With the beginning of language, adaptation to the material world and to the thoughts of others commences. Between the twelfth and eighteenth months the notion of the perceived universe as a series of inconsistent pictures declines, and a world of stable objects begins, including a fragmentary sense of self-identity. A serial-order interest emerges. This order exists exclusively one-by-one in the immediate present. Reality remains shadowy and inconstant, encompassed by omnipotence of self.

Between the eighteenth and twenty-fourth months, progressions in development include a threshold discrimination of space and form, interest in aggregate objects as opposed to single objects, an increased but still meager distinction between self and nonself, an awareness of end results and terminations with specific interest in the completion of a chain of events. At two years, the vocabulary consists of 200 to 300 words, primarily nouns, but with other parts of speech beginning to be used. This marks the onset of elementary symbolic processes.

## Egocentric or Representational Phase—2 to 6 Years

During the second to third year of life the first inconsistent evidence of the thought process begins to emerge, marked by the beginning ability to formulate a negative judgment—A is not B (Aristotelian law of identity on a subjective representational level in present experience). The use of plurals begins. Intention to action is implied by the simultaneous verbal expression of action and the action itself. Memory span lengthens to recall of yesterday. Verbally this is expressed in the present tense.

After the third year, experience is reapplied and extended. Notion of self and nonself is increased but remains imperfect with the ejection of self-mental status to others. A rudimentary awareness of future is indicated by willingness to sacrifice immediate satisfaction for near-future satisfaction. However, awareness of past and future remains meager through the fifth year.

During the fourth to sixth years, consecutive and combinative forms of thinking are displayed. Capacity for comparative judgment is not developed, but rather two consecutive judgments can be made without connection between the two. Language serves several functions including interpersonal communication, self-expression to others, and self-expression in reverie and thinking. Thought is absolute. The organism is unaware of thinking as subjective in an objective world. Symbols of objects are fused with the objects they represent. Definition is in terms of use: "a horse is to ride"; [1] "a hat is for the head." [2]

## Summary of Thought Process at Termination of Stage 1

1. Physical actions dominate mental operations
   a. Thinking is object-related rather than principle-related

[1] Gesell, A., *The First Five Years of Life*, p. 55.
[2] Cruze, W. W., *Readings in General Psychology*, p. 222.

    b. Concern with practical success of ends without consideration of means

    c. Unable to distinguish between self-action and external or objective processes

2. Undifferentiated generalizations are made
   a. Inability to organize operations in serial order
   b. Unable to conceptualize cause and effect
   c. Observes with precausal linking and random association
   d. Inability to make classifications within categories

3. Tools of organized symbolic thought are used, but symbols are frequently fused with objects represented

4. Global intuitive understanding is used in problem-solving, with a reduction of trial-and-error as a basis for problem-solving.
   a. No internalization of actions as operations

# STAGE 2

## Concrete Operational Thought—6/7 to 11/12 Years

The second stage of development marks the beginning of operational logic. An operation is defined by Inhelder and Piaget as a means of mentally transforming data about the real world so they can be organized and used selectively in the solution of problems. An operation differs from an action in that it is internalized and reversible. Reversibility, by definition of the same authors, is the permanent possibility of returning to the starting point of an operation.

Initially, during the second stage of development, there is an increase in recall of past experience. Recall of events and experience has little logical relevance. Rather, it serves the purpose of learning by absorption of the new into familiar past learning by identification, comparison, verification, and reinforcement. This quantitative learning is essential to the later formulation of logical structures.

The second stage encompasses the gradual transition from preoperational to formal logic based upon concrete structures. Two forms of logical concrete structures emerge. The first form is the logic of relations, upon which serial ordering is based. These organized systems of thought are predicated upon the direct organization of given data structured in immediate reality. The second form is the development of the logic of classes, which enables the individual to manipulate part-whole relation-

ships within categories. Concepts of the permanence of groups and qualities, differentiation, classification, and a grasp of independent variables in
a structured whole become systematized. Thought content cannot be
generalized to all physical qualities; it proceeds from one factor to another, isolating the elements of underlying principles with a limited concept of total implication. The reversibility of classes is derived from inversion, i.e., the canceling or negating of an operation which permits a
reformulation.

The logic of relations proceeds by the manipulation of objects, ordering and reordering physical relationships in serial order with a gradual
comprehension of the relating links of cause and effect. Correspondences
between two independent series are noted with understanding. The reversibility of relations is derived from reciprocity, i.e., compensating a difference by an equivalent operation. Both logic of classes and logic of relations are independently reversible on the concrete level. There is no
structure of thought present permitting integration of reversibility of the
two systems into a single system, which allows abstract reasoning.

Thought on the concrete level is marked by manipulation and conceptualization of observable elements rather than abstract concepts. There
is an extended ability to generalize, to think in terms of relations and the
causes of things not personally experienced. Symbolic processes of language are developed, and exploration of nonconcrete experience is begun.
Conceptual and abstract thought begin to emerge in the latter part of
the concrete-thought stage. Extension of the actual in the direction of
potentiality is noted. This extension is not extended into a set of hypotheses until a later point in development.

The second stage is marked by the internalization of concrete operations. Action is accompanied by an awareness of individual techniques and
coordination. The elements of underlying principles have been isolated but
cannot be verbally formulated. A concept of the permanence of groups is
established, as well as partial comprehension of relativity as compared to
the former concept of reality as egocentrically absolute.

## SUMMARY OF THOUGHT PROCESS AT TERMINATION OF STAGE 2

1. Qualitative learning is increased
   a. Increased recall of past experience
   b. Accumulation of increased direct experience
2. Operational logic develops, combining present and past experience with

a limited comprehension of potential
   a. Logic of classification
   b. Logic of relations
3. Ability develops for independent reversibility of the two types of logic without integration of systems
   a. Classification—inversion
   b. Relations—reciprocity
4. Conceptualization of observable elements and a limited concept of abstract elements begin
5. Internalization of concrete operations develops, with partial insight without the ability to verbalize concepts
6. Ideas of permanence and of relativity develop

## STAGE 3

### FORMAL OPERATIONS—11 OR 12 TO 15 YEARS

The third stage in development marks the evolvement of thinking from particular to general, from concrete to abstract, from absolute to relative, from direct to vicarious experience, and from the utilization of past and present experience to the concept of potentiality. The transition is difficult to isolate. Competencies acquired in former modes of thinking are used combinatively in formal operations. Isolated segments of the formal thought process are found in earlier forms of thinking.

During the concrete stage the human organism attempts to find relationships through an abundance of data which eventually become so complex that an exclusion of superfluous factors is necessary. The effectiveness of thinking is related to this broad language or symbol system he has developed and will continue to develop throughout his life experiences. The broad collection of data presents a problem that precedes the utilization of formal logic. Independently structured factors in observations and experiments interfere with expected results, yielding inconsistencies, contradictions, exceptions, and partial regularities. The use of independent methods of logic does not suffice. A need to develop operations that permit integration arises in order to coordinate the results of concrete operations that lack sufficient internal consistency.

The discovery of formal logic occurs by two means. It occurs with the separating of raw empirical data to coordinate the results of concrete operations in possible combinations or with the coordinated grouping of classes and structures into a systematic whole. Either method ultimately yields the utilization of formal logic in thinking.

Immediately preceding the use of formal logic, the individual has the capacity for classification on an elementary level. On this level of classification a system of class by variables is not included. To deal with the problem, a new grouping system on a higher order is needed. A combinational set of groupings emerges including all possible groupings not totally exclusive.

There are a gradual extension of the totality of possible operations and a learning by experience that variables may be interdependent and overlapping. Former learning and new learning evolve with an integration of the systems (expanded and modified) which formerly operated separately.

Thought on the formal level permits separation of variables, an ability to identify and concentrate on separate variables in complex problem consideration, analysis of associated variables, a linking of successive judgments, and interpretation of relationships. Analysis of proofs develops which can be expressed verbally. Thought at this level also includes the ability to deal critically with self-thought, to reflect the real and the possible, and to reason with reality as a function of possibility rather than with direct reality.

## SUMMARY OF THOUGHT PROCESS AT TERMINATION OF STAGE 3

1. Development of new grouping systems that are not mutually exclusive
2. Comprehension of potentiality
3. Integrated reversibility of logic of classes and logic of relations
4. Identification, separation, and analysis of variables
5. Linking of successive judgments, analyses, interpretations
6. Propositional analysis of proof, expressed verbally
7. Ability to deal critically with self-thought

## CONCLUSIONS

The thought process presented above deals with formal operations. Thought, however, does not proceed from stage to stage with the mutual exclusion of former thought structures. Formal thought utilizes earlier modes of experience. Thinking, as a process, includes:

1. Free association
2. Autistic thinking

3. Creative imagination
4. Reasoning
   a. Problem
   b. Definition of problem, isolation of data
   c. Possible solutions
   d. Evaluation of solutions, hypothesis
   e. Observational or experimental test of solution
   f. Steps b through e until solution is found

# BIBLIOGRAPHY

ALLPORT, F. H., *Theories of Perception and the Concept of Structure,* John Wiley and Sons, New York: 1955.

ARIETI, S., *Interpretation of Schizophrenia,* Robert Brunner, New York: 1955.

ASHER, E., TIFFIN, J., and KNIGHT, F., "Kinds of Thinking Activity" and "Autistic Thinking," *Readings in General Psychology,* Crow and Crow (eds.), Barnes and Noble, New York: 1954.

BIBER, B., MURPHY, L., and BLACK, I., *Life and Ways of the Seven to Eight Year Old,* Basic Books, New York: 1952.

CRUZE, W. W., "The Development of Language," *Readings in General Psychology,* Crow and Crow (eds.), Barnes and Noble, New York: 1954.

DASHIELL, J. F., "The Principal Stages in Reasoning," *Readings in General Psychology,* Crow and Crow (eds.), Barnes and Noble, New York: 1954.

GESELL, A., *The First Five Years of Life,* Harper and Bros., New York: 1940.

HILGARD, E. R., "The Thinking Process," *Readings in General Psychology,* Crow and Crow (eds.), Barnes and Noble, New York: 1954.

INHELDER, B., and PIAGET, J., *The Growth of Logical Thinking,* Basic Books, New York: 1958.

LEWIS, M. M., *How Children Learn to Speak,* George G. Harrup and Co., London: 1957.

RAPAPORT, D., *Organization and Pathology of Thought,* Columbia University Press, New York: 1951.

SARGENT, H. D., and MAYMAN, M., "Clinical Psychology," *American Handbook of Psychiatry,* S. Arieti (ed.), Basic Books, New York: 1959.

SPEIGEL, R., "Specific Problems of Communication," *American Handbook of Psychiatry,* S. Arieti (ed.), Basic Books, New York: 1959.

SULLIVAN, H. S., *Conceptions of Modern Psychiatry,* W. W. Norton & Co., New York: 1953.

WHITEHEAD, A. N., *Symbolism,* Capricorn Books, New York: 1959.

WITENBERG, E. E., RIOCH, J. M., and MAZER, M., "The Interpersonal and Cultural Approaches," *American Handbook of Psychiatry,* S. Arieti (ed.), Basic Books, New York: 1959.

# 2 THOUGHT DISORDERS OF PSYCHIATRIC PATIENTS

*Shirley W. Armstrong*

Disordered thought processes, which are reflected in language content, are major problems for many psychiatric patients. The kinds of thought disorders exhibited by psychiatric patients and methods by which nurses can assist patients to overcome or correct thought disorders are discussed in this chapter.

## DEVELOPMENT OF THOUGHT DISORDERS

Thought disorders cannot be observed directly; they can only be observed in the communication and behavior of a person. Probably the two main processes in thought are autistic invention and consensual validation. Autistic invention is the use of highly personal meanings for words and events. It is normally used by children. As the child grows and becomes socialized, autistically invented meanings are replaced by consensually valid meanings of words and events that are accepted and understood by society. Thus the foundation for the development of thought disorders is laid in early childhood. If the child is cut off or discouraged from replacing his autistic thoughts with consensually valid ones, thought disorders begin. For example, if the child is left to guess at the meanings of words and actions of the parents, this guessing will become a pattern.

Sullivan referred to the early, autistic thinking of the child as referential processes. Briefly, the development of mature thinking as outlined by Sullivan [1] was

[1] Sullivan, H. S., *Clinical Studies in Psychiatry*, pp. 13–14.

At early age of development, the child uses obscure, autistic, unrefined thinking operations in communicating with his parents, and eventually the parents come to feel, "People won't understand Willie; these statements of his don't make sense." So gradually Willie gets to know that he must always make sense, or sound like people who think they make sense. And so awareness is simply relieved of these uncommunicative processes; there is no sense in paying attention to these more primitive types of mental operations, and finally they are just confused puzzle books.

Many psychiatric patients have never learned to replace their autistic thinking with socially necessary, consensually valid thinking. Language disorders can be observed in nonpsychotic people. The term "language disorders" has been used to describe communication problems in "normal" people instead of the term "thought disorders." The difference between the "normal" and the psychotic person is that the "normal" person can correct his communication when requested to do so, while the psychiatric patient has difficulty correcting his language. For example, if a "normal" person tells a story in which he uses many pronouns, when questioned, this "normal" person can substitute a proper name for the pronoun. Many times the psychiatric patient cannot replace a pronoun with its referent.

## IMPLICATIONS FOR MENTAL HEALTH

The thought process has definite implications for mental health. Parents and schoolteachers can assist children in replacing their autistic thinking by validated thinking in several ways. Some of these ways are allowing children to ask questions, giving reasonable answers to questions, shedding doubt on autistic communication, and provoking awareness of understandable communication in the child.

## SOME TYPES OF THOUGHT DISORDERS

Some types of thought disorders and nursing intervention follow.

### USE OF GLOBAL PRONOUNS

This type of thought disorder involves the use of many pronouns without their referents. When questioned, sometimes the person is able to supply the referent and sometimes he is unable to do so. Paranoid patients, especially, often reveal this thought disorder. Example:

Patient: People think you're nuts I guess but you know yourself that you have a good idea. Something happens when you least expect it.
Nurse: You have been using the word you. To whom are you referring?

*Patient:* Like I said, I was referring to baseball naturally. (Much time had passed since the patient had last referred to baseball.)

## LACK OF DIFFERENTIATION BETWEEN FEELINGS, THOUGHTS, AND ACTIONS

This thought disorder is common to many people, psychotic and non-psychotic. Often people say they feel something that is really a thought or an opinion. The lack of differentiation among feelings, thoughts, and actions is often blatant in a psychotic patient. The patient may be able to describe his actions and thoughts but not his feelings. When asked to describe feelings, this same patient will respond by describing an action or thought. There can also be a split in awareness among thoughts, feelings, and actions. The third possibility is that the patient can remember and describe feelings and thoughts, while his actions have been dissociated. Example:

*Patient:* Silly thoughts have something to do with my being here.
*Nurse:* Tell me about your silly thoughts.
*Patient:* Well, being in here I act like everybody else.

## CIRCUMSTANTIALITY

Circumstantiality is "a characteristic of conversation that proceeds indirectly to its goal idea, with many tedious details and parenthetical and irrelevant additions." [2] Example:

*Patient:* I guess you can't remember everything. I guess little things get bigger later. Little things build and build. Big things you can see you know.
*Nurse:* I don't follow you.
*Patient:* Well when I talk like that, I am talking about baseball.

## AUTOMATIC KNOWING

A common expression that people use is "you know" at the end of a statement. Normally, little attention is paid to the "you know"; both people understand that the listener does not know the story if he is hearing it for the first time. The use of "you know" becomes pathological when a person really thinks the listener knows what is about to be said. One patient with whom the writer worked intensively ended almost every sentence with "you know." Example:

[2] English, H. B., and English, A. C., *A Comprehensive Dictionary of Psychological and Psychoanalytical Terms*, p. 88.

*Patient:* (Had been discussing sports.) All about these sports, you know.
*Nurse:* On what basis do you think I know about sports?
*Patient:* Well, everyone knows, at least a little bit.

### SPEAKING IN THE NEGATIVE

A person with this thought disorder focuses on negative feelings, thoughts, and actions in his communication. Example:

*Patient:* I don't want to remain in this stationary position.
*Nurse:* What do you want to do, Mr. D.?
*Patient:* I want to get out of the hospital and go to the rehabilitation center.

*Patient:* I didn't sleep at all that night. Not one minute. Just couldn't get to sleep.
*Nurse:* What did you do?
*Patient:* I told you—I didn't sleep a wink.
*Nurse:* You told me what you did *not* do. What was it that you *did* do?
*Patient:* I worried about my ideas. I worried that I couldn't turn my thoughts off. I had worked hard all day. I was tired. I wanted to be asleep—resting. The thoughts kept coming and I couldn't shut them off.

### SCATTERING

A common thought disorder of psychotic patients is scattering, in which the patient moves from one topic to another with no apparent connection between them. Example:

*Patient:* I went to N——— on a bus early in the morning. Eating chocolate doughnuts stands out in my mind, there must be some unknown reason. I can't make head nor tail of that situation. I don't know its connection with what a guy on the ward said. His wife came and he had his pick between three different kinds of sandwiches. There is some connection between the chocolate doughnuts and eating sandwiches, in my mind, which I can't figure out.
*Nurse:* (Elicited more description of the two situations in an attempt to clarify connections.)

### SWITCHING THE SUBJECT

In this thought disorder the person talks around and around a subject, and even though he switches topics, he keeps coming back to the original subject. Example:

*Patient:* These pills are putting on the finishing touches. I shouldn't even be here now. So if you are in another country you can take the law in your own hands, but here in the United States you have to follow a system. Like now, I really don't belong here because I am cured, but I have to wait to be notified by the rehabilitation center. If I were in another country I could just rush right in. I don't know how to say it. Now I'm getting myself all involved.

*Nurse:* (Assisted the patient to describe his feelings, thoughts, and actions in connection with hospitalization and discharge in order.)

## IMPUTING INTENTION AND/OR IDEAS TO OTHER PEOPLE

Some persons will predict what the other person thinks or intends to do without sufficient evidence upon which to base the prediction. Example:

*Patient:* Nothing can beat a profession yet. It would be nice if everyone in the world would be of a profession, wouldn't it? Well, I can't think of the words, you know. You and me having a profession, it's natural we would think everyone should have a profession. Course you and me have a different profession.

*Nurse:* My profession is nursing. Just what would you say your profession is?

## DEPERSONALIZATION

The individual's self-concept as well as a thought disorder is involved in depersonalization. Depersonalization means that the person does not see himself as a *total* person. Example:

*Patient:* I'm something.

*Nurse:* You're something?

*Patient:* I'm just taking up space. I'm just matter. Anybody that takes up space is matter. You are matter.

*Nurse:* But you are a person; I am a person.

*Patient:* But everything that takes up space is matter; everything is matter. You can't say I'm wrong.

*Patient:* (Walking in wide circle near nurse.) They won't let her do anything—they won't let her. She wants to go upstairs, but they won't let her. She doesn't bother anybody. She wants to go upstairs, she does.

*Nurse:* Who does?

*Patient:* (Pointing to her own chest.) She does.

## USE OF GLOBAL ADJECTIVES

It is culturally acceptable for people to use such ambiguous words as good, nice, bad, beautiful. However, these words convey somewhat different meanings to different people. The nurse should ask the patient to clarify ambiguous adjectives so that both patient and nurse understand the meaning the other has attached to the adjective. Adjectives can also be used by people to cover up their true feelings. Example:

*Patient:* I'm happy every second of my life.

*Nurse:* You're happy every second of your life? Is that possible?

*Patient:* Yep, thrilled and happy every second of my life. It's a good feeling. Even when angry in appearance, I'm happy.

### EXTENSIVE USE OF MODIFIERS

Some individuals are so unsure of what they are saying that they use many modifiers in order to avoid making direct statements. Example:

*Patient:* I thought perhaps I might mention going home to my mother, at least maybe I could go home for a little while.
*Nurse:* You plan to discuss going home with your mother?
*Patient:* Yes.

### AUTISTIC INVENTION

As stated earlier, mature adults replace autistic invention with consensually valid concepts. Often psychiatric patients have not learned to do this. Example:

*Patient:* I have had quite a bit of experience for my age. I just imagine that, I could be wrong.
*Nurse:* Tell me about your experience.
*Patient:* I could be wrong. Like I said I just imagine. Maybe I am just letting my imagination run away from me.

In dealing with autistic invention, the nurse would aim at assisting the patient in learning to check out his ideas with other people in order to arrive at socially acceptable formulations.

All the clinical examples above of thought disorders were abstracted from data of one nurse-patient relationship. This list is in no way complete. Other patients will have various combinations of these thought disorders, or other thought disorders.

## CONCLUSION

The nurse's therapeutic intervention depends on her awareness of the therapeutic ingredient of language. If the nurse agrees with disordered thought content or makes no response, the patient may never learn that this communication is ineffectual. The nurse must also be aware of, and correct, her own inappropriate use of language if she is to be therapeutically useful to the patient.

## BIBLIOGRAPHY

ENGLISH, HORACE B., and ENGLISH, AVA C., *A Comprehensive Dictionary of Psy-*

*chological and Psychoanalytical Terms*, Longmans, Green & Co., New York: 1958.

SULLIVAN, HARRY STACK, *Clinical Studies in Psychiatry*, W. W. Norton & Co., New York: 1956.

———— *The Interpersonal Theory of Psychiatry*, W. W. Norton & Co., New York: 1953.

# 3 VERBAL COMMUNICATION: AN ASPECT OF THE NURSE–PATIENT RELATIONSHIP

*Elizabeth P. Rosenblum*

A major aspect of the nurse-patient relationship is the communication that evolves between the nurse and the patient. An individual comes to a mental hospital with serious difficulties in his ability to communicate satisfactorily with other individuals. An important task for the nurse is to facilitate his communication. To accomplish this task, the nurse must study the verbal and nonverbal behavior of the patient and of herself in relation to the patient, for it is in these observations that the nurse can identify the behavior that will assist the patient in achieving satisfactory communication.

Many aspects of behavior must be considered in studying communication—the anxiety of the nurse and of the patient; the nonverbal gestures or feelings which are revealed; environmental effects; verbal interaction, including the content, tone of voice, and possible interpretations; and numerous other factors that influence communication between two individuals. An effective method of studying communication is through the process of learning. This approach includes the following steps: (1) observations, (2) description of these observations, (3) analysis of these collected data, (4) formulation of the meanings and relations within the collected data by using theory of behavior and communication, (5) clarification of formulations, (6) validation of formulations by discussing them with appropriate people, (7) utilization of formulations in future behavior, and (8) utilization of steps 1 through 6 to evaluate the results of behavior. This process of studying the interaction between the nurse and the patient can provide information about modes of communication that assist the patient in increasing communication.

18—

The purpose of this chapter is to illustrate the utilization of the above process in studying communication in nurse-patient relationships. This chapter is limited to verbalizations used by the nurse and their effect on communication of the patient.

## SETTING

The data in this chapter were collected during a series of individual interviews with Miss S., who was hospitalized in a large state mental hospital. The clinical diagnosis of Miss S. was schizophrenia. The nurse referred to in this paper functioned under the supervision of two nursing instructors during the series of interviews with the patient.

## METHODOLOGY

The nurse selected Miss S. and requested her permission to spend an hour with her twice a week for two months, explaining that the time would be spent with the patient talking about any experiences or problems that she wished to discuss. One limit of the discussions was that the nurse and the patient were not to talk about the nurse. The focus of the conversation was turned to the patient whenever a question was asked about the nurse. The purpose of this limit was to indicate to Miss S. that the nurse was sincerely interested in Miss S. as a person, in her experiences and her problems.

The nurse recorded the verbal and nonverbal behavior of the patient and her own verbalizations in a notebook during each interview. These data were studied by the nurse following each interview and the series of interviews, and were reviewed during individual conferences with the nursing instructors. In this study, some verbalizations by the nurse seemed to be consistently followed by a decrease in the patient's communication, while others were consistently followed by increases in her communication. The data were further studied, and the following criteria were developed to identify increases and decreases in satisfactory communication by this patient. Increases in satisfactory communication are statements by this patient which (1) express thoughts, feelings, or actions about herself or (2) clarify a preceding communication. Decreases in satisfactory communication are no response by the patient, or statements by the patient that are accompanied by an increase in anxiety and which (1) degrade her in some manner, (2) switch the focus of the conversation abruptly, or (3) provide vague information about the preceding communication. The criteria for identifying increases in anxiety were developed from observations of non-verbal behavior. Nonverbal behavior that indicates increase in anxiety of this patient is increased motor activity—swinging her leg, moving around in the chair, blinking her eyes. Speaking more rapidly also indicates increased anxiety.

These criteria of increased and decreased communications were used to select verbalizations of the nurse that were followed by increased or decreased communication by the patient. The process of learning, previously mentioned, was then utilized in studying the nurse-patient interaction in these situations.

Many factors were identified that might influence communication, e.g. words used, anxiety, tone of voice, facial expressions, and other aspects of the nurse's behavior. However, the words of the nurse were selected for study. The writer does not intend to indicate that the words are more important in communication than the nonverbal aspects of the nurse's behavior. The latter were considered by the nurse and her instructors when the nurse was planning changes in her own behavior.

The following discussions of selected interactions between the nurse and the patient will illustrate: (1) the application of the process of learning to the study of communication in a nurse-patient relationship and (2) the utilization of the information obtained in planning changes in the nurse's behavior to facilitate the communication of the patient.

## BACKGROUND OF NURSE–PATIENT INTERACTIONS

After the nurse had stated the purpose and limits of the time she would spend with the patient, Miss S. readily responded that she would like to spend the time with the nurse. The place for the interviews was selected by Miss S. She met the nurse there at the scheduled time twice a week. Miss S. was allowed to select the topics of conversation and then was encouraged in her description of these topics. The following nurse-patient interactions were selected from the series of interviews.

## NURSE–PATIENT INTERACTION I

### OBSERVATIONS

*Patient:* How are you this morning?
*Nurse:* Let's talk about you.
*Patient:* I am getting some more pills, and I think that they're helping me.
*Nurse:* Tell me about them helping you. (Pause.)

*Patient:* They have a library here, too, that we can go to. (Begins to swing leg.)

*Nurse:* Tell me about the library.

*Patient:* They have books—*Marjorie Morningstar*. They made *Marjorie Morningstar* into a movie and I read that book. Have you seen the picture?

*Nurse:* No. Let's talk about you.

*Patient:* I cut down on foods, but then I was hungry, so now I'll eat as much as I like—the only thing is that I gain weight when I eat and I should lose about ten pounds. My mouth is awfully dry. Do you mind if I go get a glass of water? (Spoken rapidly and leaves the room without waiting for a reply from the nurse. Miss S. returns to the room in a few minutes.) I almost lost you. (Sits down in the chair.) I wish I didn't have to take so many pills. I take five and I think that I should just take four. There's a few nice girls on this ward. Mrs. S. asked me if I would like to go to work in the employee's residence. They've changed Armistice Day to Veteran's Day, haven't they?

*Nurse:* Yes.

*Patient:* Mrs. R., what do you do during your vacation? Do you work?

*Nurse:* I am here to talk with you about your problems.

*Patient:* I had a fight with a girl about a silly thing. She took my bobby pins.

*Nurse:* Tell me about it.

*Patient:* (Silence.) I thought Miss R. just comes in the afternoons. (Silence.) I have to write a letter to my sister.

*Nurse:* Tell me.

*Patient:* Because I need some money to get my mother a present. (Continues talking about sisters, other family, and self.)

## DESCRIPTION OF OBSERVATIONS

An increase in anxiety and a decrease in communication are observed in Miss S.'s behavior—swinging her leg, rapid speech, abrupt and frequent shifts of topic, and periods of silence. This interaction occurred at the beginning of the hour, and the communication during the remainder of the hour was more satisfactory, with discussions of experiences by the patient. Are the verbalizations of the nurse increasing the anxiety of the patient during this period and disrupting, rather than facilitating, communication?

## ANALYSIS

After the nurse directed the conversation to Miss S., she talked about her medication. The nurse attempted to encourage description, but in the following statement, the patient shifted the focus of the conversation. Did the words used by the nurse influence this shift? The nurse used the indefinite pronoun *them*, which could refer to anything helping Miss S. The following statement by the patient could be an attempt to explain the *them* who are helping her: "*They* have a library here, *too*, that we can go to."

The nurse encouraged description of the library, and communication by the patient increased.

When Miss S. turned the conversation to the nurse with a question, the nurse abruptly shifted the focus to the patient. An increase in the patient's anxiety is observed, as she spoke rapidly and left the room. Did the verbalization by the nurse increase the patient's anxiety? In the verbalization, the nurse focused on the question by Miss S. and abruptly shifted the focus of the conversation to the *patient*, rather than encouraging description of the topic she was discussing. This maneuver would indicate that the patient's topic is not acceptable for discussion. This implication would lower the patient's self-esteem and increase her anxiety. The sudden shift by the nurse would also cut off communication about the topic. This verbalization by the nurse increased anxiety and decreased communication of the patient.

When Miss S. returned to the room, she spoke rapidly and shifted from topic to topic in her conversation, indicating that her anxiety was still increased. In response to a direct question about her life, the nurse indicated an interest in the patient's problems, and Miss S. spoke about "a fight with a girl." The following verbalization by the nurse contained the indefinite pronoun "it," and communication was decreased with a silence and a shift in topic. The nurse did not respond to the comment about another nurse, but then, she encouraged Miss S. when she spoke about "a letter to my sister." Communication was increased as Miss S. clarified the previous statement and continued to talk about her family and herself.

### FORMULATION

The use of indefinite pronouns and an abrupt shift in the focus of the conversation by the nurse resulted in a decrease in the patient's communication. In two instances, when the nurse responded to a question about herself by returning the focus of the conversation to the patient, communication was increased. The verbalization, "Tell me," was also followed by an increase in communication.

### UTILIZATION OF INFORMATION

The nurse will attempt to (1) clarify her communication by using definite names rather than indefinite pronouns; (2) maintain communication by focusing on the topic of the conversation, rather than rapidly shifting the focus; and (3) encourage communication by returning the focus to the patient after a question about the nurse and by using "Tell me." The following observations show the nurse's attempts to implement these plans.

## NURSE–PATIENT INTERACTION II

### OBSERVATIONS

(Silence. Miss S. is blinking her eyes, looking at the nurse and the floor, and moving around in her chair.)
*Nurse:* Are you uncomfortable?
*Patient:* Well, I don't feel like talking today. I was hoping I'd get a new dress so I could wear it to church.
*Nurse:* Tell me about it.
*Patient:* (Moving in chair, sighing, and swallowing.) It's a hard life being put away like this. (Pause.)
*Nurse:* Go on.
*Patient:* I gained a pound. (Holding her hands tightly clasped, blinking her eyes rapidly, moving in the chair.)
*Nurse:* Are you uncomfortable?
*Patient:* Yes.
*Nurse:* Tell me about it—being uncomfortable.
*Patient:* Maybe it's because I haven't had a shower in two days.
(Following this interaction, the patient begins to talk about the hope that she will go home for a visit.)

### DESCRIPTION OF OBSERVATIONS

The nurse again used an indefinite pronoun, a shift in the patient's conversation occurred and was followed by an increase in the patient's anxiety. When the nurse encouraged description of the patient's discomfort, clarification of the pronoun was followed by an increase in communication.

### ANALYSIS AND FORMULATION

The use of indefinite pronouns decreases the communication of this patient, while a clarification of a pronoun is followed by an increase in communication.

## NURSE–PATIENT INTERACTION III

### OBSERVATIONS

*Patient:* You know, Mrs. R., I think that I'm the average. The people here aren't sick. I don't know why they don't go home. Why is that?
*Nurse:* Tell me about average.
*Patient:* It's silly.

*Nurse:* No.
*Patient:* I just don't think that people who are feeling well should be here.
*Nurse:* Tell me about feeling well.
*Patient:* Well, some of them are as healthy as you and I.
*Nurse:* Tell me about you.
*Patient:* I wasn't feeling too well for the past couple of months, but now I think I'm getting out of it.

### DESCRIPTION OF OBSERVATIONS

The nurse attempted to understand the communication of Miss S. by focusing on the statement about herself. The patient moved to discuss other people, and the nurse encouraged description of the phrase describing people. Following the patient's next statement, "as healthy as you and I," the nurse encouraged Miss S. to talk about herself, and communication by the patient about herself was increased.

### ANALYSIS AND FORMULATIONS

When the nurse focuses on the theme of the conversation, rather than the final words of the patient, communication is maintained and increased.

## SUMMARY

The application of the process of learning in studying communication in a nurse-patient relationship has been demonstrated. By using this approach, the nurse was able to identify aspects of her own verbalizations that were followed by increases or decreases in satisfactory communication by this patient. Although only selected examples from the data are presented, the nurse, in her studies of the series of interviews, was able to identify numerous problems in her own verbalizations and found important aspects to consider in communicating with this patient. This information can be utilized in several ways in the task of facilitating the patient's communication. First, the nurse learns ways of manipulating her own behavior so that the patient can more easily communicate with her. Second, the nurse can assist the patient in observing and understanding his own difficulties in communicating with other individuals. Third, the nurse can also utilize her formulations by assisting other personnel to identify and understand their problems in communication with the patient.

Although this chapter shows selected nurse-patient interaction, the same criteria of increase and decrease in communication and the utilization of the process of learning were used briefly to study data from other nurse-patient relationships. When the nurse used indefinite pronouns or abruptly shifted the focus of the conversation, the satisfactory communication by the patient was decreased. The use of "Tell me" and shifting the focus to the patient after a personal question to the nurse continued to increase satisfactory communication by the patient. These similar results indicate that principles of communication in nurse-patient relationships can be developed when these studies are done on a larger scale. These principles would be helpful in assisting nurses to develop their communication skills.

This writer anticipates that nurses will use the process of learning to study many aspects of communication in nurse-patient relationships. From this study of communication, principles and concepts can be formulated that will guide nurses in the major task of facilitating each patient's satisfactory communication.

[The unprecise use of pronouns in verbal content, as noted above, frequently leads to an entirely different problem in the nurse-patient interaction, which may be called "assuming comprehension." This occurs frequently during the orientation phase of the nurse-patient relationship when the patient repetitiously uses plural pronouns, and the nurse fails to elicit clarification.

A nurse was assigned to interview for one hour daily, for four days, a multigravida postpartal patient. Excerpts from the data follow:

*Patient:* We always go shopping together on Friday evening. See, the stores are open later and with seven mouths to feed, buying food takes me some time. We enjoy getting out of the house for awhile too. It's about my only time away from the kids, kinda like a short vacation. Sometimes we do some window shopping too. Then, we stop in for a soda or something before we go on home.
*Nurse:* What else do you do together?
*Patient:* Oh—not much I guess. Sometimes when there's someone around to look after the younger kids we get out for a short ride. Not often though.

Note, in the above excerpt the frequent use of the plural pronoun "we" by the patient. The nurse failed to elicit the name of the other participant(s) in the activities. What the nurse knew, presumably, from her knowledge of grammar, was that "we" means "I and one or more others."

When the data above were reviewed in seminar, the seminar leader inquired about the other person who with the patient comprised the "we" of the pronoun. The interviewer stated that it was the husband. The seminar discussion follows:

*Nurse:* (Read the data.)
*Leader:* In the exchange which you have just read, who were the participants in the patient's "we"?
*Nurse:* What?
*Leader:* "We" is a plural personal pronoun. "We" equals I and someone else or many others. The activity mentioned was done by the patient and whom else?

*Nurse:* Her husband.

*Leader:* Where is the evidence in the data?

*Nurse:* It had to be her husband. She said, "We always go shopping together on Friday evening."

*Leader:* Did the patient say that the other person in the "we" is "my husband"?

*Nurse:* No. But it was.

*Leader:* What data have you to support your assumption that "we" equals I (the patient) plus my husband? Where in the data do you find substantiation for your belief that the patient means "We equals my husband plus I"?

*Nurse:* Who else could it be?

*Leader:* It?

*Nurse:* We—who else could "we" be?

*Leader:* Part of the task of the nurse is to assist the patient in clarifying the plural pronouns. The inquiry you choose to use, namely, "What else do you (plural) do together?" provides the patient with the right to believe that you know of whom she speaks without her having to tell you. I think you will find substantiation for this factor in subsequent verbalization by the patient. Is it not a fact that the patient persisted in her use of the plural pronoun "we"?

*Nurse:* Yes. But it has to be her husband.

*Leader:* Patient plus husband equals we is certainly a possibility. Will you ever, though, really know unless you ask the patient?

*Nurse:* I guess not.

The nurse assumed comprehension beyond the data. She failed to seek clarification of plural pronouns until the last interview with the patient. Her comment, once she sought and received person identification of the plural pronouns was: "Imagine my chagrin! All that first and second hour Mrs. A. was talking about her nineteen-year-old daughter! I swear, though, I was *sure* she meant her husband!"

One of the cardinal principles of the nurse-patient relationship can be stated: As the nurse is precise in her use of language, and as she assists the patient to be precise in his use of language, the patient is free to correct other aspects of his pathology. The patient will rarely be more precise in his use of language than is the nurse.]

# BIBLIOGRAPHY

ELDRED, STANLEY H., *et al.*, "A Procedure for the Systematic Analysis of Psycho-therapeutic Interviews," *Psychiatry*, 17:337–45, 1954.

MAY, ROLLO, *The Meaning of Anxiety*, The Ronald Press, New York: 1950.

PEPLAU, HILDEGARD E., "Therapeutic Concepts: Aspects of Psychiatric Nursing," *The League Exchange*, No. 26B, National League for Nursing, New York: 1957.

RUESCH, JURGEN, and BATESON, GREGORY, *Communication: The Social Matrix of Psychiatry*, W. W. Norton & Co., New York: 1951.

SULLIVAN, HARRY STACK, *The Psychiatric Interview*, W. W. Norton & Co., New York: 1954.

TUDOR, GWEN E., "A Sociopsychiatric Nursing Approach to Intervention in a Problem of Mutual Withdrawal on a Mental Hospital Ward," *Psychiatry*, 15:193–217, 1952.

# 4 AUTISTIC INVENTION: A NURSING PROBLEM IN COMMUNICATION

*Shirley W. Armstrong*

When a person is admitted to a psychiatric hospital, he becomes essentially isolated. His avenues of communication with the outside world are limited to hospital personnel, visitors, letters, and for some patients, home visits of varying lengths. Even things taken for granted by most people, such as newspapers, television, and radio, may not be available. How does the patient obtain information? What is the role of the nurse in supplying information to patients? When patients are not given explanations, they will make up a personal reason, which more often than not is erroneous.

Peplau [1] describes psychiatric hospitals as

> . . . specialized educational institutions set up by the community to assist the patient to learn about living—learning which did not occur sufficiently prior to hospital admission. The patient needs to develop his abilities to use reason to describe, to analyze, to formulate, and to validate the meaning of experience with other persons. The patient may also need to learn social and vocational skills essential for productive living. All of these learnings are primarily the responsibility of other existing social institutions —the family, school, church, community centers, and the like. But when these institutions have failed and the individual has therefore not succeeded in securing the competencies he needs for living comfortably and productively with people, then the psychiatric hospital, as a specialized educational institution, offers specialized techniques for promoting such learning at a later date in the life of a person.

What is the role of the nurse in the psychiatric hospital's specialized educational function? One aspect of this role is that the nurse can con-

[1] Peplau, H. E., *Therapeutic Concepts*, p. 28.

—27

tribute to the patients' learning process by such a simple thing as supplying sufficient, valid information, and assisting patients in obtaining valid information instead of resorting to autistic invention.

Autistic invention is normally a phenomenon of childhood and is characterized by events taking on a highly personal meaning to the child.[2] Sullivan[3] defines autism as

> . . . a primary, unsocialized, unacculturated state of symbol activity, and later states pertaining more to this primary condition than to the conspicuously effective consensually validated symbol activities of more mature personality.

Peplau[4] adds,

> The child will communicate the feelings that he has if he feels free to do so, and if he perceives that his expressions will be accorded proper respect. If they are laughed away and he is chided for entertaining thoughts that have not occurred to adults around him he may find it necessary to continue to interpret events on his own, without validating them with others.

There are probably various reasons why the psychiatric staff, and here the author refers to the entire hospital staff, puts the patient in a position to make up his own reasons for his experiences. One of these reasons may be contempt and/or lack of respect for the patient as an individual. Another reason might be "passing the buck" to another staff member, as illustrated by the following clinical example:

*Patient:* (Tells about a problem.)
*Staff Member:* Tell the doctor your troubles.

The nurse may give an explanation to the patient at a time when the patient is too anxious to hear what has been said and refuse to repeat the given explanation.

*Patient:* (Asks a question about ward routine.)
*Staff Member:* I told you what the ward routine was when you first came to the ward.

The chances are great that the patient was anxious when he arrived on the ward. If he has just been admitted to the hospital, he is in a totally new environment. If he has been transferred from another ward, the physical environment may not be too new, but certainly there is a whole new set of people, both patients and staff. The patient, in any case, does not yet know what these people expect of him or how they will accept him.

Information may not be given to the patient because the staff member does not have the information available.

2 Peplau, H. E., *Interpersonal Relations in Nursing*, p. 196.
3 Sullivan, H. S., *Conceptions of Modern Psychiatry*, p. 17.
4 Peplau, H. E., *Interpersonal Relations in Nursing*, pp. 196–97.

*Patient:* What about these foster homes that people refer to?
*Staff Member:* I don't know anything about foster homes. (Walks away.)

Another reason for not giving explanations to patients might be that the personnel consider themselves too busy to respond to the patient's inquiry:

*Patient:* (Query about electric shock.)
*Staff Member:* Can't you see I'm busy with inventory and cleaning? If you want to do something, help me.

In the preceding example, the patient needed an answer, was cut off by the staff member, but was then asked to give help.

A patient's use of autistic invention became clear to the writer while working with individual and groups of patients. Throughout a 30-hour nurse-patient relationship, the patient insisted that a doctor had come from the hospital with an ambulance, forced her into the ambulance, and brought her to the hospital. Dissociation and electric shock treatments made it difficult for this patient to remember the events of hospitalization, and the patient's family and the hospital staff gave no explanation for the hospital admission. Her attempts to obtain information were futile, as shown by the following extraction from nurse-patient data:

*Patient:* I lived with my mother and husband. My mother didn't know how I got here either. (According to the chart, the mother and husband had been active in the committment procedure.) I just wrote and they found out I was in ——— (name of hospital).
*Nurse:* They didn't know before that?
*Patient:* No, they didn't know where I was.
*Nurse:* Have you asked anyone about these circumstances of getting here?
*Patient:* No. The doctor asked me and when I told him, he just laughed.

Patients' use of autistic invention is often labeled guessing or imagination by them. It can cover a wide range of experiences, from the food they eat to the reason for hospitalization. In a hospital where patients are moved from ward to ward, the reasons for these transfers become an area of speculation in which patients may help each other find reasons for the move. The following is an excerpt from a group session in which a nurse was the leader. One patient had been speculating for several sessions about her move to a new ward:

*Leader:* You say that you still don't know why you came? Could you check with the head nurse, Miss V.?
*Patient 1:* She can rest.
*Leader:* This is guessing. What other way is there to find out?
*Patient 2:* They wouldn't give me information. Maybe they are not supposed to give information. I asked when I could go home. They seemed they didn't like me questioning them. Suppose she says, "I can't give you information"?

The unmet need for information increases the person's level of anxiety. The patient invents a reason that functions to meet the need and reduce the anxiety to a more tolerable level. Personal explanations, the autistic invention of reasons, probably do not alleviate the anxiety completely, since the patient can never be certain that the reasons he has invented are accurate. The pattern for autistic invention is laid down in early childhood, and perhaps hospital admission can be considered an analogous situation. Sullivan says that the child "adds an autistic element to take the place of that which cannot be inquired about." [5] That is, if the person learns that he will not receive adequate answers to his questions, he will soon stop asking questions and resort to his imagination for answers. Patients will ask for information when this is not discouraged. The following excerpt from a group meeting clearly illustrates this point:

> Patient 1: How come A. did not pass staff?
> Leader: I do not know. (Turning to Mrs. A.)
> Patient 2: I don't know, didn't ask anyone.
> Patient 3: Why didn't I pass staff?
> Leader: Could you ask someone?
> Patient 3: No.
> Patient 1: You must not have failed because you go home on visits.

Nurses can intervene in the pathology of autistic invention. Information can be given in language understandable to the patient. Questions can be answered. However, this must be done at a time when the patient's anxiety level is such that the patient can hear the information being given. In order for the nurse to observe and evaluate the patient's level of anxiety, the concept must be clear in her own mind. There are four easily recognizable levels of anxiety. The first level is characterized by increased perceptual awareness. A person having this mild degree of anxiety is alerted, sees, hears, and grasps things more readily than previously. In the second level of anxiety, a person's perceptual field is narrowed. He sees, hears, and grasps less than when in mild anxiety, but can attend to more when directed by someone to do so. The nurse can offer such direction. Learning can take place in these mild and moderate stages of anxiety. The observable behavior in the third stage of anxiety is that the perceptual field of the person has narrowed so that he focuses on a detail or many scattered details. This detail or details that have been focused on in the third stage become "blown up" in the fourth stage, and the person experiences panic, including the feelings of awe, dread, and/or uncanniness. It is impossible for learning to take place in these last two levels of anxiety (see p. 326).

The nurse, having observed the anxiety level of the patient, can take

[5] Sullivan, H. S., *The Interpersonal Theory of Psychiatry*, p. 221.

the direction of helping the patient to reduce his anxiety. Once the anxiety has been reduced to the mild or moderate levels, the nurse can proceed with giving information and/or assisting the patient to obtain the answers to questions.

The nurse can encourage and assist the patient in finding information about himself that the nurse does not possess. Perhaps the patient must learn some particular piece of information from his family or the doctor. A useful tool of psychological development that normally is learned initially in the preadolescent period is consensual validation. This concept involves talking things over with others—comparing notes with another person or persons and coming to an agreement with that person about the contents discussed. As the patient learns to replace autistic invention with consensual validation, he develops a technique for working out solutions to problems that have led to his hospitalization.

## BIBLIOGRAPHY

PEPLAU, HILDEGARD E., *Interpersonal Relations in Nursing,* G. P. Putnam's Sons, New York: 1952.

———— Therapeutic Concepts: Aspects of Psychiatric Nursing," *The League Exchange,* No. 268, National League for Nursing, New York: 1957.

SULLIVAN, HARRY STACK, *Conceptions of Modern Psychiatry,* W. W. Norton & Co., New York: 1953.

———— *The Interpersonal Theory of Psychiatry,* W. W. Norton & Co., New York: 1953.

# 5 DISGUISED LANGUAGE: A CLINICAL NURSING PROBLEM

*M. Phyllis Hurteau*

Well, some have a lot and throw off in a loud voice and still nothing will satisfy them and their speech and talk is useless and nothing.[1]

What can a nurse do to help a patient give up socially useless language and restore his verbal communication to a level of comprehension? What can she do when she cannot understand the patient's language—when it makes no sense to her? The patient's words, though they sound familiar, have a strange grammatical sequence. Sometimes the words themselves hold no intelligible meaning, and the nurse as a listener is at a loss in terms of response.

Potential responses to uncommunicative or "disguised language" are many and varied. Some known responses are suppression of the patient's autistic speech (i.e., personally useful, but socially useless words); mimicking the responses of others; laughing or restraining laughter; going along as if the listener understood; ignoring the words; embarrassment, annoyance, helplessness; exploitation of the patient in the cause of clinical teaching. There are numerous other responses peculiar to the individual nurse.

When the nurse "suppresses" the autistic speech of the patient, she follows the pattern of meaningful past people in the patient's life. Parents, teachers, and other representatives of the social order, in teaching the child dictionary meanings of verbal terms, "suppress" the child's autistic words. In this process of acculturation and learning, the child does not transpose autistic words into new words. The words disappear from awareness, but

[1] Richter, D., "Teaching a Concept of Anxiety to Patients," p. 72 (quoting patient data).

32—

continue to be available as types of the referential and thought process. Sullivan [2] refers to this when he writes of the schizophrenic person:

> Now the Schizophrenic is . . . essentially characterized by the fact that his self system has lost control of awareness so that it cannot exclude these earlier processes and restrict awareness to late, highly refined types of thought (and language). By the time one becomes schizophrenic, the self is in such a critical position that these earlier types of mental processes receive more or less the same representation in awareness that they did in late infancy or early childhood; but that does not remove from them all the values—crazy, impractical and so on—which have been attached to them in early years, and which are the reason for denying them consciousness whenever possible.

It is not only in the diagnosed schizophrenic person that one sees a resurgence of autistic language. Anxiety can call forth the phenomenon in all persons in varying degrees (see p. 326).

The nurse adds to the disorientation of the patient if she mimics responses which she, herself, does not understand. The patient gets caught up in the dilemma of the nurse who laughs, restrains it, and then feels embarrassed. This response serves to lower the already low self-esteem of the patient.

If the patient assumes that he is understood by the nurse when he is not, there is little reason for him to change. His pathology is supported by such a response.

The feeling of isolation a patient has can be enhanced when the nurse ignores him. Annoyance on her part can effect the same result. Also, annoyance expressed by the nurse can give the patient a psychological weapon with which to drive her away. Helplessness offers the patient an added burden.

Finally, exploitation can elicit painful recall of significant situations and figures in the patient's past. A significant situation for one person was the time when his play-yard peers did not understand his "very own word" for something that his mother thought so cute and acceptable.

## POSSIBLE REASONS FOR NURSE'S RESPONSE

Possible reasons for the behavior of nurses in relation to the problem, again, are many. Anxiety is basic to all of them (see p. 324). The nurse's anxiety can be converted to withdrawal in the sense of total avoidance—a defensive measure. Anxiety is increased when prestige needs and/or status needs are not met in a situation. It is detrimental to precise communica-

[2] Sullivan, H. S., *Clinical Studies in Psychiatry*, p. 24.

tion. When the nurse experiences an increased level of anxiety, often her own language fails to signify what she means to say. Many nurses have experienced the serious ramifications of communication breakdown in the hospital situation. The same nurse's language is adequate without this stress. Some nurses are more highly skilled in verbal communication than others. Yet, even with these people, under stress the potential for breakdown in transmission of communication exists.

## A METHOD OF DEALING WITH THE PROBLEM

Using the assumption that the unintelligible language of the patient is a sign of anxiety, the nurse can develop the ability to reduce the amount of this language. Through this reduction of anxiety level, a restoration of comprehension is probable. This process involves a complex two-way interpersonal relationship. The process, once learned by the nurse as a therapeutic agent, can be transmitted to others and used consistently in dealing with other patients having the problem.

The following is an example of one such therapeutic attempt at solution: The nurse was in the process of learning therapeutic psychiatric nursing skills. The patient was diagnosed as schizophrenic for the past twenty-six years. The initial encounter of nurse and patient elicited "autistic language" in the patient. Both nurse and patient resorted to "referential processes"—the patient to those of early childhood, and the nurse to those of earlier psychiatric nursing experience. The patient said, "I lost my angel." The nurse did not know what to say. She could not think immediately of the words that would tell the patient she didn't understand. In retrospect during seminar, the nurse recognized two features basic to her response: (1) increased anxiety and (2) the resultant verbal ineptness of the nurse. Examples of the patient's use of autistic language follow:

### EXAMPLE I

*Patient:* No pay comes into this house, ya know.
*Nurse:* I don't follow you.
*Patient:* No hot toast comes into this house.
*Nurse:* Is this a house, Miss M.?
*Patient:* I think this is a house—I think so.
*Nurse:* (Sat quietly and looked at the patient.)
*Patient:* It's a little house on the road—you're 'spose to get hot toast and cornflakes.
*Nurse:* Is this a house on the road?
*Patient:* (Nodding yes.) Isn't it?

*Nurse:* Is it?
*Patient:* It's a hospital, isn't it?
*Nurse:* Yes.

In the preceding example, the nurse was guided by the following psychiatric nursing principles: In the counseling role, the nurse takes the direction in communication easiest for the patient to follow. The nurse helps the patient to describe and clarify the comments of her chosen direction in the topic. The nurse assists the patient in hearing and noticing what she said: the words "house" and "a house on the road." The nurse is cautious that she does not embarrass the patient by an attitude relative to the irritationality of the statement, "I think this is a house." The patient really did think the hospital was a house. The nurse allowed the patient to arrive at more accurate description at the patient's own pace. The nurse then validated the correct description—*Patient:* "It's a hospital, isn't it?" *Nurse:* "Yes." By doing this, the nurse helps the patient capture lucid moments and make use of consensual validation.

## EXAMPLE II

*Patient:* When I was going in this house, ya know, I saw a fire—I tried to put it out. Are you supposed to put it out?
*Nurse:* Help me to understand what you're saying—I don't understand.
*Patient:* Huh?
*Nurse:* Help me to understand what you're saying—I don't understand.
*Patient:* I'm talking about something burning down. Have you got that down? I don't feel sorry for the boys—the firemen—you know—it was a good building.
*Nurse:* (Sat quietly and looked at the patient.)

In example II, the nurse repeats carefully her own words when the patient says, "Huh?" The patient's response here is indicative of selective inattention found in anxiety states (see p. 326). The nurse then avoided increasing the patient's anxiety (shown by verbosity) in that she waited for and did not push the patient too hard in order to elicit description and observation (see p. 333).

The use of disguised language by the patient decreased gradually in the fourth, fifth, and sixth sessions to abatement in the seventh and eighth sessions. Analysis of the verbatim data indicated that a therapeutic working relationship had been established at this point. Since relationships are stressful to people diagnosed as schizophrenic, it was not surprising that the patient in the ninth session used five incomprehensible statements.

By this time, however, the nurse was comfortable with verbal maneuvers selected to elicit observation and description by the patient (see p. 334). She had integrated these into her verbal communication. This skill in eliciting description of observations facilitated her dealing with an emergent change in the patient's speech pattern from the scattered type, the two quoted examples, to a repetitive type (e.g., "I, I, I, I, I, I" and "Poochy, poochy, poochy, poochy, pooch"). This latter type of speech pattern occurred in the thirteenth, fifteenth, and seventeenth sessions.

During the nineteenth session and thereafter, the patient relinquished the use of disguised language in talking with the nurse. Later, the patient was included in one of the nurse's groups. She used her "old way" of relieving anxiety only in the first few meetings. When the other patients in the group used the verbal behavior of the nurse as a model in response to disguised language, this patient did likewise.

With a nurse's help, a patient moved from an earlier developmental method of speaking to an adult level of verbal communication.

## BIBLIOGRAPHY

RICHTER, DOROTHEA, "Teaching A Concept of Anxiety to Patients," master's thesis, The Graduate School, Rutgers, The State University of New Jersey, 1957.

SULLIVAN, HARRY STACK, Clinical Studies in Psychiatry, W. W. Norton & Co., New York: 1956.

# 6 NONVERBAL COMMUNICATION

*Shirley A. Smoyak*

In the area of interpersonal relationships, what is *not* said is equally important to, if not more important than, the spoken words. Ideas and emotions can be effectively communicated through gestures alone. Gestures, when used in conjunction with verbal language, serve to emphasize and clarify the content of what is said. They may do just the opposite. Gestures may serve to indicate that the person does not really believe or feel what he has said.

Critchley,[1] who defines gesture as "a kind of italicized speech," has made a comprehensive study of gesture, including its early roots, its place in literature, and present-day studies concerning its relation to personality. He points out that elaborations of gesture include the following: [2]

1. Mimicking, pantomime and the dance.
2. Religion, with its extensive rituals and symbology.
3. Conventional gestures, i.e., those that have been "curtailed, stylized, abbreviated and later have passed into the common currency of ordinary usage." Examples are the handshake, military salute and kiss.
4. Systems of sign language that may be utilized to the total exclusion of spoken speech, such as the flag signals used at sea and the systems used by deaf-mutes.

Critchley reports on studies by Oseretsky, Ruttman, Allport, and Vernon on the correlation between personality and gesture. In considering postures that are inexplicably assumed and maintained, as in catatonic schizophrenia, Critchley[3] says, "It is probable that all these attitudes and

[1] Critchley, M., *The Language of Gesture*, p. 128.
[2] *Ibid.*, p. 10.
[3] *Ibid.*, p. 31.

mannerisms possess meaning which, though obscure, may nevertheless yield to the psychological methods of study."

In reporting on the sign language of secret societies, Critchley states that among members of a Chinese secret brotherhood, there is even a code of rules for handling inanimate objects, a walking cane, for instance. By the particular way that one handles such objects, he can be recognized in public by other members of his society. This is similar to the codified behavior at tea parties, wherein the method of handling a cup and saucer gives clues as to one's upbringing.

The following is among Critchley's examples of gestures used throughout the world in religion, the theater, and literature. This Hindu tale is about Naran, a rigidly chaperoned princess, who signals from her balcony to the minister Ssaran. She holds up one finger and encircles it with her hand; then she clasps her hands together and separates them. After that she places two fingers together and points toward the palace. The interpretation of this symbolism is: upraised fingers, a tree; the encircling action, a wall; clasping and unclasping the hands, an invitation to enter the flower garden; and the juxtaposition of two fingers, she would welcome a visit.

Frequently, in these ancient tales, and in the Bible, the sign language is very difficult for the layman to interpret, and he goes to a seer or a prophet for aid. A present-day analogy might be drawn—frequently bizarre movements or gestures are beyond the person's understanding, and he goes to a psychiatrist to have them interpreted.

Critchley allows that there is individual variation in the degree of use of gesture, but also holds that there is a nationality factor. Mediterraneans are notorious for their propensity to gesture, whereas Nordics are taught to restrain tendencies toward gesture and emotional display of all kinds.[4]

Critchley quotes Quintilian's Institutes of Oratory (A.D. 40–99): "If our gesture and looks are at variance with our speech; if we utter anything mournful with an air of cheerfulness or assert anything with an air of denial, not only impressiveness is wanting to our words, but even credibility." The truth of this last statement has been witnessed by all persons at one time or another.

Krout[5] reported the use of a hypnoanalytic technique aimed at testing the reproducibility of autistic gestures in studying the problem of gestural consistency. The experimental findings reveal that autistic gestures frequently cannot be interpreted, even though they are consistent in reap-

[4] Ibid., pp. 87–88.
[5] Krout, M., "Autistic Gestures."

pearance. He suggests that gesture analysis may be applied to personality study.

Critchley expressed the opinion that there is a universality of certain emotional movements and gestures, and that these are recognized readily by all. He offers proof for this hypothesis by relating the incident of several deaf-mutes from many different countries meeting on one occasion and being able to communicate with each other with little or no difficulty, whereas, if verbal communication were used, understanding would be impossible.

Pei [6] disagrees with this contention of universality of gesture. He states that sign language is no more truly international than speech. He shows how gestures vary in meaning and method from country to country.[7] In Italy, the gesture of stroking the chin means, "I'm so bored that I'm growing a beard." In Brazil, the same gesture means, "It's in the bag!" For protection against bad luck you would touch an iron object if you were Italian, or knock on wood if your mother country was the United States.

Critchley's statements about the universality of gesture sound something like the theory of the "racial unconscious." Both theories, when examined and tested, however, seem to lack evidence. If there were such a universal understanding, it would seem that UNESCO's project on a highway-symbol system for motorists of all languages would be a waste of time.

Birdwhistell [8] is studying the science of "kinesics," body motions as a form of communication. He is especially interested in television and states, "The T.V. performer's body is often more outspoken than the spiel itself." He thinks that Elvis (the Pelvis) Presley is the most conspicuous United States body manipulator and that "Presley's wiggles seem almost an imitation of an imitation of being sexy. That's why so many in the audience laugh and Puritans react so violently."

Ruesch, a psychiatrist, and Kees, a poet and film producer, combined authorship to explore nonverbal communication.[9] Self-expression, unintentional communication, purposeful manipulation, and group interaction are treated by pictorial illustrations and discussions. In proposing a comprehensive theory of communication, they explain two methods of codifying information.[10] The first, analogic codification, constitutes a series of sym-

[6] Pei, M., *All About Language*, p. 186.
[7] *Ibid.*, "Gesture Language."
[8] Birdwhistell, Ray L., "Listen to the Body Bird."
[9] Ruesch, J., and Kees, W., *Nonverbal Communication*.
[10] *Ibid.*, p. 8.

bols that in their proportions and relations are similar to the thing, idea, or event for which they stand. People who "think in pictures" use this system. This system, however, is difficult in communicating interpersonally. Thus one must learn to use digital codification, which deals with discrete step intervals, as in the numerical system and in the phonetic alphabet. Some of the difficulty in the communication between a mental patient and a therapist lies in the area of the patient's trying to reproduce experiences which were analogically perceived into digital codification or verbal expression. As he becomes better able to cross this gap and use verbal description, he moves closer toward mental health.

This hypothesis of theirs is applied to psychosomatic disorders, in which "organ language predominates, with action language secondary and verbal language employed least of all. As the patient improves during therapy, the language spectrum shifts to a predominance of action language. . . . Finally, . . . patients eventually grow to use verbal and gestural language appropriately." [11]

Many authors write of the importance of nonverbal communication. However, nowhere in the literature are specific suggestions spelled out for arriving at an understanding of gesture or for investigating their meaning in a psychiatric setting.

Sullivan includes gestural aspects of communication in a discussion on various diagnostic signs.[12] He describes three major divisions

    1. Stereotyped getures—the person recurrently makes the same movement in the most incongruous situations.
    2. Mannerisms—peculiar body movements are made which are not the usual accompaniments of certain thoughts.
    3. Tics—certain groups of muscles seem, as it were, to perform with complete disregard of everything else that is going on.

He states that any of these signs may appear in patients with mental disorders, but that they also may appear in any of us.

In another book, Sullivan [13] discusses the learning of gesture, in which he includes the learning of facial expressions. This learning occurs well before the first birthday, but Sullivan adds, "I might suggest that the acquisition of mannerisms through trial-and-error learning by human example is by no means confined to early life. The number of chronologic adults who are big chunks of mimicry, particularly regarding the gestural aspects of speech, is amazing. Psychiatrists often find that patients begin to sound like them. . . ."

[11] *Ibid.*, p. 166.
[12] Sullivan, H. S., *The Psychiatric Interview*, pp. 193–95.
[13] *Ibid.*, *The Interpersonal Theory of Psychiatry*, pp. 178–80.

In the clinical area, two graduate fellows carried on individual nurse-patient relationships on an almost entirely nonverbal level for a period of four months. They spent two hours per week with their respective patients.

One patient, Mr. G., during all this time, never spoke directly to his nurse. He was described by ward personnel as "very disturbed" and "quite sick." When the head nurse was leaving, she commented, "Mr. G. won't miss me. He doesn't notice what's going on." This patient paced the corridor and hallucinated for the majority of the day. When the nurse approached Mr. G. for the orientation, he quickly walked away from her. The nurse attempted to give Mr. G. this orientation and setting of limits piecemeal whenever he stayed near enough to her to make verbal communication possible.

This nurse attempted to gain an understanding of Mr. G. through observing his gestures, describing them in seminar, analyzing them, and then arriving at a formulation of their meaning. Here the learning process stopped, however, since she was not able to validate the meaning with the patient. It is not possible to work with concepts via gestures; there must be validation on a verbal level.[14] The nurse noticed that Mr. G. would make many attempts during the hour to sit next to her, but he apparently found this move very difficult. He would almost sit, but then hesitate and turn away, only to start back again. The nurse used the gesture of pointing out a chair next to her where he could sit. The nurse thought that Mr. G. understood this gesture, since this was the chair he would move toward. The nurse, observing this hesitation, vacillation, and indecision, deduced that the concept of conflict might apply here, but was not able to discover the two opposing goals and validate them with the patient. Toward the end of the relationship, Mr. G. was spending more and more time pacing closer to the nurse, or even sitting next to her for a few minutes.

Mr. M. also maintained silence for the majority of this four-month period. From time to time he answered questions in a monosyllabic fashion. His nurse attempted verbal observation of his gestures as a point from which to help the patient speak. She thought that many times he almost would say something, but he never quite got the words past some unknown barrier. This nurse was able to move a step further than the nurse in the first situation described. With Mr. M. she was able to validate the meaning of some of his gestures. For example:

[14] Perhaps the exception to this is in the case of the mother-infant relationship, where validation is done nonverbally. Both experience satisfaction when the infant's needs which, expressed nonverbally, are correctly interpreted and relieved or met by the mother.

*Nurse:* I have noticed that sometimes you shake your foot more than at other times. Perhaps this is when something I do makes you more uncomfortable.

*Mr. M.:* (Nods head "Yes," and utters deep sigh.)

The nurse noticed that as she became more anxious, Mr. M.'s anxiety seemed to increase, and his leg and foot motions increased proportionately. This motion was a fairly accurate measurement or indicator of his anxiety level. One interesting comment about this relationship that is not related to the subject of gestures is that although the nurse began to doubt if Mr. M. would ever speak to her, he spoke "several paragraphs worth" during the last few minutes of the last hour.

In another nurse-patient relationship, gestures were used frequently by both the nurse and the patient, although verbal communication was also used to a large extent. Again, gestures served as accurate indicators of anxiety on the part of both nurse and patient. When Mr. T. became anxious, he moved around in his seat, crossed and uncrossed his legs, ran his fingers through his hair or over his top lip, or when very anxious, got up and went to the bathroom. When the nurse became anxious, her hands became cold and perspired, she stopped taking notes, chewed on her pen, or sat forward in her chair. At one particularly anxious moment, the nurse moved forward in her seat, and then the patient also moved forward. The nurse advanced forward more, as did the patient until finally they were so far forward on their chairs that a slight nudge would have sent them sprawling on the floor. At this point the patient got up and went to the bathroom. That these gestures are indicators of anxiety has been validated by the nurse and the patient. For example:

*Mr. T.:* (Crosses and uncrosses legs.)

*Nurse:* (Following the movement with her eyes.) You're feeling uncomfortable?

*Mr. T.:* Yes, very. I guess my legs gave away my secret again. (Smiling and sitting back in chair.)

Mr. T. interpreted many gestures of other people autistically, and described how he did this. Working with the nurse, he arrived at an explanation of the process. For example:

(Preceded by discussion of other people being against him.)

*Mr. T.:* They would "shoe" this person.

*Nurse:* I don't understand what you mean by "shoe."

*Mr. T.:* They would lift their shoe and put it down again. That's all the sympathy they had.

*Nurse:* How did you arrive at that?

*Mr. T.:* At what?

*Nurse:* That, "That's all the sympathy they had."

*Mr. T.:* Well, in my mind, it's a way of saying "that's that!"

*Nurse:* You mean something like—"putting your foot down"? Are shoe and foot connected?

*Mr. T.:* That's right. I say it my way. I used to imagine other mannerisms —like when you're rubbing your eyes means you're staring too hard, or when you're folding your arms across your chest means, "Keep away from me," and when you're putting your hands behind your back means "I'm open."

At several points in the relationship Mr. T. brought books to the hour and told the therapist "stories." At first the nurse therapist tried this approach: "Shall we talk about you or O. Henry?" Mr. T. was able to use his imagination and always came up with proof that the story really concerned him, so he and the nurse were, in fact, talking about him. The nurse then tried a new approach. When Mr. T. began to discuss literature, she closed her book, put her pencil down, and looked around in a bored fashion at the ward and out the window. From time to time she glanced at Mr. T. to see if he was still on the same subject. The first time this technique was used, Mr. T. gave a twenty-minute monologue on the current book and then said, "Well, now I'll tell you about a fight I had yesterday." The second time this technique was used, the therapist had just put down her pencil when Mr. T. said excitedly, "Okay! Okay! Let's talk about me. I know I've changed the subject."

Mr. T.'s father, according to the patient, was quite concerned with the "sickness" of some of his son's gestures. It appears that lay persons have definite thoughts about what kind of gestures can be labeled sane or insane. Mr. T. stated that his father became very angry when he saw him gesturing oddly with his hands or sticking his tongue out a bit and wiping his lips before he spoke. Mr. T. said his father "yells at me and says 'Stop that! That's a sick way of using your hands and tongue. Stop it this minute! Do you want to make yourself sicker?'"

Learning the meaning of gestures is as valuable in group work as it is in working with individual patients. Watching the group as a whole, or individual members within the group, will help the group leader ascertain the general feeling of a group or their reaction to a particular area of discussion.

A husband and wife group-leader team met with a group of teen-age girls for one hour each week. The husband is a psychiatric technician with training in group work. The wife is a nurse. Frequently, during the hour, the husband and wife exchanged eye signals which said, "Well, are you going to pick that subject up or shall I?" On several occasions, group members noticed this gesture and commented on it. One fifteen-year-old girl said, "Say, Mr. M., are you making out with your wife with that look or just what does it mean?" This opportunity was used to validate the gesture with the patient, and an explanation like this was given: "No, we weren't 'making out,' but just checking to see who was going to speak." This handling of the matter puts the facts on the table, where they can be examined and validated.

These leaders found that the teen-agers were very aware of gestures and quick to ask for validation on a verbal level. As one girl told a tale of her exploits of prostitution and alcoholism, she was stopped by one of her peers who asked, "Are you fidgeting, sweating, and turning red because you're lying or because you're ashamed of what you have done?"

Two graduate fellows led group sessions weekly for three months at a county mental institution. Almost all the patients in the group had been hospitalized for many years. Only two patients in the group of fifteen women were verbal at the outset of the group. The nurses found that this principle applied: In a working relationship phase of group work, the members will take on the manner of operating that the leaders use. If the nurses questioned and investigated the meaning of nonverbal communication, the members later initiated these investigations and inquiries on their own. For example, the nurses observed that about five women in the group slept at intervals during the hour. They pointed this out to the group and invited them to take a look at it and analyze it. Suggestions by the group were that the sleepers were not interested, had had too much Thorazine, were very tired, or were troubled for some reason or another. After further discussion, they formulated that the sleeping was an escape when the content of the discussion caused them discomfort or anxiety. One patient, who sometimes slept during the hour, described it this way "Sometimes I get very upset and then I feel just plain knocked out—wish I could go to sleep for days." This technique of inviting the group to examine nonverbal as well as verbal communication was used during all the sessions.

In order to understand nonverbal communication, the conceptual framework of the learning process may be used. The tasks and questions are presented according to the operations of this concept and process. These are—

1. Observing what is going on: facial expression, posture, body movement, etc.

2. Describing the observation correctly and accurately.

3. Analyzing the nonverbal communication: What does it accomplish? Is it saying something? How does it operate?

4. Formulating an explanation: What is the message of the nonverbal communication?

5. Validating this formulation with at least one other person.

6. Using this formulation as foresight.

These steps were carried out in the group at the county mental institution in regard to sleeping during the hour. In subsequent hours, when a patient started to go to sleep, one of the members would say, "Oh, oh. She must be getting upset. I wonder why?" These steps could not be carried out in the case of Mr. G., since consensual validation was not possible.

## SUMMARY

1. Nonverbal communication is as valuable as, if not more valuable than, verbal communication in the therapeutic psychiatric setting.

2. The use of gestures in the therapeutic situation is most valuable when validation of meaning is possible.

3. The theory of the universality of gestures seems to lack adequate proof.

4. Gestures can serve as accurate indicators of anxiety.

5. Your gestures may "give you away" by contradicting what you are trying to communicate verbally.

6. The study of nonverbal communication as a science is new; much research, especially in the clinical area, is needed.

## BIBLIOGRAPHY

BIRDWHISTELL, RAY L., "Listen to the Body Bird," *Time*, 70:68, July 15, 1957.

CRITCHLEY, MACDONALD, *The Language of Gesture*, Edward Arnold & Co., London, 1939.

KROUT, MAURICE, "Autistic Gestures," *Psychological Monographs*, Psychological Review Company, Vol. XLVI, No. 4, 1935.

PEI, MARIO, *All About Language*, 1st ed., J. B. Lippincott Co., Philadelphia and New York: 1954.

———— "Gesture Language," *Life*, 28:79–80, January 9, 1950.

RUESCH, J., and KEES, W., *Nonverbal Communication*, University of California Press, Berkeley and Los Angeles: 1956.

SULLIVAN, HARRY STACK, *The Interpersonal Theory of Psychiatry*, W. W. Norton & Co., New York: 1953.

———— *The Psychiatric Interview*, W. W. Norton & Co., New York: 1954.

# 7 TOWARD A STUDY OF SILENCE

*Shirley E. Davis*

Many people have been told at one time or another that "silence is golden." Is it? If so, for whom is silence golden? How powerful silence can be is determined by the power given to it. An individual can be intimidated by silence or make it work for him.

The problem of silence can be approached via the concept of anxiety. According to Peplau,[1] "anxiety is a response to unknown danger that is felt, experienced as discomfort, and that arms the human organism for mobilizing resources." One of the characteristics of anxiety is that as the discomfort increases, the perceptual awareness decreases. The nurse who is aware of the foregoing as she perceives the patient's discomfort can use this natural response to advantage in problem-solving as she assists the patient in the reduction of the anxiety.

> I distinguish this tension of anxiety from the sundry tensions already called needs by saying that the relaxation of the tension of anxiety, the re-equilibrium of being in this specific respect, is the experience, not of satisfaction, but of interpersonal security.[2]

Sullivan further writes of his formulation of the theorem of escape:

> The self-system from its nature—its communal environment factors, organization and functional activity—tends to escape influence by experience which is incongruous to its current organization and functional organization.[3]

[1] Peplau, H. E., *Interpersonal Relations in Nursing*, p. 127.
[2] Sullivan, H. S., *Interpersonal Theory of Psychiatry*, p. 42.
[3] *Ibid.*, p. 190.

As discussed in this chapter, silence is an escape from a threat to the self *for those persons capable of speech.* Silence is a manifestation of the self's need for security. It is characterized by a period of time without verbal communication.

Assuming that all behavior is meaningful, another question arises. What are the various meanings of silence? Some of these meanings can be abstracted from the clinical practice of nursing. Various nursing situations follow wherein the meanings of silence are speculated about or have been validated by the person or persons who used the maneuver. The implications of the various meanings of silence are anything but unique to nursing situations. Silences occur in any type of interpersonal setting or situation.

The first interaction example is one in which the meaning of silence is unvalidated by the person who used the silence. A nurse-patient relationship had been initiated through mutual decisions of both persons involved regarding the expenditure of time. The patient verbalized for several sessions. Then, he became silent. The nurse had expected this patient to verbalize, and her own anxiety level increased during these silent times with the patient. She was increasingly concerned with the reduction of her own anxiety. She related to her colleagues, "As I became comfortable in the silence, I became aware of what was going on around me." She decided to "sit this one out." Seven weeks went by, and still the patient did not talk. Thereupon, the nurse decided that anything that happens in the situation, even silence, can be discussed. During the eighth week, she broke the silence by verbalizing her thoughts and feelings to the patient so that he would know the nurse's view of the situation.

*Nurse:* I have the feeling that you get pretty uncomfortable.
*Patient:* (Silent. Movement of extremities.)
*Nurse:* You may say something if you like.
*Patient:* (Silence.)
*Nurse:* I get uncomfortable when you and I sit in silence. I feel helpless. I would like to learn how to help you, but I don't know how to go about it. You and I have one more session on Thursday.
*Patient:* (Silence.)
*Nurse:* Good-bye.

The final session began, as usual, in silence. Thereupon, the following occurred:

*Nurse:* I have the thought that you want to talk. Correct me if I am not right. You seem to be able to talk to others on the ward. I thought you might be angry with me.
*Patient:* (Shakes his head to signify "No.")

*Nurse:* I wouldn't have known if you hadn't told me. This is our last meeting. (Pause.) What are your plans for Christmas?

*Patient:* Well, I'm going to be invited out to dinner. . . . (Verbalizations continued to the end of the session and the good-byes were said.)

The most valid explanatory theory is anxiety. This theoretical explanation was validated by one of the two persons—the nurse. The nurse had a cue to the anxiety in the patient. She herself expressed awareness of her own anxiety. The patient may have felt this anxiety of the nurse, even though he may not have been aware of it at the time. The concept which explains the transfer of feelings between two persons is empathy. Peplau [4] writes, "Empathy refers to an ability to feel what is going on in a situation without specifically being able to discuss and to identify elements of it into awareness." Each person may have reinforced the other's anxiety. Once the nurse had her own anxiety under control, the patient's anxiety from empathy was not reinforced. She was able to help to reduce the patient's discomfort by the innocuous question, "What are your plans for Christmas?"

No one can say precisely and validly just why the patient was silent. He was the only one who knew and would be able to validate the nursing formulations. The only analysis possible is in the realm of speculations rather than explanatory concepts. He may have perceived himself as being unworthy, unimportant, and/or unable to talk with an authoritative figure in the hospital setting. His thoughts may have been perceived as being personal and/or too precious to himself to share with others. He may have had experiences in the early weeks of the nurse-patient relationship with which he could not cope. The manner in which the social system and other elements of the hospital impinged upon this patient in the early weeks of relationship with the nurse is another area for many speculations.

Review of the clinical and learning experiences of nurses reveals several meanings attributed to silence by the person or persons involved. These meanings, in all probability, are an incomplete listing. The author believes that the interpretation a person places on his own silence is the one in which he perceives the silence of others.

In the general hospital, as well as in the psychiatric hospital, nurses have had recurring experiences with patients who are silent upon admission. There seems to be fear of the unknown that makes patients experience an increase in anxiety. This increase in anxiety may result in the use of silence as a maneuver to obtain some comfort. When a person enters

[4] Peplau, *op. cit.,* p. 173.

a general hospital, he is there due to a defect in organic make-up. His self-picture is changed. The silence is a maneuver that partially hides *the discomfort*. One of these persons in a general hospital described his reason for silence thus:

> *Patient:* I didn't know what was going to happen to me. I was afraid I was going to die. (Brief pause.) The operation seems so simple now that you [nurse] have explained what is going to happen to me. I wish someone had told me sooner; I wouldn't have worried so much.

A second meaning of silence is inherent in the manifestations of anxiety. People have become "speechless" by some shock to the self-system, as in awe, dread, utter despair, grief, anger, hostility, helplessness, feelings of failure. All of the foregoing are manifestations of anxiety. The ability to communicate verbally undergoes considerable alteration by these specific manifestations of anxiety and by anxiety in general. The resulting silence is usually not in the awareness of the individual.

A third meaning of silence is *thought*. During a teaching seminar, the topic of silence was brought to the student's attention by the faculty member. The question of why some group members were silent and others were not was raised. One of the replies is significant to this meaning of silence. "Someone else always says what they have to before I formulate an answer to the problem and present it." This student apparently considered statements of other persons prior to making her own formulations and verbalization. This silence appears to be a strategic withdrawal maneuver which is consciously used to collect one's thoughts. This reply negates the possibility that silence always means the absence of thought or intelligence. Silence can be constructive. Clark's study [5] indicates the constructive use of silence. The subjects of this study were asked to solve problems without consciously making use of any explicit form of behavior. Images were substituted when thinking was baffled or when precepts would have ordinarily been of use. The individual was found to be noticeably quiet when actually thinking. Movement was usually apparent just before the thinker indicated that he had resolved the problem.

Some persons seem to verbalize more rapidly following stimuli than do other persons. Not all persons think by using pictures or images. Some persons seem to transfer their thoughts immediately into words which appear to facilitate verbal communication.

A fourth meaning of silence is inherent in the silent *way of life* of the Trappist monks. Wiesman [6] writes: "To them silence is a means of tem-

[5] Clark, R., "An Experimental Study of Silent Thinking."
[6] Wiesman, G., "Silence and Psychotherapy," pp. 241–60.

porary rejection of the goals and appetites of the world in order to establish direct communication with higher and more abiding powers."

A fifth meaning of silence is the *comfort* experienced in the silences of friends and marital partners. Communication has been established via other modes such as nonverbal communication—i.e., gestures, movements, etc.—and empathic communication.

Silence is the absence of verbal communication. However, it does communicate to other persons. One of the problems of silence is the distortion inherent in the assumption that silence has one meaning—that of the person making the assumption.

# BIBLIOGRAPHY

CLARK, RUTH, "An Experimental Study of Silent Thinking," *Arch. Psychol.* Vol. 11, No. 48, April, 1922.

PEPLAU, HILDEGARD E., *Interpersonal Relations in Nursing,* G. P. Putnam's Sons, New York: 1952.

RUESCH, JURGEN, and BATESON, GREGORY, *The Social Matrix of Psychology,* W. W. Norton & Co., New York: 1951.

SULLIVAN, HARRY STACK, *Interpersonal Theory of Psychiatry,* W. W. Norton & Co., New York: 1953.

WIESMAN, G., "Silence and Psychotherapy," *J. Study Interpersonal Processes,* pp. 241–60, August, 1955.

# 8 THERE ARE NO MUTE PATIENTS

*Gloria Oden*

[Mutism, as used by this writer, is a manifestation of a functional dis-order. Nurses realize, generally, that there is mutnesss due to organic prob-lems. The writer quickly acknowledges that there are aphasics. Patients who have aphasia are of two different types. There are those who, due to con-genital anomalies or defects of the speech organs or organic damage sus-tained at a preverbal age, have never used spoken language. There are other patients who have been verbal and who later, due to some anatomical change, have lost their ability to speak.

This paper is not concerned with the aphasic patients, however. It is concerned with a functional problem, aphrasia. Aphrasic patients have the capacity for speech, the ability to speak, but do not, for various reasons, use their capacity. A more accurate term might be "low verbal productivity" or "nonproductive verbally." The choice of the term used herein, however, was made by the author of the chapter.]

There is no such thing as a mute patient. The writer saw the applica-tion of this concept by a clinical specialist in psychiatric nursing and then tried it herself.

What are the dynamics of nonverbal behavior? The psychotic patient experiences severe anxiety because of lack of satisfaction and security in interpersonal relationships. Internally, the self-concept is extremely low. Externally, the ability for socialization is limited. Attempts to meet in-ternal and external stress result in the devolpment of defensive patterns. The defenses prove inadequate, anxiety increases, and a vicious circle of failure followed by more limitïng patterns of defense emerge. Eventually the high degree of anxiety and the repeated failure of defensive patterns result in an episode of panic. The personality disorganizes, then reorgan-izes along pathological lines. Psychotic reorganization is marked by disturbances in reality relationships, with changes in thinking, affect, and behavior.

The mute patient appears to withdraw completely from reality relationships, cutting off all communication with others. Avoidance of all relationships reduces anxiety to a level that is tolerable. There is, however, a healthy aspect of the patient's personality that leans toward contact with others, for "we are all much more simply human than otherwise," [1] with a need for relationships with others. This conflict between the desire for interpersonal relationships and the desire to avoid all contact with others is the initial problem to be solved. Nursing intervention can assist the patient in resolving this conflict by movement toward health.

The nurse, too, has problems in the situation. She attempts to establish a relationship with the patient and to communicate verbally with him. Frequently, her efforts are met by silence. The nurse's anxiety increases because of repeatedly unsuccessful attempts to communicate (she, too, has a self-concept), and the nurse withdraws from the situation. It then becomes a problem of mutual withdrawal. This, in turn, is reinforced by other staff members and patients on the ward who anticipate silence from the quiet patient. [2]

This chapter deals with nursing intervention to establish verbal communication with the quiet patient in a group-therapy setting. It consists of two approaches which operate concurrently—the establishment of a one-to-one relationship with the nurse outside the group setting and the establishment of multiple relationships in a group. This combined approach affords maximum opportunity to motivate the quiet patient to verbalize with one or more individuals, according to his ability at a given point in time.

Hurteau [3] has done extensive work with quiet patients in the nurse-patient relationship. The results have been rewarding. Using principles and techniques cited by Hurteau in her H-SET, [4] the writer has modified them for application in a group setting. The following describes the basic principles and techniques used. Examples have been culled from actual data of group and individual meetings.

The group consisted of six schizophrenic patients with no organic bases for their muteness. One patient was classified as mute by ward personnel, the second as rarely speaking. The remaining four patients were verbal and in good contact with reality. The four verbal patients lived in

[1] Sullivan, H. S., *Conceptions of Modern Psychiatry*, p. 16.
[2] The writer will henceforth refer to the nonverbal patient as the quiet patient.
[3] Hurteau, Phyllis, "The Psychiatric Nurse and The Mute Patient."
[4] Hurteau's Speech Eliciting Technique (H-SET), *Ibid.*, pp. 57–58.

the same ward; the quiet patients were selected from other wards in the hospital.

Group meetings of thirty minutes' duration were held twice a week. Before and after each group meeting the nurse spent ten to fifteen minutes with each of the quiet patients on his own ward. Initial responses were made by the quiet patients in the one-to-one relationship with the nurse. By the fifth meeting, both quiet patients were giving limited responses at the group meetings.

INDIVIDUAL MEETINGS

The basic principle used by the nurse in initiating verbal communication with the quiet patient was that the patient could and would speak. She approached the patient with a quietly optimistic attitude. Her choice of simple, precise communication which required an answer added impetus to her belief that the patient would respond.

Persistence was found to be essential. Each question was stated slowly. Adequate time was allowed for the patient to respond. The same question was asked repeatedly. The nurse limited the introduction of new topics to assure consistency within the interview.

Orientation was a part of each interview. At the onset the nurse stated, "I will be here for fifteen minutes to talk with you." Five minutes before leaving, the nurse told the patient, "There are five minutes left for you to talk with me today." During the latter part of the interview, the nurse queried, "What will you do after I leave?" Immediately before termination, the nurse oriented the patient to her return by saying, "I will return to talk with you tomorrow morning at ten-thirty."

[The choice of the preposition used by this nurse, and others, is of considerable importance. Note that the preposition selected was "with" rather than such words as "to," "at," or "for." The word most frequently used by novice interviewers is "to." Implicit in the preposition as used, "I will be here for fifteen minutes to talk *to* you," is the idea that the nurse will talk and the patient will listen.

When the nurse's statement is altered, the implication is modified. The nurse's statement, "I will return to talk *with* you tomorrow," implies that both parties, the nurse and the patient will participate in the interaction. Reciprocity is conveyed by the use of the preposition "with," so that the patient is able to grasp the intention of the nurse that he, too, will talk.

One of the difficulties experienced by novice interviewers is grasping the subtleties of the spoken language. In social conversation, the preposition chosen in the above statements, "with," "at," "to," etc., are of less consequence than the precision required in the counseling role of the nurse.

During the interview, the questions formulated could not be answered by a "yes" or a "no." All statements pertained to the present or referred only to the immediate past or future. Such questions as "What were you doing before I came?" "What do you see (down the hall, outside the window, etc.)?" or "What will you do after I leave?" were found to encourage a verbal response.]

Initially, conversation was directed toward eliciting descriptions of actions rather than of thoughts or feelings. This approach is least threatening to the patient. Both quiet patients responded verbally during the first nurse-patient interview and continued to speak during every subsequent interview.

GROUP MEETINGS

All the group members were invited to participate at the group meetings and had agreed to do so. The quiet patients were particularly anxious during the early meetings of the group. While the nurse encouraged the quiet patients to remain for the entire meeting, she passively allowed them to leave the group if they desired to do so. During the first three meetings, the quiet patients left before the conclusion of the meeting. After the third meeting, the quieter of the two patients was able to remain for the entire meeting, while the second patient again left before the meeting terminated.

The quiet patients were treated in the same manner as the verbal patients during group meetings. The only modification of this principle was that the nurse consistently directed a question to each of the quiet patients to include them in each topic under discussion. If the quiet patient did not respond, the nurse repeated the question. The nurse acted as a model for the group by her attitude of expectancy that the quiet members would speak. In addition, the nurse did not avoid discussion of the quiet patients when their silence was mentioned by other group members.

During the fourth group meeting, the nurse asked a quiet patient several questions but received no response. The nurse heard the other group members whispering such comments as "She's a mute," "She won't talk," "Boy, that nurse is patient," and "She never talks." The nurse responded with a matter-of-fact, "Miss K. is able to speak. She often talks with me. Miss K. will talk in the group meetings when she is ready. Were any of you other group members quiet when you came to the hospital?" Mrs. M., who was particularly talkative, responded with, "Oh, yes, I was. I could hear everything that was being said. Sometimes I would shake my head when somebody talked to me, but that's all I did."

There were much laughter and good-natured teasing following this statement, whereupon the group decided that Miss K., would speak.

Until this time the group had tended to exclude the quiet patients. After Mrs. M's description of her past experiences, the group began to include the quiet patients in the conversation. The following excerpts from the data are indicative of the change of attitude within the group.

Mrs. C.: C'mon, Dorothy, you can talk. Answer the question. We want to know if you have any brothers and sisters, too.
Miss K.: (Looked down, frowned, and did not answer.)

(Later, during the same session, the following occurred.)
Mrs. C.: Do you leave the ward for activities, Dorothy? Dorothy? Huh, Dorothy? Answer the question.
Miss K.: (Raised her head, looked at Mrs. C., moved her lips for several seconds and replied.) No.
Mrs. C.: She talked!
Mrs. J.: That's good, Dorothy. You can talk to us.
Nurse: Yes, Miss K. can talk. She will talk even more when she's ready.
Mrs. M.: Yes, she will. I used to be like that. I didn't talk. Look at me now.
(The group laughed.)
Mrs. J.: Boy, that's hard to believe. You sure are a gabber now.
Mrs. M.: I know it, but it's true.

The combined individual and group approach to the quiet patient enables the nurse to foster dependence, independence, and interdependence concurrently. In the individual phase of nursing intervention, the nurse allows the patient to be dependent upon her. She encourages independence, however, by permitting the patient to do whatever she is able to do for herself. The nurse avoids manipulating the patient into complete dependence upon the nurse. Interdependence is developed in the group setting. As soon as the quiet patient responds verbally to the nurse, the nurse encourages the patient to "tell the entire group." On the quiet patient's ward, the nurse brings a third person into the relationship. This person is usually a staff member who is interested in the patient. By using additional personnel resources, continuity of nursing intervention is attained.

A dual approach to the problem of mutism, including individual and group contacts, appears to be an effective method of nursing intervention. It enables the nurse to form a one-to-one relationship with the quiet patient, while avoiding the possibility of the formation of a symbiotic relationship. By providing opportunity and encouragement for the quiet patient to form single and multiple relationships, movement toward socialization can progress according to the ability of the individual.

The techniques described above were successful with the patients discussed in this chapter. They remain very ill. They have, however, made the first difficult stride toward health by establishing relationships with others through verbal communication.

[The editors recently supervised a student as she worked with a verbally nonproductive patient. The reasons for failure or refusal of patients to speak are numerous. Some are noted above. A unique reason for functional mutism by the patient was stated directly by the patient when he resumed his use of spoken language. An excerpt from the nurse-patient data follows. These statements were made during the seventeenth interaction session.

*Nurse:* Patients decline or refuse to use speech for various reasons. Something is accomplished by the behavior. What purpose did silence serve for you?

*Patient:* (Laughed. Moved about in chair. Seemed reluctant to answer the question.) What did I get out of it? You wouldn't believe it if I told you. They have all kinds of kids—students you know—on this ward. Nurses, practical nurses, aides, trainees of all kinds. Well, this will sound silly, but I used to talk. They have a man down here who don't talk. Those students have got some kinda idea about figuring out—or outfiguring—that old guy. It was really funny, now I think about it. This old guy used to sit there and the kids would walk over. So he'd look kinda down and they'd say such things as "Do you want a drink?" "Do you want an orange?" "Do you want a cigarette?" "Do you want some candy?" Stuff like that. Well, he don't answer "yes" or "no," so they all keep supplying him with stuff. They all feel good cause they figure they've "read him" and he's making out.

I got no family to supply me with money and stuff so when the next kids come on the ward, I figured to try it too. I made out. I got stuff you wouldn't believe—even money once—and the girls got pleased 'cause they thought they could figure what I wanted or needed. The whole thing went so good I found I could get more for nothing—which was what I had, nothing—by silence than by asking. I told you you wouldn't believe it.

You ought to come around where there are students and watch the silent patients make out. What they have handed to them, you won't believe. Now I talk to you and I got no more suppliers. Guess they figure I can ask for what I want. I used to do better with the guessing-what-Joe-wants game, though. Maybe I'll go back to it—who knows.]

# BIBLIOGRAPHY

HURTEAU, PHYLLIS, "A Proposed Nursing Intervention in Mutism," unpublished thesis blueprint, Rutgers, The State University of New Jersey, 1961.
——— "The Psychiatric Nurse and the Mute Patient," *Am. J. Nursing,* 62:55–60, 1962.
POWDERMAKER, F., and FRANK J., *Group Psychotherapy,* Harvard University Press, Cambridge, Mass.: 1953.
SULLIVAN, HARRY STACK, *Conceptions of Modern Psychiatry,* W. W. Norton & Co., New York: 1953.

# SECTION

# II

## SOME ADDITIONAL PROBLEMS MANIFESTED IN INTERPERSONAL RELATIONSHIPS IN NURSING

# 9 ROLE TESTING IN A PSYCHOTHERAPEUTIC NURSE–PATIENT RELATIONSHIP

*Anita M. Werner*

The necessity for an awareness and identification of the roles enacted by a nurse and patient is an important aspect of the psychotherapeutic nurse-patient relationship. The nurse needs to know in what role she perceives the patient in order to facilitate the accomplishment of the therapeutic goals of the relationship.

Stanton and Schwartz [1] define role as an "organization of human behavior" which is recognizable and identifiable and which must satisfy certain needs of the individual. Lindesmith and Strauss [2] further define role as something learned, involving verbal communication. They also stress the important point that roles are not isolated but must be related to counterroles.

The process of role enactment is spelled out by Lindesmith and Strauss: [3]

    1. An identification of self
    2. Behavior in a given situation which is appropriate to this identification
    3. A background of related acts by others which serve to guide specific performances
    4. An evaluation by the individual and by others of the role enactment

There exist certain expectations of the roles of the nurse and of the patient. Role expectations, according to Parsons,[4] grow out of "an organ-

[1] Stanton, A., and Schwartz, M., *The Mental Hospital*, p. 472.
[2] Lindesmith, A. R., and Strauss, A. L., *Social Psychology*, Ch. 12, pp. 371–410.
[3] *Ibid.*, p. 8
[4] Parsons, T., *Towards a General Theory of Action*, pp. 13–16.

ized system of interactions between ego and alter [which leads] to reciprocal expectations of each other's actions and attitudes."

For purposes of this chapter, a role is defined as a learned and organized pattern of social interactions. These interactions are based upon reciprocal expectations of actions and attitudes.

A psychotherapeutic nurse-patient relationship, according to Peplau,[5] involves intervention by the nurse to facilitate the development of learning products in another person and to provide "opportunities and setting for experimentation in the use of new patterns of relating to people based upon such learning products." A nurse-patient relationship of this type is used in this chapter to analyze role testing.

Miss C. is a thirty-two-year-old woman, diagnosed as schizophrenic, who had been hospitalized four times during the past ten years. She had been in a large state hospital for a period of four months when the nurse-therapist began working with her.

Miss C. had in the past been in therapy with a psychiatrist. Because her ability to understand the nurse's behavior was limited by her past experiences in similar relationships, e.g., her experience with the psychiatrist, she immediately placed the nurse in the role of a psychiatrist. In the first four interviews, she related, without prompting, what she called her "case history." This "case history" was typical of that expected and asked for by a psychiatrist on a routine admission to a mental hospital. She told the nurse such information as:

> *Patient:* I had double pneumonia. I also had whooping cough. My brother and I heaved over the banister. Maybe my illness had something to do with it.
> *Nurse:* With what?
> *Patient:* I just mention it to let you know I had the ordinary childhood diseases.

She later validated the nurse's speculation about this particular role by asking the nurse if she were studying to be a psychiatrist.

The question of the difference between a nurse-psychotherapist and another kind of a psychotherapist might be raised at this point. Do the functions differ, and if so, in what ways? According to Peplau, the nurse-psychotherapist functions similarly to other psychotherapists, but in a different situation, that is, the nursing situation. "The fact that the psychotherapist's role is merely one among several sub-roles is one principal difference between the practice of psychoanalysis and the practice of nursing." [6]

[5] Peplau, H., "Therapeutic Concepts," p. 2.
[6] *Ibid.*, p. 21–22.

Miss C. had also, in the past, related with social workers. She spent several interviews in which she talked about her job history and her work skills and capabilities:

> . . . So that about is the job situation. That's my capacities. I'm not an office worker. That's very important to me. There must be something I can do well.

Analysis of these data supported the awareness of the nurse that the patient was placing her in the role of a social worker.

At one time she saw the nurse as a peer or a chum and tried to relate to her as if she were her girl friend. She mentioned several times the similarities between the nurse and her "other girl friend." Both were people who showed an interest in her and with whom she felt free to talk about things that were intimate to her. An important aspect of a chum relationship is the expectation that the needs of both parties will be considered and that there will be a mutual sharing of intimacies. The relationship between the nurse and Miss C. was different in that the nurse expected the needs of the patient to be the primary focus of the relationship.

The patient's beginning awareness that the relationship with her nurse therapist was a different one came in a disguised form in the fourth interview, in which she related a childhood experience about a baseball game:

> I used to play baseball. That was new to me. I felt like a real hick. But I hit the ball. I felt so awkward. All eyes are on you if you're new. By accident, I hit the ball, so I wasn't so much an object of attention. So it pays to hit the ball.

To interpret this symbolic material, the nurse used a method of decoding, i.e., picking out the key concepts in the data, transposing them by use of synonyms and reclassifying them in relation to other concepts or, as in this case, in another context. The decoded meaning was restated as follows:

> I used to act in an interview which was new to me. I felt uncomfortable, but I hit upon the method of the interview. I felt incompetent. The nurse's eyes are on me if I'm uncomfortable. By chance, I hit upon the method of the interview. So I wasn't so much an object of the nurse's attention. So it is worthwhile to hit upon the method of the interview.

In a later session, the sixth interview, the patient indicated that her awareness of the necessity to learn a different role was even clearer.

*Patient:* You start over at anything.
*Nurse:* Who starts over?

*Patient:* We do. Even if it's an interview, anything you attempt to do is new anyway. Every interview is different.

In learning this new role, she distorted the nurse's role into that of mother-surrogate and acted with feelings of helplessness, expressing in indirect ways a desire to be cared for. The role of mother-surrogate can be therapeutic if it provides a mothering experience which the patient has not had. "It requires sensitive observation and awareness, disciplined by the use of concepts which help explain what is observed, to transform the role-action of mother-surrogate into vehicles for psychotherapeutic intervention." [7]

During the initial interviews, the nurse saw the patient in the counter-role of a stranger, whom she was gradually getting to know and to understand. When the patient, however, began to express a need to be cared for, the nurse responded by seeing the patient as a child. By so doing, she increased the patient's dependency. When the nurse became aware that she saw the patient as a child, she was able to evaluate the patient's need for dependency and begin to help her progress toward a state of inter-dependency and, finally, independence. Then both patient and nurse saw each other as adults and cast each other in roles peculiarly individual to each of them.

## SUMMARY

The foregoing analysis presents role testing as it relates to a psychotherapeutic nurse-patient relationship. It illustrates the roles in which a patient and a nurse cast each other in the process of therapeutic nursing intervention.

## BIBLIOGRAPHY

LINDESMITH, A. R., and STRAUSS, A. L., *Social Psychology*, Dryden Press, New York: 1956, Ch. 12.

PARSONS, TALCOTT, *Towards a General Theory of Action*, Harvard University Press, Cambridge, Mass.: 1951.

PEPLAU, HILDEGARD E., "Therapeutic Concepts: Aspects of Psychiatric Nursing," *The League Exchange*, No. 26B, National League for Nursing, New York: 1957.

STANTON, ALFRED, and SCHWARTZ, MORRIS, *The Mental Hospital*, Basic Books, New York: 1954.

[7] *Ibid.*, p. 10.

# 10 SUPPORT: A LAY CONCEPT IN NURSING

*Elizabeth W. Carter*

In nursing schools "support" floats around in informal gab sessions and in formal class periods, surreptitiously avoiding definition or investigation. In conversations among graduate nurses it continues to be an all-pervading, mysterious, undefined term. For example, it is frequently associated with such phrases as "meeting all the needs," "understanding the patient," and "accepting the patient as he is." What do these phrases mean? Support is discussed by nurses who may know what they mean when they say the word; however, since it is not defined, in such circumstances each person who hears the word attaches his own connotation, regardless of the original intention of the speaker or the content of the discussion.

In eliciting several nurses' opinions, this writer found that nurses understand support as an innate, intuitive quality possessed by "good" nurses. When asked if nurses give support to patients, the answer received was unanimously affirmative. However, when asked to define support, the answers, given more thoughtfully, were extremely varied and frequently difficult to follow. The most frequent thought expressed was that this "support" is something that cannot be taught or learned; either a nurse has it or she doesn't. Furthermore, on the basis of possession or nonpossession of this apparently unique quality or ability, nurses are often judged "good" nurses or "bad" nurses.

In reviewing many of the recent nursing journals and textbooks, this writer found the word "support" used in nearly every article in which the nurse is involved in interpersonal situations with patients or other members of the health team. It was included in every nursing care plan read. Only one definition (taken from the dictionary) was found in the material reviewed. This was, "To support means to keep a person from fainting, sinking, yielding; to comfort or strengthen." [1] Another definition taken from lecture notes of a training school in Ireland during World War II is, "Support is doing what comes naturally in whatever way seems best."

This lack of clarity points out a need to define this term upon which so much of nursing is based. Only after support is defined can nursing look more clearly at its techniques and determine whether the care being given is based on a professional therapeutic concept or whether, as is this writer's thesis, this is a lay concept utilized primarily to reduce the nurse's anxiety.

Support is an interpersonal lay concept which is utilized to reduce anxiety of the patient and/or the nurse by adaptive maneuver(s). Support is defined operationally in this way.

1. A person perceives another person as having an unmet need. This unmet need may or may not have been perceived correctly.
2. There is an increase in the anxiety level of one or both persons.
3. This increased anxiety is empathized by the other individual.
4. One of the two persons utilizes adaptive maneuver(s).
5a. If the adaptive maneuver(s) is (are) successful, both persons experience a decrease in levels of anxiety.
5b. If the adaptive maneuver(s) is (are) not successful, anxiety levels of both persons continue to increase toward the level of panic.

In the initial step the nurse's perception may be distorted in one of several areas. The patient may not have an unmet need; the unmet need of the patient may not be perceived accurately by the nurse; or the need which is unmet may be the nurse's and not the patient's. In Step 2 the anxiety or lack of comfort is experienced due to the tension of the unmet need of the patient or the nurse. If a distortion is involved in the nurse's assessment of the patient's needs, this, too, will increase the level of anxiety. In Step 4 the nurse utilizes adaptive maneuvers to decrease her anxiety. For example, a concrete physical task is carried out. The nurse may initiate physical contact with the patient. She may use a common cliché which says little and means less, such as, "Everything will be all right" or "I understand." If these techniques are successful in creating a more comfortable environment, the anxiety of both the patient and the nurse will be decreased.

To comprehend this concept more fully, the definition of adaptation must be considered. Adaptation is the process by which an individual re-

[1] Hart, B. L., and Rohweder, A. W., "Support in Nursing," p. 1399.

duces felt needs by using automatic behavior patterns without experiencing learning. In the process of learning, the patient and the nurse explore the unmet need carefully by proceeding through the steps of observation, description, analysis, formulation, validation, and integration of thoughts, feelings, and actions. Thus, when a nurse utilizes adaptive maneuvers, the patient may experience "a relief from the initial tension or anxiety, connected with the felt difficulty without understanding what happened or developing foresight which would enable the person to meet similar situations in the future without anxiety or with less tension." [2]

To illustrate the concept of support as an interpersonal lay concept, the following verbatim nurse-patient data is presented.

*Nurse:* (Making rounds in the early morning, finds the patient crying with the sheet pulled over her head.) There, there, Mrs. G., whatever is troubling you?

*Patient:* (Sobbing.) I had such awful pain all night. I was sure I was going to split open or die or something. No one came when I pushed my light. They left me to die.

*Nurse:* (Pushes light and sees that the bulb is burned out.) Dear, dear, Mrs. G. Look here. We need a new bulb. I'm awfully sorry you had to wait so long. I'll run now and get you something for your pain. You know, if I were you I would have shouted for someone long before this. Hold on now. I'll be right back.

Another illustration is:

*Patient:* (Diagnosis—bilateral lung abscesses, tuberculosis.) Miss C.! Come here! How was Dr. W.'s lecture yesterday? (Dr. W., chief chest surgeon and consultant.)

*Nurse:* Oh, my, very, very interesting. I took notes like mad and really learned a lot.

*Patient:* Then tell me if you think I'll ever get well enough to get out of here walking instead of in a box feet first.

*Nurse:* Oh sure you will. Dr. W. showed us x-rays of lots of cases worse off than yours, and some of them recovered. You shouldn't worry. Worry prevents you from getting well.

If maneuvers oriented to the concept of learning had been applied in these two situations rather than adaptive maneuvers, a more psychotherapeutic nursing intervention would have resulted. The patients' fears of death would have been explored and discussed instead of avoided in each instance—in the first by a physical nursing task, and in the second by the use of a meaningless cliché. Both maneuvers cut off further related conversation. In each situation the operational steps of support can be followed sequentially. In each situation it can be speculated that the nurse's

[2] Peplau, Hildegard E., "Therapeutic Functions," p. 24.

anxiety was decreased by her maneuver, which avoided the anxiety-producing theme of death.

Nursing needs to sharpen up its concepts and techniques—to stop talking in generalities such as, "accepting," "understanding," and "meeting patients' needs." Let's start by looking more closely at this phrase "giving support." These situations can be experiences of learning for both the patient and the nurse.

## BIBLIOGRAPHY

BURD, SHIRLEY F., "An Operational Definition of Support," unpublished definition, College of Nursing, Rutgers, the State University of New Jersey, 1961.

HART, BETTY L., and ROHWEDER, ANN W., "Support in Nursing," *Am. J. Nursing*, Volume 59, No. 10, October 1959.

PEPLAU, HILDEGARD E., "Therapeutic Functions," paper prepared for Eastern Regional Conference of the National League for Nursing, Washington, D.C.: April 1956.

# 11 WAITING: A CONCEPT IN NURSING[1]

*Dorothea R. Hays*

There are many concepts which, if more clearly understood by the nurse, can become helpful tools in the care of the sick. One concept which has many meanings, which explains behavior and, therefore, is important to nursing practice, is waiting.

The three most frequently encountered aspects of this concept are the acts of *waiting for, waiting on,* and *waiting with* a person (or persons): A patient may be waiting for an operation, a nurse may be waiting on a patient, or a nurse may be waiting with a patient for a doctor. In each case, the roles and expectations of the persons involved differ. Thus the nurse may be a participant in the acts, as in the second and third examples, or she may be a spectator. The concept of waiting also is closely related to other concepts that help to explain its operations—expectation, time, readiness, and power.

Several dictionaries, in defining waiting as "staying or resting in expectation till the arrival of some person or event, being in readiness to perform services for someone, calling upon or visiting, and remaining neglected for a time," show the varieties of meaning generally connected with the word and indicate the necessity of reducing the concept into its subdivisions. These subdivisions each fulfill a part of the definition.

The subconcept *waiting for* can be defined as "staying or resting in expectation till the arrival of some person or event." Here a person is stationary, his attention directed toward a distant object or person moving through time toward him. Examples are the antepartum patient waiting for labor to start and the patient waiting for the nurse to care for her.

[1] Originally published in *Nursing World*, Vol. 132, No. 5, June, 1958.

The subconcept *waiting with* is closely related to the preceding sub-division. In this situation, two or more persons are "staying in expectation till the arrival of some person or event." This person or event may concern one or both, part or all, of the waiting persons; it may even affect them in varying ways. Here two or more people are stationary, with their attention focused in two directions: toward the approaching event and toward each other. Students waiting together for an examination to start or a nurse waiting with a dying patient for death are two instances of this subconcept.

The definitions "being in readiness to perform services for someone" and "calling upon or visiting" apply to the subconcept *waiting on*. Here the actor is willing—and ready—to move toward a person to fulfill certain needs. For example, a mother waits on her very young infant, the circulating nurse waits on the scrubbed nurse during surgery.

These variations of waiting become more meaningful when seen in relation to other concepts that have a part in their operation. Expectation, time, readiness, and power are concepts that should be considered. Because they relate to the different roles assumed by different actors in the process of waiting, they help to explain some of the relationships among the persons involved.

Expectations can be defined as "the looking forward to or anticipation of an event that is believed to be about to happen." A person develops a notion, through repeated experience, by accepting the word of an authority, or by an autistic invention, that certain events will usually be followed by certain other happenings. When a patient rings a bell, he expects a nurse to appear or that someone will talk to him over an inter-communication system. On the other hand, a nurse may expect a patient to wait patiently until she gets around to care for him. Thus we see there is a possibility of conflicting expectations in the process of waiting.

The concept of time involves the duration between the first moment of expectation and the fulfillment of the expectation. The time element may be known or controlled by one or both of the actors. In some instances, neither party knows or controls the time.

A lady-in-waiting expects to be called by her queen, but only the queen knows and controls the time—when she will call the lady-in-waiting and how long she will need her services. Or a group of students is waiting for class, knowing it will start in ten minutes. Or a patient in labor and her nurse wait for the third stage of labor, neither of them knowing exactly how long it will take. When an infant cries for food, its mother knows how long it will take to heat the meal.

To be prepared, i.e., equipped with what is needed and willing for what one is about to do or experience, is to be in readiness. Readiness, like time, may be available to all, one, or none of the participants. It also may be found completely or only in parts: A nurse may be ready to listen to a mentally disturbed patient, but she has to wait until the patient is ready to talk. Or a nurse and patient, both ready for their roles in surgery, are waiting together for the surgeon to get ready.

Power, the ability (as well as the force) to act and to make decisions, may refer to a person's own decisions and to those of other people. Power, as it relates to waiting, may be found in any, all, or none of the concerned persons; it is relative in quantity and application. An infant waiting to be comforted by his mother is powerless to supply the comfort; he can only cry—which may not even achieve the desired result. The mother here is all-powerful in supplying or withholding comfort. In a nurse-patient relationship, the patient may have the power to control the waiting time for the nurse by having an attack of dyspnea or vomiting when the nurse does not appear immediately.

Some of these examples indicate how and when the concept of waiting and its related concepts fit into nursing practice. Being able to wait comfortably and understanding the situation of waiting for, with, and on patients are important functions of the nurse.

The ability to wait must be acquired as part of the development of the personality. The child must learn to understand and cope with the various waiting situations, and he probably learns to wait for, with, and on, in that order. At first the child is capable only of expectation: When he cries he expects relief of hunger and discomfort. The mother has to be ready; she controls the time element and has the power to take care of the infant's needs. As the child grows older, he has to assume part of the readiness—especially if the mother has other obligations. He must be ready to be nourished when the family eats, or to go for a walk when the mother has time. Here the mother still controls the time and power elements.

Next, the child learns to lengthen the time interval when waiting from "after you finish the game" to "next Christmas" to "when you are grown up." He develops patience and the ability to delay satisfaction—he learns to wait for events and people—as he becomes more aware of his own personality and the distinct personalities around him.

While he may be still perfecting his ability to wait longer and longer, he starts to partake in the role of waiting with others. There may be brothers and sisters who are more or less ready for an awaited event. He can share his experiences and feelings and validate some of the things he has learned, as they relate to waiting; he can validate his expectations with his peers.

Finally, he learns to assume the role of one who waits on others, first by fulfilling the immediate expectation of others. He brings an empty dish when his mother asks him; he learns to be ready to help whenever called upon. Eventually he anticipates the needs and expectations of others over a long period of time. Once he has learned to expect certain events and to be ready for them, he learns to assume power and to control time in coping with many of his own waiting situations. Having developed the ability to wait, he may choose to delay earning money by waiting until he has had an extensive education.

Nursing students have more or less completely undergone the foregoing development and experiences. Yet incompleteness in this developmental process may carry over into (and complicate) student nurse–teacher relationships; if not recognized here, it may follow into nurse–patient relationships. Several patterns can be observed in the student which may be helpful in explaining the student's readiness to take different roles involving waiting and guessing possible deficiencies in this area of learning. Suppose the student shows an ability to wait for, with, and on people. This means that her personal development in this area has proceeded well.

But if a student shows frequent signs of impatience when waiting for others, it indicates that she never had the experience of having someone waiting for her. She may have a great, although unrecognized, need to be waited for. Another student may be impatient waiting for others but can comfortably wait on patients. This student may have had an impatient mother and may be rebelling against her, trying to be a better mother figure. A student who waits comfortably for and on others but feels uncomfortable in sharing a waiting situation with others may have difficulties in other areas involving situations which call for sharing. This points to a need to develop skills in interpersonal interaction.

In nursing practice there are times when the nurse becomes aware of a feeling of annoyance when a patient makes excessive demands on her services. But this feeling of annoyance, if it is recognized and if it leads the nurse to explore the nurse-patient relationship, can be useful. Either the nurse, the patient, or both, may have a lack of ability to wait. The nurse, if she is able to observe and examine what occurs between herself and the patient just before she felt annoyed, may be able to validate her conclusions with the patient. A patient, who became very anxious in a nurse-patient relationship when the nurse had expected her to move ahead faster than she was able to at the time, expressed relief when the nurse finally recognized what was happening and expressed her willingness to wait and to proceed at the patient's speed.

Many unformulated connections interfere with effective nursing, but often these connections are not clearly understood. A nurse may have a need for approval, and having someone wait for her may be tied up with feelings of worthiness.

In our culture some forms of the term "waiting" may have emotional connotations to some nurses. Two such forms are waiter and lady-in-waiting. Both call pictures to our minds that may be emotionally charged according to the degree of identification and the degree of prestige we associate with these occupations. For instance, a nurse may resent performing such services as fetching things and running errands for a patient, functions which the nurse may feel are more those of a waiter than of a nurse. She may feel that the patient needs a lady-in-waiting or personal maid, not a nurse. The question then arises: "What are the needs of this particular patient and how can they be fulfilled in the most therapeutic way?" But in order to investigate the patient's needs, the nurse must first recognize and understand her own feelings toward the patient and the particular situation which involves waiting on others.

The concept of *waiting for* is also involved in cultural patterns of interaction related to levels of prestige. The higher the prestige of a person, the more valuable his time is, the more he expects others to be ready for him. This reasonable expectation sometimes becomes distorted. Instead of serving expedience only, waiting becomes an index and indication of self-esteem, as in the case of the doctor who becomes very annoyed when he has to wait for a nurse; he may consider the delay a threat to the prestige accorded to his person and position.

Patients, too, often connect waiting with prestige and personal worth. Some patients in a large, but small-staffed, mental hospital who were required to wait in line for certain services, such as receiving medication or taking showers, expressed feelings of unworthiness because of this waiting. They felt that they were the lowest prestige group in the hospital because they had to wait for everyone else. Some of these patients may have had people waiting for and on them before their hospitalization and have built up the expectation that others wait for them. They did not realize that waiting is related to expediency.

Another distortion of the concept of waiting is related to the feeling of abandonment seen when a student nurse feels very anxious if a teacher or patient or doctor does not wait for her. This feeling may be related to an experience in early childhood when the child could not keep up with the pace of an adult and lost contact and sight of him temporarily at an age when the child was not yet able to find his own way.

Waiting can also be part of the pattern of helplessness often found in psychiatric patients. The patient is able to wait for someone else to do things for him, but he feels helpless to do those things himself. He may need help to develop the ability to wait with and on others as well as the capability of helping himself.

The concept of waiting can be usefully incorporated into nursing education as a tool that can facilitate interpersonal interaction. Students can be helped to examine the concept of waiting. By observing and analyzing their own feelings and actions in situations involving aspects of waiting, they can learn about and examine their own patterns of waiting and the extent of their ability to wait for, with, and on others, especially in nurse patient situations.

Next, students can observe and study inabilities to wait as developmental problems of some patients. This involves a study of the tasks of waiting as they are learned in childhood and the reactions exhibited to incompletely understood waiting situations as they are observed in children. A two-month-old baby can become very restless and cry pitifully if a feeding is unusually delayed, because he has not learned to wait for food, nor does he understand what is involved in getting the food ready. He does not understand why it does not come as it usually does when he is hungry. The same pattern or a modification of it, and possibly crying, can be observed in a patient who has no understanding of what is involved in a situation of waiting for a person or event.

Finally, students can develop ways to help patients develop an understanding of the concept and the ability to deal more satisfactorily with waiting situations. The patient may need an interpretation of the realistic aspects of the waiting situation. He needs an understanding of his expectations, of how and why they did not correspond with the events. He needs to understand how he felt about the situation and how he reacted to it, as well as how this affected others involved in the situation.

Out of an understanding of his patterns of reaction to waiting situations, the patient may be helped to develop new and more satisfactory ways of waiting for, with, and on others.

# 12 LEARNING TO TRUST

*Anita M. Werner*

Trust is an essential component of a healthy interpersonal relationship. Without the ability to trust, man is isolated, lonely, and anxious. This chapter examines trust, its development in the normal person and lack of development in the person diagnosed as schizophrenic. Some formulations concerning the remedy of mistrust in the person diagnosed schizophrenic, supported by clinical examples, are presented.

Erikson [1] developed the concept of basic trust. He explained trust as "an attitude toward oneself and the world derived from experiences of the first year of life. By trust I mean what is commonly implied in reasonable trustfulness as far as others are concerned and a simple sense of trustworthiness as far as oneself is concerned." Baldwin [2] defines trust more specifically as "a global undifferentiated attitude, a contentment and confidence which stems from a deep assumption that life is pleasant and will not become unmanageable." Trust develops from the experience the child had with his mother, providing that experience was satisfying. If his needs were met in a manner relatively free from undue anxiety and in a manner that communicated trust and respect, the child will in turn trust and respect himself and others. Trust, like other attitudes, is learned by empathic communication from the mother to the child. Arieti [3] describes this communication as follows:

> There is a reciprocal trust that things are going to be well, that the child will be capable of growing up to be a healthy and mature man. The child

[1] Erikson, E. H., "Growth and Crises of the Healthy Personality," p. 190.
[2] Baldwin, Alfred, *Behavior and Development in Childhood*, pp. 547–48.
[3] Arieti, S., "What is Effective in the Therapeutic Process."

perceives this faith of the mother and accepts it, just as he used to accept the primitive responses to the usual stimuli. He finally assimilates this trust of the significant adult, and he trusts himself.

The child expects satisfaction and security in his relationship with his mother. Feelings of expectancy, euphoria, and trust result when his needs are met. These feelings are vague and indefinite until the child, at a later age, learns to formulate them. Later, the child expects not only his physical needs to be met, but also his social and psychological needs. He expects approval, that is, the child trusts that the adult will trust him.[4]

In the childhood of the person diagnosed as schizophrenic this trust is defective because the mother is either rejecting or extremely anxious. Instead of an atmosphere of trust, there is an atmosphere of anxiety, which is likewise communicated to the child. The child learns that he is a person who is mistrusted and disapproved. Sullivan[5] speaks of the difficulty this person has in developing a favorable self-system because "early in life the idea was in some way conveyed inescapably to him that he was relatively infrahuman, a burden of sorts." The person who is diagnosed schizophrenic thus becomes distrustful, suspicious, and hostile, and withdraws from relatedness with other people.

It is the purpose of psychotherapy to restore this trust by reaching these persons in specific ways and, in so doing, helping them to learn to trust themselves as well as others. The therapist cannot love the patient like a mother loves a child, but he can have faith in the patient's potentialities toward health. By conveying an attitude of hopefulness concerning the patient's potential for returning to a meaningful existence, the therapist will be doing immeasurable good in facilitating the therapeutic process. The essence of therapy is the establishment of an interpersonal relationship via communication, primarily verbal communication. Sullivan[6] states that "the principal problem of the therapeutic interview is that of facilitating the accession to awareness of information which will clarify for the patient the more troublesome aspects of his life." But in order for such information to be brought into awareness, it must be communicated in some way to the therapist. Before such communication can occur, the therapist must create an atmosphere which is nonthreatening enough that the patient's feeling of security increases, his mistrust lessens, and he talks with the therapist. The following illustration will serve to clarify the above concepts.

[4] Arieti, S., "Introductory Notes on the Psychoanalytic Therapy of Schizophrenics," p. 76.

[5] Sullivan, H. S., Clinical Studies in Psychiatry, p. 364.

[6] Sullivan, H. S., Conceptions of Modern Psychiatry, p. 185.

A nurse-therapist worked for a short time with Mrs. A., a patient diagnosed paranoid schizophrenic. Mrs. A. had been in the hospital only a few days when she was seen for the first therapeutic interview. She was suspicious and frightened, and her angry, assaultive behavior had led to her becoming virtually isolated from the other patients and the staff. She had driven others away by her stony silence and her obviously seething anger. As she withdrew into her loneliness and isolation, others withdrew from her to prevent the discomfort that contact created. During the first interview and for many subsequent interviews, Mrs. A. said nothing to the therapist. She merely sat and stared in an angry silent manner. The therapist interjected remarks occasionally conveying her wish to understand the patient and requesting her to share her thoughts. Mrs. A. persisted, however, in her silence, and the anxiety in both the patient and the therapist increased. The patient withdrew even further from a situation which had become intolerable to her and spent the time allotted for the therapeutic interviews away from her room and the therapist, watching television. Although the therapist continued to see the patient, she became aware of her own increasing feelings of discomfort and fear of the patient's assaultiveness. When these feelings were recognized, explored, and resolved, the therapist was able to approach the patient with feelings consistent with the trust she wished to convey to the patient. The therapist made a point of explaining to the patient that she had been afraid of her but no longer felt this way and wished to continue seeing her in her room as before. This time Mrs. A. came to her room and proceeded to discuss her problems and to reveal her great fears of people. When the therapist trusted the patient and communicated that she actually did believe in her, the patient was able to trust herself and the therapist enough to communicate her thoughts and to begin to work therapeutically.

Patients frequently verbalize in some way, in the beginning of a therapeutic relationship, their fear and mistrust. The therapist needs to be alert to such communications so that the patient can be assisted in describing and exploring his feelings.

Mr. B. was a patient, diagnosed schizophrenic, who had been hospitalized for several years on one of the back wards of a large county hospital. When the nurse-therapist began working with Mr. B., he was disheveled, silent, and highly anxious. The therapist was aware of the patient's tremendous mistrust and fear that another human being wanted to establish contact, and so took efforts to be as nonthreatening as possible. This was achieved partly by assuming an attitude of expectation that the patient would talk when he felt more comfortable, by refraining from demanding anything from the patient, and by making description-eliciting comments concerning nonthreatening topics. In the second interview he began to talk in a soft whisper about games that were being played on the ward. In the middle of this discussion he said, quite clearly, "I can't give you anything. Oh, if we could have something together. There are too many questions of importance." The therapist replied, "Tell about the questions of importance." Mr. B. said, "I'm scared of what might come out if I talk." With clarity, he verbalized his mistrust of the therapist and his fear of talking. He gradually became more comfortable and was eventually able to talk quite freely.

Trust is not an attitude that is learned quickly. In the growing child it takes several years to develop. Likewise, in the person diagnosed schizophrenic it may take years of intensive therapy to help this person learn to trust.

The foregoing is a presentation of some general considerations concerning trust. The clinical examples serve to illustrate in a concrete manner material which is highly abstract.

## BIBLIOGRAPHY

ARIETI, SILVANO, "Introductory Notes on the Psychoanalytic Therapy of Schizophrenics," in *Psychotherapy of the Psychosis*, Arthur Burton (ed.), Basic Books, New York: 1961, pp. 69–89.

—— "What is Effective in the Therapeutic Process," *Am. J. Psychoanal.*, 17:30, 1957.

BALDWIN, ALFRED, *Behavior and Development in Childhood*, The Dryden Press, New York: 1955, pp. 547–48.

ERIKSON, E. H., "Growth and Crises of the Healthy Personality," in *Personality in Nature, Society and Culture*, Clyde Kluckhohn and Henry Murray (eds.), Alfred A. Knopf, New York: 1953, pp. 185–225.

SULLIVAN, HARRY S., *Clinical Studies in Psychiatry*, W. W. Norton & Co., New York: 1956.

—— *Conceptions of Modern Psychiatry*, W. W. Norton & Co., New York: 1953.

# 13 THE QUESTIONING PATIENT

*Betty H. Newsom*

Schwartz and Shockley [1] point out the necessity for nurses to maintain effective communication with patients. Part of this communication process involves the questioning patient. At this time, nurses must concern themselves with questions on their own part, such as "What is the basis for the question the patient asks?" or "When is it therapeutically feasible for me to answer his inquiries?" Many of the answers to the nurse's perplexity come in the verbatim data given by the patient. It is up to the nurse to evaluate the data in order to make her own decisions.

In psychiatry, nurses work with the person who is diagnosed schizophrenic and who lives in his self-created image of reality. The real world is so anxiety-producing that he creates his own image of how the forces around him should be. To be sure, reality, whether he is confined in an institution or not, constantly impinges upon his daily activities.[2] He handles the inconsistencies of life frequently through the process of autistic invention. Sullivan speaks of this process of thought stating that "things are manifested in the interview situation by peculiar misunderstandings and mistakes—for example, the person may hear something which the interviewer has not said, and has not meant to say." [3] The reasons for the development of this particular communication disturbance date back to when the patient first began to speak to significant persons around him. In some manner, adult invasion into his private world as a child had a profound

[1] Schwartz, M., and Shockley, E. L., *The Nurse and the Mental Patient,* p. 243.
[2] Sullivan, H. S., *Clinical Studies in Psychiatry,* pp. 25, 26, 331, 332.
[3] Sullivan, H. S., *The Psychiatric Interview,* p. 192.

effect on his habit of communication.[4] Possibly the significant persons involved did not aid the patient in making logical connections. To aid this process, the person must be comfortable enough to ask questions and to have these inquiries answered in a valid and direct manner.

During the therapeutic relationship of the nurse and the patient, part of the nurse's goal is to allow the patient to become comfortable enough with her to relate all the fears and the anxieties that the patient encounters. Each and every relationship must go through the orientation phase of the stranger-to-stranger atmosphere that prevails.

When a new person is met in a social setting, this "getting to know each other" phase may consist of a rapid and superficial rundown of each of the persons' life experiences, awkward silences, and/or possibly a pleasant exchange of the knowledge of mutual friends or acquaintances. However, in the therapeutic setting, the nurse participates in this exchange only to the extent that she elicits the patient's thoughts, feelings, and actions of his experiences. The nurse is involved with this communication only insofar as the relationship itself brings forth the patient's difficulties in relating with people.

During the orientation phase, seldom does the patient ask questions of the nurse that concern him therapeutically. If questions do arise during this period, generally, two types of questions can be categorized.

The first type of questions has to do generally with the patient's role in the relationship. For example, "What am I suppose to do here?" "How will this talking help me?" "Am I talking too much?" or "To whom do you tell this information that I give you?" This type of questioning has to do with the patient's unsureness in this new one-to-one situation. Time, honesty, and consistency on the part of the nurse help him over this hurdle.[5]

The second type of questioning has to do with the patient's mechanism of defense—avoidance. Usually the patient has impulsively related to the nurse a secret desire, wish, or confidence. The patient, overwrought with anxiety of what this confession might do to him, then attempts to switch the conversation to the nurse by questioning her. For example, "How old are you?" "Where do you live?" "Are you married?" "What religion are you?" "Are your parents still living?" "I've been talking with you now for five interviews; why can't you get me out of here?" The nurse asks the patient the basis for his interrogation and then reflects the interview topic back to the patient and his problems.

But as the patient moves along in the relationship and his trust and

[4] *Ibid.*, p. 190.
[5] Schwartz, M., and Shockley, E. L., *op. cit.*, pp. 241–42.

confidence in the nurse become stronger, another type of questioning arises. If the nurse will keep in mind the patient's level of development, she will observe that the patient is not interested only in himself, but his interest also extends to the world and the events around him and how they are related to him. This writer has found that the patient has a desire to learn the meaning of current events, and that the patient has attached a personal meaning to the topics.

Frequently, too, the nurse might take a look at the actual schooling experienced by the patient and see if he had an adequate education. If the patient has had the benefit of a better-than-average education, the nurse may begin to question just how much the patient, with his habitual inability to handle his anxiety, grasped during that time.

The patient who is motivated to get well is inquisitive. Many questions arise in his mind that require an answer. When the nurse has determined that his questions do not evade the interview topic at hand, she answers him straightforwardly.[6] The following clinical situation is an example.

While the patient was on leave, he and his uncle had a discussion about the Red Chinese government and Cuba. The patient admired this uncle and wanted to contribute something to the discussion. That week end the patient began reading in the newspaper about the political crisis of Cuba. He asked no questions about it while at home. During the following interview session with the nurse, the patient talked about the incident.

*Patient:* . . . Oh, the Red Chinese government in Cuba. He [the uncle] told me not to worry about it . . . well, I was all excited . . . this in Cuba . . . Tell me, is Cuba part of South America or not?
*Nurse:* Tell me why you want to know.
*Patient:* Some people say it is and some say it isn't. I don't know.
*Nurse:* Have you seen a map?
*Patient:* No, I don't know. I don't have one.
*Nurse:* At the next interview, I shall bring one to answer your question. But go on about your discussion of you and your uncle.

At the next interview session, the nurse brought a world map for the patient to see. He carefully looked at it, asked to see where Cuba was and then stated, "There's really nothing worse than stirring up people." He went on to talk of his discomfort when he heard or read about unpleasant or hostile actions.

In the following example, the patient used value judgment terms, such as "good," bad," "awful," "terrible." The nurse, attempting to elicit further description of these terms, frequently asked the patient for an ex-

[6] Wolberg, L. R., *The Technique of Psychotherapy*, p. 303.

ample of the words used as each related to him. Several interviews followed with seemingly unfruitful results. Finally, the patient asked the nurse, "What is an example?" Further examination of the patient's question elicited data that told the nurse that this patient did know the meanings of many words that are used during the daily course of living. Subsequently, a careful, precise explanation of the words used by the interviewer was always given to the patient.

Theoretically, as the patient learns to question the nurse about matters of the world in which he lives, the nurse encourages him to seek out his own answers. This seeking-out on the part of the patient is in the form of widening his circle of interpersonal contacts to satisfy his curiosity about reality, the people who form a part of this reality, and how it all relates to himself.

In summary, during the therapeutic nurse-patient relationship, the patient will ask specific questions of the nurse. The nurse must determine the basis for the patient's interrogation. When it has been established that the patient seeks clarification of the world around him, the nurse gives valid, direct answers to his questions.

## BIBLIOGRAPHY

SCHWARTZ, MORRIS, and SHOCKLEY, EMMY LANNING, *The Nurse and the Mental Patient*, Russell Sage Foundation, New York: 1956.

SULLIVAN, HARRY STACK, *Clinical Studies in Psychiatry*, W. W. Norton & Co., New York: 1956.

——— *The Psychiatric Interview*, W. W. Norton & Co., New York: 1954.

WOLBERG, LEWIS R., *The Technique of Psychotherapy*, Grune & Stratton, New York: 1954.

# 14 WHAT IS AN OBSESSIVE-COMPULSIVE NEUROSIS?

*Alice A. H. Hadley*

At a party, a girl was observed to be neatly lining up several pretzels in her hand. She made sure the ends nearer her were even and then carefully graduated the pretzels according to length. Someone observed her doing this and announced, "Say! You're compulsive!" It seemed to the writer that possibly a great many people make this, or the rather similar admonition, "Oh, you must have been toilet-trained early," when they possess only a cursory knowledge of what obsessions and compulsions are. The purpose of this chapter is to point out the definitions that various medical and nursing experts give to obsessions and compulsions, to indicate what treatment is used, and to show the implications of theory for nursing care. A clinical example will be used for illustration. An operational definition of the obsessive-compulsive neurosis will summarize the chapter.

Sullivan [1] sees the obsessional dynamism arising from a very early, if not lifelong, condition of profound insecurity. In discussing the development of the problem he writes,[2]

> The obsessional neurotic . . . plucks out of the tissue of autistic speech of early childhood certain words, phrases, or sentences, and uses them as points of preoccupation. . . . In the pursuit of security, the obsessional person regresses in certain cognitive operations—knowing operations—to the stage of quite autistic speech.

He clarifies this further by saying that he feels that children who later become obsessional are reared in homes where there is no open expression

[1] Sullivan, H. S., *Conceptions of Modern Psychiatry*, p. 113.
[2] *Ibid.*, p. 29.

of hostility, but rather where family members give recourse to noble ethical principles and moralistic statements. Gradually the child learns "verbal propositions" that prevent the descent of anxiety or punishment that would otherwise result from his actions or misdeeds. However, things are still never quite right in the situation between the child and the significant person, and the child retains a low-grade anxiety. In Sullivan's words [3] the child, "learns that a great many things do not quite work with anybody, and yet they are better than nothing." The child does not have the high educative effect of sharp failure with verbal magic. He retains this primitive formula, or it becomes a relatively fixed way of handling threats to his security. Thus, Sullivan warns that although much of the obsessional thinking and many of the obsessional rituals sound all right, it must be remembered that these props to adjustment were fixed in childhood when the referential meaning of words was much more autistic and that what obsessional people really think is anything but as obvious as it may sound.[4] Finally, he says that obsessional people do not magically achieve security by their operations; they are insecure, but they would feel much less secure without their obsessional content.

Peplau [5] states, "Obsessions are usually thought of as ideas that dominate and limit the possibility of new experiences bringing about a revision in thinking." She thinks that obsessions may indicate needs or longings, and that there is always limited recognition in awareness of these "barriers to further growth," so that their expression is generally indirect. What can be observed are the actions or compulsive acts that provide a way of managing the unacceptable obsessive thoughts. Obsessions and compulsions usually are seen together,

> . . . the obsession being an idea or feeling that must be avoided at all costs in order to feel safe. . . . A compulsive act is the ameliorative activity performed to manage the anxiety that would arise if the forbidden thoughts or feelings gained entrance into awareness.[6]

Peplau, like Sullivan, states that the compulsive act is an adaptation that was "required and reinforced" in childhood when the child was dependent on significant persons for satisfaction and security. If wishes and satisfactions were not permitted, then the child included other acts that seemed to ensure safety.

Masserman defines obsessions as "urgent ideas or impulses that remain

[3] *Ibid.*, p. 231.
[4] *Ibid.*, p. 29.
[5] Peplau, H. E., *Interpersonal Relations in Nursing*, p. 151.
[6] *Ibid.*

in consciousness despite their recognized irrationality and unwelcome obtrusiveness." [7] He writes,[8]

> Clinically, obsessions appear most frequently as disguised reaction-formations to unconscious impulses which also give rise to defensive patterns of external behavior called compulsions; these compulsive acts then deviate the energies of the repressed impulses into relatively harmless, but typically stereotyped and ritualized behavior.

Masserman agrees that compulsive acts are performed "on pain of anxiety" should they be omitted.[9]

Matheney and Topalis [10] see compulsive acts as methods "of handling the problems of interpersonal relations through rigidly ritualistic behavior designed to retain control over a situation and keep anxiety at a minimum." For all these authors, control over the situation is an essential base of security.

Wolberg [11] writes in psychoanalytic terms that he believes that reconstructive therapy may not be successful because in the obsessive-compulsive, the ego is usually too weak to handle the anxiety that would be released.

Many authors agree that obsessive thoughts and compulsive acts are a matter of degree. All individuals make use of these mechanisms at some time during life and in some degree. Masserman [12] outlines how Western culture condones ritualized behavior in dress and eating habits.

Another point on which many authors agree is that patience and great amount of time are needed for treating the obsessive-compulsive. Wolberg, Sullivan, Masserman, and Matheney and Topalis, using different terms, describe the verbal or intellectual insight the patient develops without an accompanying emotional insight. Wolberg refers to the problem as an "isolation" of the intellectual process from the emotional content; the attitudes of the patient toward the therapist may be so ambivalent that a working relationship may never develop. Sullivan [13] writes, "Under therapy, the obsessional neurotic actually goes through the motions of operations that look as if he is getting absolutely panicky at the prospect of having something formulated clearly in the realm of his personal problems." The general thinking seems to be that a change in the patterning of the pa-

[7] Masserman, J. H., *Principles of Dynamic Psychiatry*, p. 42.
[8] *Ibid.*, p. 42.
[9] *Ibid.*, p. 169.
[10] Matheney, R., and Topalis, M., *Psychiatric Nursing*, pp. 54–55.
[11] Wolberg, L., *The Technique of Psychotherapy*, p. 604.
[12] Masserman, J. H., *The Practice of Dynamic Psychiatry*, p. 163.
[13] Sullivan, H. S., *Clinical Studies in Psychiatry*, p. 240.

tient's behavior is usually provocative of anxiety. Change is strongly resisted by the patient, particularly when this change means giving up any secondary gains of his neurosis and using new and hopefully more useful ways of interacting.

In discussing his techniques of therapy, Sullivan writes that it is futile to inquire about compulsive rituals. The patient only knows that he performs these acts because they make him feel better. In the area of the doubts of the obsessional, Sullivan believes the problem to be one of seeing around the doubts to what the patient is doing. He believes that doubting is part of the obsessional's pattern of being unclear about things. According to Sullivan, the obsessional uses doubt to place the burden of his neurosis on the environment, that is, he asks the environment for reassurance and advice. Another technique that Sullivan uses is not giving any interpretation of a particular life situation to a patient until the interpretation has become almost self-evident. He believes that, in this way, the obsessional goes over the content again and again, but each time it becomes a little clearer to him. Generally, Sullivan says he does not find a direct attack on the patient's self-esteem useful.

Some techniques which Wolberg has found useful with obsessive-compulsive patients are reassurance, guidance, and support. Both Sullivan and Wolberg think that for some people, there is a bridge between the obsessive-compulsive neurosis and schizophrenia. A person who has an obsessional way of handling life may, under pressure of anxiety, move to a schizophrenic way of handling life.[14] When the pressure is diminished, he may return to the obsessional pattern. Some patients shift back and forth between the obsessional and schizophrenic processes. Sullivan believes that there is no particular difference in the obsessional neurosis that progresses into schizophrenia and the one that does not.

Nurses, student nurses, and attendants working with obsessive-compulsive persons can use several useful techniques. First, they can study the way in which these coping mechanisms, obsessions and compulsions, operate. Second, nurses can develop ways to help patients feel safe with them. If nurses know how these mechanisms operate, they understand that if they attack these defenses of the patient, the patient will feel more anxious. Peplau says that by permitting the patient's mechanisms to operate, possibly his feelings of security will become strong enough that that he will feel safe to doubt what he is doing.[15] "When doubt comes from the patient it is his feeling, and he will initiate actions in accord-

[14] Ibid., pp. 257–64.
[15] Peplau, H. E., Interpersonal Relations in Nursing, p. 155.

ance with it; when doubt is initiated by the nurse it may function as another barrier, requiring redoubling of his efforts towards security." [16]

Nurses can also introduce new experiences carefully to the patient, since they may pose a threat. Matheney and Topalis suggest that since one of the purposes of ritualistic behavior is to relieve the patient of the necessity for making decisions, the nurse can be therapeutic by providing a sufficiently controlled environment to relieve the patient of as many decisions as possible. Since ritualistic behavior is time-consuming, the patient needs to be allowed adequate time without any sense of pressure or criticism. Where limits must be drawn on carrying out the compulsive act, as in serious interference with maintenance of the patient's health, the limits need to be consistently enforced. Measures such as tube feeding need to be done on schedule. The nurse may need to plan for avoidance of fatigue when the patient's behavior is so elaborate and involved that it exhausts him. This plan, like tube feeding, needs to be consistently carried through. The patient may have physical needs of adequate food and fluid intake or of skin care resulting from his compulsive acts. Matheney and Topalis also suggest that encouraging the obsessive-compulsive patient to participate in group activities is an important nursing function. They recommend starting the patient in some activity where he already has some skill and interest.

The usefulness of some of the above-mentioned nursing skills can be conceptualized by the reader when reading a statement of the problems of Judy E. Judy was fourteen years old, five feet seven inches tall, and weighed 76 pounds when she was admitted to a small, intensive-treatment psychiatric hospital. Judy had gradually decreased the kinds and amounts of food she consumed, so that her weight had dropped in a two-year period from about 120 pounds to 76 pounds. She never sat down, even while eating, and she stood in one spot for long periods, so that she had stasis of blood in her legs and skin breakdown of her ankles. Because of her poor nutrition, she also had thin, dry hair and sores where her glasses touched her ears and nose. Her standing to play cards, plus her emaciation, made her very noticeable in the group. Every morning and night Judy performed an elaborate and time-consuming grooming ritual. She spoke in a very soft voice which required very close attention on the part of the listener, and she asked the same questions about the ward routines every day.

In conclusion, the following definition is the author's view of the emerging operations of an obsessive-compulsive neurosis:

[16] *Ibid.*, p. 155.

1. An individual has a wish to or a desire to act.

2. This wish or desire is seen as unacceptable by significant persons, usually because it is related to hostile or aggressive feelings.

3. The unacceptability of the wish becomes a barrier to the individual's carrying out his wish or desire.

4. The individual feels this barrier of unacceptability as a threat to personality.

5. The individual experiences an increase of anxiety which occurs because the personality is threatened.

6. The individual develops adaptations to reduce or avoid the anxiety. These adaptations are routine or stereotyped ways of thinking and acting (obsessions and compulsions).

7. The original wish or desire to act is dissociated; the individual has the illusion of security.

8. These routine or stereotyped ways of thinking and acting are repeatedly reinforced in the process of growing up and maintain the illusion of security.

9. Ultimately, these routine and stereotyped methods of thinking and acting represent a denial of self.

# BIBLIOGRAPHY

MASSERMAN, JULES H., *The Practice of Dynamic Psychiatry*, W. B. Saunders Co., Philadelphia: 1955.

———— *Principles of Dynamic Psychiatry*, W. B. Saunders Co., Philadelphia: 1946.

MATHENEY, RUTH, and TOPALIS, MARY, *Psychiatric Nursing*, C. V. Mosby Co., St. Louis: 1957.

PEPLAU, HILDEGARD E., *Interpersonal Relations in Nursing*, G. P. Putnam Sons, New York: 1952.

SULLIVAN, HARRY STACK, *Clinical Studies in Psychiatry*, W. W. Norton & Co., New York: 1956.

———— *Conceptions of Modern Psychiatry*, W. W. Norton & Co., New York: 1953.

WOLBERG, LEWIS, *The Technique of Psychotherapy*, Grune & Stratton, Inc., New York: 1954.

# 15 REJECTION AND THE INTERPERSONAL RELATIONSHIP

*Theo J. Umland*

With increasing emphasis being placed on the formation of interpersonal relationships with her patients, the nurse needs to reinforce and add to her understanding of the bases for such relationships. The psychiatric nurse, particularly, finds herself in the position of having to know and comprehend the various ways in which a patient may relate to others, be it the nurse, the physician, or other patients.

One facet of any relationship is the possibility of rejection by one of the participants. As no relationship can be formed between two persons if one rejects the idea, the nurse must be able to understand and recognize rejection, its causes, development, behavioral manifestations, and the possible ways in which she may deal with it. Then, too, the nurse must understand her own feelings when rejection of a relationship occurs.

Why does a patient reject the nurse's offering of assistance in relating to others? The reason for rejection by an adult may have its roots in childhood experience with one's parents or parentlike authority figures. The child, during the same period in which he is adding substantially to his self-concept, seeks acceptance, closeness, and affection from his parents, especially his mother. For some one of many possible reasons, the mother rebuffs the child or pushes him away, in other words, rejects him. The child represses or suppresses the resulting frustration, hostility, and/or fear which he feels and redoubles his efforts to gain his mother's approval. His efforts only succeed in redoubling the number of times he is rejected as well as the amount of frustration, hostility, and/or fear which he feels.

With continuation of this pattern of denial by others, the child develops the thought that he is worthless and bad, because even the people who are nearest to him do not accept and love him. Such a blow to one's self-concept, reinforced by repetition in childhood and/or in adult life leads to a self-picture that contains little more than self-abasement, discouragement, hostility, and flight. Consequently, the person manifests rejection and denial of other people in order to prevent himself from being rejected.

The anxiety generated by the circumstances described above is disorganizing to the personality and, hence, may result in mental illness. Such was the case of Mr. C., a patient on a psychiatric ward. This patient, disheveled in appearance, struck out at attendants and asked to be restrained because of his actions. During such episodes he repeated several times, "I'm no good. See what I did? Even God thinks I'm beyond help. I'm not worth it. Just tie me down to the bed."

He persisted in this behavior for about one week, during which time the head nurse on the ward, a male attendant, and the graduate fellow [1] talked with Mr. C. for short intervals, but regularly each day. This was to indicate to him that he was worth their attentions.

When approached by anyone, Mr. C. inevitably said, "Why bother with me? Help others. I'm beyond human help. Everything's lousy. I'm no good." Because the head nurse, the attendant, and the clinical specialist continued to "waste" their time from the patient's point of view, he resorted to testing their acceptance with behavior which one person described as "the ultimate in human degradation." He ate feces and drank urine. He refuse to eat and could not make decisions of any kind because he said, "I've no right to decide anything." To complete this picture of total rejection, Mr. C. avoided all contact with other patients.

The nurse's role in dealing with such a patient as Mr. C. is an important one. She must plan a course of action for working with this patient. All nursing personnel must be familiar with the plan of care so that the patient is dealt with consistently. Then a persistent relationship must be set up with the patient on a regular schedule.

In the case of Mr. C., the head nurse told the patient each time she met him that she accepted him as an individual, even though she did not always approve of his actions. Furthermore, the attendant used the same approach when he attempted to get Mr. C. to eat. The graduate fellow, as well as functioning in the planning phase of Mr. C.'s care, provided

[1] Graduate student in the graduate program in advanced psychiatric nursing at Rutgers, The State University of New Jersey.

time in which Mr. C. could talk about his thoughts and feelings regarding the relationships others had set up with him.

Over a period of six weeks, Mr. C. became able to talk comfortably with nursing personnel. He was observed talking with other patients and attended a dance in the recreation hall. He still did not seek the company of others, but he did not refuse to take part when others came to him. He began to make small decisions—about his clothing, whether or not to shave, and whether or not he would keep an appointment with the graduate fellow.

Because of many other complicating factors in his illness, Mr. C. did not become a happy, well-adjusted person during this time. However, he came to realize that at least three persons in his acquaintance found him worthy of a relationship in which he was accepted as an individual. With these three persons he did not have to protect himself from being hurt by running away from the offered relationships, nor did he have to fear that they would reverse any decisions he made. Although he did not become mentally healthy, he took one step in that direction.

In summary, rejection is one aspect of an interpersonal relationship with which the nurse needs to be familiar. In understanding the causes for a patient's refusal to accept her interest, she can plan a more effective course of action for establishing therapeutic rapport with the patient. Accepting the patient is not a cure, but it may give the patient some motivation for wanting to be well.

# BIBLIOGRAPHY

JENKINS, RICHARD L., Breaking Patterns of Defeat, J. B. Lippincott Co., Philadelphia: 1954.

KALKMAN, MARION E., Introduction to Psychiatric Nursing, McGraw-Hill Book Co., New York: 1958.

MATHENEY, RUTH V., and TOPALIS, MARY, Psychiatric Nursing, C. V. Mosby Co., St. Louis: 1957.

MULLER, THERESA G., The Foundation of Human Behavior, G. P. Putnam's Sons, New York: 1956.

SEARS, ROBERT R., MACOBY, ELEANOR E., and LEVIN, HARRY, Patterns of Child Rearing, Row, Peterson, and Co., White Plains, New York: 1957.

SYMONDS, PERCIVAL M., Dynamics of Psychotherapy, Grune and Stratton, New York: 1957, Vol. II.

# 16 THE PATIENT'S GIFT

*Janice Clack*

Gift-giving in the nurse-patient relationship can lead to one of two outcomes: experiential learning or reinforcement of a problematic pattern. The particular outcome is determined by the way the nurse handles the situation. It is not enough for the nurse to solve the conflict of whether to accept or to reject it. Experiential learning for the patient, i.e., understanding and changing of behavior, can only occur when the nurse talks through the gift-giving situation with the patient.

An extensive review of nursing literature revealed minimal information about gift-giving in the nurse-patient relationship. The author hopes to fill this gap of needed information in three ways: (1) to inform the reader that the patient's giving and the nurse's receiving of a gift can be problematic, (2) to describe some of the varied needs and expectations of patients and nurses in the gift situation, and (3) to propose a therapeutic nursing intervention for the working-through of the gift situation. Through the knowledge and application of this intervention, the nurse's hesitation, vacillation, or anxiety can be eliminated when the nurse is faced with the offer from the patient. The nurse's energy, instead of being converted to anxiety, can be channelized toward facilitating therapeutic benefits for the patient.

The nurse is first confronted with the gift-giving situation as a student. An instructor may discuss the situation in class. In nursing schools, statements are often made in the guise of principles that are supposed to guide the student in the working-through of various situations. Such a "principle" might be stated: When a patient offers the nurse a gift, it is more

90—

helpful if the nurse does not accept the gift. What is the theoretical basis for this "principle"? Does the student understand why she should act in the prescribed manner? In order to meet the varying gift-giving situations, the student must understand the behaviors involved in the dyadic relationship of patient and nurse. Therapeutic nursing intervention is built on learned theory, not accepted advice.

Nursing was once considered a charitable service. Over a period of time and progress, nurses learned to consider themselves professional practitioners who receive financial benefits for their work. However, some patients tend to cling to the old viewpoint, still thinking of the nurse as a charitable worker. Perhaps this viewpoint is a basis on which some patients give the nurse material repayment in the form of a gift.

In general and in psychiatric hospitals, patients often become aware, through direct observation or from other patients, that it is customary to give the nurse a gift. Some nurses expect these gifts as an expression of the patient's appreciation of the nurse's efforts to help. The giving patient receives a barrage of thank you's and smiles as he is discharged. If the gift is presented during his hospitalization, he buys extra attention through his own manipulative act of giving. The nurse is obligated to the patient; this obligation influences her future behavior. When the nurse accepts the patient's gift, she is rendering herself powerless in the relationship with the patient, who becomes powerful.

When the nurse receives the patient's gift without exploring the meaning of the gift, she communicates to the patient understanding and approval of his behavior. The nurse has sanctioned an overt pattern, giving, without any validated knowledge of the meaning of this behavior to the patient. The nurse is the model for the patient, the one with whom he identifies. She sets the pace of her relationship with the patient; her act of receiving the patient's gift can lead to a problematic relationship. Peplau [1] says, "This pattern may be said to be problematic when participation in this expression of the illness, by receiving what is given by the patient, reinforces and thus strengthens the needs and problems of the patient which are symbolized in the recurrent act of giving."

When the nurse refuses a patient's gift without exploring with the patient the meaning of this behavior, the patient may become anxious. He may have expected the nurse to take the gift; his expectations were not met. He may feel ashamed or think he is misunderstood. He may experience a number of different kinds of thoughts and feelings.

What is giving? Giving is a symbolic act of communication; the act

[1] Peplau, Hildegard E., "Giving," unpublished paper, p. 1.

meets the needs of two persons (the patient-giver and/or nurse-receiver). Operationally defined, giving involves these steps:

1. An individual (patient) has a need.
2. Need tension is felt.
3. Giving is a way to meet this need.
4. The individual (patient) chooses another person (nurse) as a recipient.
5. The individual (patient) offers this other person (nurse) a gift.
6. The gift is received.
7. Need tension decreases.
    or
7. The receiver (nurse) performs the expected reciprocal action(s).
8. Need tension decreases.
    or
7. The receiver (nurse) *does not* perform the expected reciprocal action(s).
8. The giver experiences an increased level of anxiety.

The patient's anxiety may be converted to aggression, withdrawal, somatization, or *learning*.

The needs and expectations of the patient who is giving are not known to the nurse. The giving may be a personal overture for closeness, a repayment, a bribe for some future nurse behavior, a way to rid oneself of something undesirable, or an act in accordance with cultural standards. The gift may be used to emphasize or substitute for a verbalization. If it is the latter, the nurse may be reinforcing a nonverbal pattern by accepting this gift. By accepting the gift, she communicates that she understands the gift meaning; there is no need for the patient to talk with her. Another patient may hope to gain recognition, favor, or prestige by imparting a gift to the nurse. The gift may symbolize an attempted maneuver to change the nurse's status to that of a friend or of a servant.

The nurse who spontaneously accepts a patient's gift is indicating that this gift meets some need of her own. Sometimes, the nurse's curiosity leads her to accept the gift. Often, she accepts because she thinks refusal of a gift signifies rejection of the patient. Perhaps a gift meets the nurse's needs to be liked and appreciated.

It is evident that many needs and expectations are involved in the patient's giving to the nurse. Peplau [2] says that the nurse must have an understanding of the needs and problems involved in this pattern. With this understanding as a basis, the nurse's interaction with the patient can be beneficial in solving the underlying needs and problems.

As a staff nurse, the author was involved in the following gift situation:

[2] *Ibid.*, p. 1.

A psychiatric patient ordered an expensive box of candy for the ward personnel. The gift was received; verbal appreciation was expressed to the patient. Two more boxes of candy were given to personnel by this patient. The personnel reciprocated in the same manner as before. The motivation of the patient's giving became evident when the patient laughingly and revengefully said that she was getting back at her husband. He was unware that the patient, his wife, was charging the gifts to him. He would have to pay for them. The nurses had participated in the patient's manner of expressing anger. There was no intervention or attempt to understand the basis for the giving and receiving of the gift of candy. There was no experiential learning for the patient.

Another patient said, "I wasn't supposed to smoke one time. Then she gave me a cigarette to keep me from dying." This patient data point out that the meaning of a gift cannot be assumed by the nurse.

Patients do expect some reciprocation from the nurse who receives their gift. One patient in group therapy told the nurse leader, "If you give things away, you can't find them later. You give and you don't get back."

Because of the varied needs and expectations involved in giving and receiving gifts in the nurse-patient relationship, there must be nursing intervention so that the meaning of the gift will be understood. The nurse first intervenes by stating to the patient the limitations involved concerning the acceptance of the gift. An example of setting these limits is found in these nurse-patient data:

Patient: And here is something I wrote about the problem. Would you care to take it with you.
Nurse: The paper?
Patient: Yes. This little bit of writing I did.
Nurse: I will talk about the papers with you while I am here.

The nurse rejected the gift. She did not reject the patient, but stayed to talk over the situation with the patient. If the nurse is unable to stay at the time the patient offers or asks for a gift, the nurse tells the patient when she will come to talk with him. The nurse keeps her appointment.

In talking with the patient, the nurse facilitates the patient's experiential learning about his behavior in the gift-giving situation. Statements of the nurse to the patient are made to facilitate observation by the patient of his own behavior. He learns to observe what is going on in the situation, exactly what he is doing or what he has done.

Some nurse-patient data will exemplify the different phases of talking over the gift situation with a patient.

*Patient:* Got any extra paper?
*Nurse:* Yes (writing on a pad).
*Patient:* Can I have a sheet?
*Nurse:* What for?
*Patient:* To play tick-tack-toe.
*Nurse:* You want to play games?
*Patient:* Yes.
*Nurse:* Now?

In these data, the nurse made statements to elicit the patient's observation of what was going on in the immediate situation. This patient had frequently requested paper from the nurse, even though the patient had paper. She gave various reasons for needing the paper, and when the request was not granted, she became angry with the nurse. This episode led to further exploration of one of the patient's basic difficulties, anger.

In order for the patient to understand the basis of his behavior, he must be able to describe the details of his behavior and the circumstances of the particular situation. The nurse can elicit this description by such statements as "what," "where," "when," "which," "who," "go on," "so," "tell me an example." The following is an example of a nurse leader eliciting description in a group-therapy meeting:

*Patient:* Will you give me a cigarette? Can't I have just one more, then I'll settle down.
*Nurse:* You said if you could have one cigarette, you would settle down. Tell the group more.

This patient requested a gift from the nurse. Fulfillment of this request would have reinforced the patient's bribing behavior. The nurse, by eliciting description from the patient, allows him to recall more, to focus on related and enumerated details of an event, and to provide the data needed for the analysis of his behavior.

When the patient has accomplished the tasks of observing and describing the details and circumstances of his behavior in the gift-giving situation, he is ready to analyze the situation. It is only in the analysis step of experiential learning that the nurse asks "why" or asks for the basis or direct process of some behavior. The patient has the materials needed, observation and descriptive data, to explain the reasons for his behavior, to make comparisons, and to evaluate his actions, thoughts, and feelings. Since he is prepared for these statements from the nurse, he will be less threatened by them. Two excerpts from these data are analysis situations.

*Patient:* Can I have your paper? I can talk better if I take notes.
*Nurse:* You can talk better if you write?
*Patient:* Yes.
*Nurse:* In what way?

This nurse and patient had discussed the paper request in previous sessions. Here the nurse asks for the process by which the patient will be able to talk better.

> Patient A: Sometimes it's real that patients have no family. I want to give them gifts and I can't.
> Patient B: Good thing you realize this. You'd just be getting them indebted to you.
> Nurse: What are some other ways beside giving gifts to show what you feel?

These data show that these patients expect reciprocation from the receiver of the gift. The nurse's statement requires that the patients know what they feel and know that the gift is a way of communicating this feeling. The patient must recall, compare, and substitute another way of expressing the same feeling.

After the patient has analyzed a situation, he must formulate the conclusions of his analysis. Then he, too, must talk over what has happened, how and what he has formulated with another person. When this situation validation is completed, the new learned product becomes integrated with other knowledge. The nurse needs to set up situations wherein the patient can test his new learning and understanding; he will use this learning, since it is a part of him.

It has been shown that the gift-giving situation in the nurse-patient relationship can be handled therapeutically whenever the nurse talks over the situation with the patient. The phases of experiential learning—observation, description, analysis, formulation, validation, testing, using—are used by the nurse as her guide for what to say to the patient. The gift-giving can be a learning experience for the patient. Talking about this situation may lead to areas other than the gift situation that need exploration. When the nurse is aware that her behavior may communicate many things to the patient regarding the gift-giving, she may be therapeutic in following the intervention spelled out in this chapter.

## BIBLIOGRAPHY

PEPLAU, HILDEGARD E., "Giving," unpublished paper read at Group for Advancement of Psychiatry, Asbury Park, N.J.: Nov., 1957.

# 17 RESISTANCE

*Alice Stueks*

Knowledge of a concept of resistance can be useful to nurses in any inter-personal situation, regardless of the clinical setting or the level of practice. Resistance is frequently noted, for instance, in patients who have medical problems for which antibiotics are prescribed. When the patient fails to respond favorably to such treatment, it is frequently because the infecting organism is penicillin-resistant. Were the same patient, in subsequent years, to be exposed to the same organism, he might be said to have a resistance to it due to an acquired immunity, as seen for example, in measles, scarlet fever, and mumps. The body has, in any given time, both natural and acquired resistances, or immunities, to invading organisms, but the degree of such resistances will depend, in part, on the health of the body. Such factors as fatigue, malnutrition, or a previous illness tend to decrease the body's potential to ward off infections. One might then say the body resistance is lowered, and the potential for infection is increased.

While resistance is a concept useful in all areas of nursing practice, the term is most frequently attributed to the specialty of psychiatric nursing. In psychiatric nursing practice, resistance is noted in the behavioral methods the patient employs, either wittingly or unwittingly, but more frequently the latter, to ward off or avoid anxiety provoked when the security operations are attacked. Resistance and repression are terms used extensively in Freudian theory and are said to be the primary tenets of psychoanalysis.[1]

[1] Puner, H. W., *Freud, His Life and His Mind*, p. 91.

The importance of the concepts of resistance and repression, considered together, are noted in the literature as follows:

> The fact that a patient . . . was unable to recall significant and emotionally charged events in the waking state, whereas under hypnosis such material would, with encouragement, make its appearance gave rise to the psychoanalytic concept of resistance which opposed such recall, and which was lessened by the hypnotic procedure.[2]
>
> Resistance refers to all the conscious and unconscious impulses, emotions, activities, motives, etc., in the patient which are in opposition to the aims of psychoanalytic therapy. Resistance is essentially an operational term and indicates the opposition of some aspect of the patient toward the aims and motives of analysis.[3]
>
> Everything that has been forgotten had in some way or other been painful; it had either been alarming or disagreeable or shameful by the standard of the subject's personality.[4]
>
> [Resistance is] opposition to any attempt to lay bare the content of the unconscious. The strength of the resistance is a measure of the repressing force. Resistance is always found in analysis.[5]

Since resistance is a defensive mechanism, used by the patient to avoid pain with its concomitant anxiety, some mention of the concept of anxiety seems essential. Sullivan [6] defines anxiety as the uncomfortable and most unwelcomed feeling which arises when an individual's self-security or self-esteem is threatened.

Every individual, from infancy on, has developed certain security operations or defensive mechanisms which are used to keep the self in a state of well-being.[7] When these security operations fail, the state of well-being becomes nonexistent and is replaced by anxiety.

The psychotic patient, who from early infancy has found his needs unmet or has constantly received disapproval from significant figures in his life, has gone to extreme lengths to develop an elaborate, detailed, and complex system to ensure his security. In the nurse-patient relationship, any attempt the nurse makes to help the patient to elucidate his problems, to explore his feelings and patterns of behavior, or to examine his relations with people may be viewed by the patient as dangerous, provoke excessive anxiety, and will require the patient to employ means to protect himself. Little or no self-worth, a feeling of shame concerning previous thoughts and actions, hostility and aggressiveness are only a few of the many reasons

[2] Abse, D. W., "Hysteria," p. 281.
[3] Greenson, R. R., "The Classic Psychoanalytic Approach," pp. 1399–415.
[4] Puner, op. cit., p. 91.
[5] English, H. B., and English, A. C., A Comprehensive Dictionary of Psychological and Psychoanalytic Terms, p. 460.
[6] Sullivan, H. S., The Interpersonal Theory of Psychiatry, pp. 20–24.
[7] Sullivan, H. S., Conception of Modern Psychiatry, pp. 158–71.

a patient may avoid discussing his life's experiences with the nurse. The patient fears that such revelations may lower his esteem in the eyes of the nurse. Resistance serves as a means of protection for the patient. Considering all this, it is remarkable that the patient approaches the nurse-patient relationship at all, since each new interpersonal relationship is fraught with potential danger.[8]

Resistance is manifested in many ways. A few examples, with clinical instances excerpted from nurse-patient data, are the following:

### 1. FAILURE TO APPROACH THE INTERVIEW SITUATION [9]

Mr. H. had been meeting with the nurse regularly, as scheduled, for six sessions. In the sixth hour, he initiated a discussion about his difficulties with his older brother, who had had the patient committed to the hospital. Mr. H. evidenced increased anxiety, with its energy converted into psycho-motor activity, almost simultaneously with the introduction of this particular subject. Each subsequent reference to his brother during the hour was accompanied with the slamming of his right fist into his left hand. The next hour, the patient was not available for interviewing. For the next four scheduled sessions, Mr. H. refused to meet with the nurse despite repeated invitations. The relationship was then terminated by the nurse, since she was in the relationship as a learner. Learning, for the nurse, was restricted in the absence of the patient.

A second example of this type of resistance was noted in another nurse-patient relationship. Mrs. M. had been chosen by the nurse as the patient with whom she would meet for counseling. After the patient had agreed to meet with the nurse, the patient got up from the chair and began to walk about the ward. Attempts by the nurse at an orderly orientation of the patient to the relationship were fruitless. One might say the orientation information was given "on the run" or on a "catch as one can" basis as the patient passed by the areas selected for the interview. Since the patient had given her consent to meet with the nurse, the nurse went to the chosen area on each scheduled day at the designated time. For seven weeks (fourteen interview sessions) the patient persisted in her refusal to sit down and talk with the nurse. At the fifteenth session, the nurse informed the patient that it was to be the last hour allocated to her. Throughout the hour, the patient continued to walk in a broad circle about the chair on

[8] Wolberg, L. R., *The Technique of Psychotherapy*, p. 463.
[9] Menninger, K., *A Psychiatrist's World*, p. 218.

which the nurse sat. At the end of the session, the nurse closed her note-book, put away her pencils, and stood up to depart. At that time, the patient came to the nurse and talked rapidly, coherently, and used five minutes to explain that she was so preoccupied with her problems that she had been unable to spare time to talk with the nurse. Here, the resistance persisted until the scheduled time of departure of the nurse.

## 2. PATIENT FOCUSES ON SUPERFICIAL CONTENT

The patient may talk about current events, ward decor, staff, and the like rather than about himself.[10]

*Nurse:* (Opening notebook.) I am ready, Mr. A.
*Patient:* I see in the paper that taxes are going up again. Something about property re-evaluation.
*Nurse:* Are you a property owner?
*Patient:* No. I thought you'd be interested in the subject of taxes for today.
*Nurse:* Talk about you.
*Patient:* Looks like it will be a nice day today. Some of the fellows are going down to the field and play ball. Good day for a ball game. You can do so much more in good weather. You can go fishing, to ball games, swimming, all that stuff.
*Nurse:* What about you?
*Patient:* Like I said, it's a good day for a ball game. Maybe you'd like to hear about the dance. That's a pleasant subject. Now, see, all the patients go—men and women—and there's music and dancing. Men dance with women and students, too. Is that a good idea?
*Nurse:* What do you think?
*Patient:* I want you to tell me.
*Nurse:* This hour is for you to talk about you, Mr. A., not for me to talk about me.
*Patient:* Where do you come from? I mean, what town?
*Nurse:* My, my, is it possible that you would find it easier to talk about the weather, baseball, or me than to talk about you?
*Patient:* I have nothing to say. I can't think of a thing.
*Nurse:* Is it possible that anyone could live for forty years and have nothing to say?
*Patient:* (Laughing.) Guess it did sound ridiculous. No—it isn't possible. I just hate to talk about all that—my past and all. If I talk about me, I have to get to Ruth [patient's wife] and that is hard to do. If I could talk about my life and leave her out, it'd be okay—but that can't be done.
*Nurse:* I'll wait until you think of something that concerns you.
*Patient:* I can talk about my brother.
*Nurse:* Tell me about you *and* your brother.
*Patient:* All right. Mike—he's my brother—is two years younger than me. When I was ten and Mike eight, we used to play at ———— Park. . . .

[10] Wolberg, *op. cit.*, p. 466.

## 3. PATIENT AVOIDS DISCUSSING MATERIAL THAT PROVOKES ANXIETY

The patient had broached the subject of her unstable childhood in the previous hour. This was a woman who had moved from foster home to foster home during her childhood. Chart history yielded the information that the patient had made repeated efforts to be reunited with her mother, and that fostering families petitioned the board of guardians to have the child placed elsewhere because she was a "habitual runaway." As the patient began to discuss the situation late in one session, she became anxious and retreated to a discussion of other patients. She did, however, agree to discuss her relationship with her mother at the next session. That session was as follows:

*Nurse:* Good morning, Mrs. J.
*Patient:* Hi. I'm here because the nurse said I had to come.
*Nurse:* Oh?
*Patient:* Yeah. I told her I was too tired and should be in bed.
*Nurse:* You were planning, as I recall, to talk about your relationship with your mother today.
*Patient:* Yeah, but I'm too tired to talk to you or anybody else. I can't sleep laying down—my asthma—it's bothering me lately.
(Patient yawned, curled up in her chair, and either slept or feigned sleep for the entire session.)

## 4. PATIENT MAKES A "FORCED FLIGHT INTO HEALTH" [11]

He attempts to convince the nurse that he is well and no longer needs counseling. Wolberg [12] points out that this form of resistance is usually associated with the need to maintain a rigid watch over everything one says for fear control will be lost or minimized.

*Nurse:* You were talking about your difficulty with Dr. F. at the end of the last hour.
*Patient:* Oh, yes. Well, that's all taken care of. I saw him Tuesday and he now agrees with me that I've improved. I'll be staffed next week and will go home at the beginning of next month. Tell you, I think you should get a new patient now because I'm all better now, and since I'm going home and all, you should get someone new. I don't need help now, see—'cause I'm going home since I'm okay so get another one of the guys. I'll tell you—I think you should pick Andy because he's sick and I'm not. You could help Andy, but now I'm well, I don't need help. Hey, Andy—come here and take my place with the nurse. She'll talk to you because I'm going to be going home.

[11] *Ibid.*, p. 465.
[12] *Ibid.*, p. 465.

The relationship with this patient was maintained for an additional seventeen hours, since the patient remained in the hospital. Subsequent data, introduced by the patient after the declaration above, led to the speculation that this patient was reluctant to discuss some aspects of his past relationships with male friends. During one of the last sessions, the patient discussed with the nurse a homosexual experience which occurred when the patient was about fourteen years of age. The patient eventually validated the nurse's speculation that he was reluctant to divulge some of his past experiences and said, "I was afraid you'd be shocked and leave me, so I thought I'd take advantage of the opportunity to leave you. Some girls get all shook up when they hear about sex. Besides, I thought you'd think much less of me when you knew about all that."

### 5. PATIENT EXPRESSES FEAR OF, OR CONTEMPT FOR, HEALTH [13]

The idea underlying this form of resistance might best be stated: "If Im sick, I'll stay sick, because to be well again requires change, and to change I must experience anxiety and possibly failure."

*Nurse:* Good morning.
*Patient:* Look, I just read about ———— in the paper. A politician throwing money around when people in his own district are hungry. He's "normal" —right? An' if he's normal, I don't want to be. You think all the nuts are in here? You're crazy if you do. The sick people are out there (pointing out the window) taking advantage of the little slobs. (Patient's voice is indicative of anger.) I'd rather stay right here than act like that. "Well?"—nuts! Those "wells" send fellas off to wars to get killed and all while they sit home and get fat watching their old ladies knit bundles for Britain. Go find yourself another boy who want to join them nuts outside, and I'll sit right here till I croak. That's the way to get out with the "wells"—in a long black box.
*Nurse:* You sound angry today.
*Patient:* Yer darned tootin! Who wants to get back to that stinkin' rat race? Not me! And that's all I have to say to you today.
(Patient got up and left the interview situation.)

### 6. PATIENT USES RATIONALIZATIONS WHEN THE NURSE POINTS OUT EVIDENCES OF RESISTANCE

*Nurse:* I was here on Wednesday, but I didn't see you on the ward.
*Patient:* Yeah. I was at the clinic.
*Nurse:* I thought you were avoiding me. You did before, as I recall, when you had started talking about your father's death.
*Patient:* That's right. It's hard to talk about death.
*Nurse:* This time you didn't come on Wednesday, and last Friday you had

[13] *Ibid.*, p. 468.

been speaking of your prolonged separation from your husband while he was in service.

*Patient:* It could be, but that wasn't it. My eyes had been tearing.

*Nurse:* Crying?

*Patient:* No. I don't cry. It's my glasses. I need to have my glasses changed. My eyes are weak.

*Nurse:* Tell me, then, about your separation from your husband.

(Patient resumed the subject at the point where she had ended the previous meeting with the nurse. She then began to cry.)

*Nurse:* You must have felt pretty helpless. I notice that you are crying now as you talk about that long separation.

*Patient:* I'm not crying. I wasn't helpless. The only help I need is to get my glasses changed. (Patient continued to weep noisily.) [14]

## 7. PATIENT MANIFESTS "INTELLECTUAL INHIBITIONS"

Included among the inhibitions manifested by patients during the counseling hours are breaking appointments; arriving late for the sessions; forgetting to mention significant events and occurrences; daydreaming during the session; a high distractability; failing to concentrate on the task at hand; and a mental fogging which is also manifested outside the interview situation.[15]

*Patient:* (Hurrying to the interview fifteen minutes late.) Is this really Friday? I thought it was Thursday. That's why I'm late. If the cook hadn't told me, I wouldn't have come at all.

*Nurse:* This is really Friday. While I was waiting for you, the nurse did say that you might be delayed somewhere because you now have a privilege card which you got last week.

*Patient:* Oh, yeah. Forgot to mention it when you were here. Is that a mirror that guy's hanging up there? We need a mirror around here. Did you say something just now?

*Nurse:* No. You were talking about your privilege card.

*Patient:* Yeah. (Patient lapsed into silence for approximately five minutes.)

*Nurse:* What are you thinking about?

*Patient:* Oh—I dunno—about being out of here. I'd like to be married to a rich man and live in a big house—bigger than Dragonwyck. Have servants. You know—a rich lady. I'd like to be a lady.

*Nurse:* I wonder if there are some subjects you feel anxious about discussing with me?

*Patient:* No. Why?

*Nurse:* The other day you were talking about your children, and then you changed the subject. Then today you were late—almost didn't get here I think you said. Now you are using the hour to dream of wealth. Is the subject of your children difficult for you to discuss with me?

*Patient:* No. I can talk about anything. Even my kids.

*Nurse:* Some women have relationships that arise out of loneliness. They

[14] Acknowledgment is made of the invaluable data supplied by colleagues of the writer, especially Claire Griffin.
[15] Wolberg, *op. cit.*, p. 465.

then hesitate to talk about the subject for fear of disapproval. Was this your experience? (This patient had three illegitimate children after her husband's death.)

*Patient:* Well, I guess it could happen, but I don't want to talk about such things. I'd rather talk about that thing that lady is sewing over there.

(The patient did not discuss her experiences with her illegitimate children until about six weeks after this particular interview.)

## CONCLUSION

These, then, are a few of the many manifestations of resistance. The literature and clinical practice suggest several others. Since resistance is noted in almost every counseling relationship, it would be helpful to have a technique for intervening when resistance is noted. One such technique, with its developmental phases, is noted by Wolberg [16] and has been useful to this author in working with patients who manifest resistance. It is as follows:

1. Call the patient's attention to the resistance itself and explore the possible reason(s) for resistance
2. Point out the possible reason(s) for resistance
3. Reassure the patient, in a tangential way, about that which he is resisting
4. Bring the patient's attention to the material against which the resistance is directed
5. Work through the resistance

Wolberg [17] offers a word of caution for those counselors who prefer to terminate the relationship when resistance is encountered, particularly in those instances where the presenting symptoms are intensified. "An explanation that the patient may possibly get worse before he gets better is often a safeguard against interruption of therapy."

In summary, then, resistance is a defensive mechanism utilized by most patients during nurse-patient counseling to avoid anxiety. Resistance is manifested in various ways and must be recognized in order that a technique to counteract it may be employed. Resistance and repression, which seem to be related in many instances, are the primary tenets of psychoanalysis and are noted particularly in the theoretical framework of Freud.

## BIBLIOGRAPHY

ABSE, D. WILFRED, "Hysteria," in *American Handbook of Psychiatry*, Silvano Arieti (ed.), Basic Books, New York: 1959.

ENGLISH, HORACE B., and ENGLISH, AVA CHAMPNEY, *A Comprehensive Dictionary*

[16] *Ibid.*, pp. 463–87.
[17] *Ibid.*, p. 464.

*of Psychological and Psychoanalytic Terms,* Longmans, Green and Co., New York: 1958.

GREENSON, RALPH R., "The Classic Psychoanalytic Approach," in *American Handbook of Psychiatry,* Silvano Arieti (ed.), Basic Books, New York: 1959.

MENNINGER, KARL, *A Psychiatrist's World,* Bernard H. Hall (ed.), Viking Press, New York: 1954.

PUNER, HELEN WALKER, *Freud: His Life and His Mind.* Dell Publishing Co., New York: 1957.

SULLIVAN, HARRY STACK, *Conceptions of Modern Psychiatry,* W. W. Norton & Co., New York: 1953.

———— *The Interpersonal Theory of Psychiatry,* W. W. Norton & Co., New York: 1953.

WOLBERG, LEWIS R., *The Technique of Psychotherapy,* Grune and Stratton, New York: 1954.

# 18 AVOIDANCE

*Gloria Oden*

One of the common problems of the nurse-patient relationship with schizophrenic patients is avoidance on the part of the patient. What is avoidance? What underlies this behavior pattern? What purpose does avoidance serve for the patient?

The dictionary defines avoidance as "the act of keeping away." [1] Avoidance, in the nurse-patient relationship, is an action, verbal or nonverbal, by which the patient keeps away from the counseling situation. Is this simple conceptualization appropriate to patients in the nurse-patient relationship in the light of the patient's total behavior? Consider the descriptions of the initial hours of the nurse-patient relationship in the following cases:

*Case 1.* Mr. A., a 36-year-old patient, diagnosed as "schizophrenia: catatonic type," agreed to participate in a nurse-patient relationship. After the second interview hour, the patient could not be found on the ward during the scheduled interview hour. Ward personnel reported that the patient's pattern of behavior had changed. Prior to his meetings with the nurse, the patient had spent most of the day on the ward. He now left the ward several hours before the interview hour was scheduled and did not return until at least one hour after the nurse had left the hospital for the day. The nurse was unable, at any time, to locate the patient.

*Case 2.* Mr. D., a 29-year-old patient, diagnosed as "schizophrenia: chronic undifferentiated type," agreed to participate in a nurse-patient relationship. Mr. D. frequently failed to arrive at the appointed hour. He occasionally missed the entire interview.

*Case 3.* Mr. R., a 25-year-old patient, diagnosed as "schizophrenia: undifferentiated type," agreed to participate in a nurse-patient relationship. He

[1] Barnhart, C. L., and Stein, J. (eds.), *The American College Dictionary*, p. 86.

—105

arrived promptly for the appointment. He talked readily, but his communication with the nurse was marked by avoidance of topics relating to himself and by abrupt changes of topic at any time that he gave information about himself.

Each of the patients described utilized avoidance as a pattern of behavior. In Cases 1 and 2, avoidance was predominantly nonverbal. In Case 3, the avoidance pattern utilized by the patient was verbal. Do all these cases accurately fit the definition of avoidance, of keeping away? Case 1 does. Mr. A., by his absence, obtained his goal of complete avoidance. The behavior of the patients in Cases 2 and 3 does not completely fit the definition of "keeping away" in terms of the patients' total behaviors.

In examining the total picture, opposite goals, or conflict, appear to be in operation. These goals are approach and avoid. According to Peplau, "conflict can be said to be present only when tendencies for avoidance are present." [2] Avoidance, then, can be termed an action to delay or to take no part in resolution of the approach-avoid conflict. In terms of the diagnosis of the schizophrenic patient, avoidance of or withdrawal from interpersonal relationships is understandable. In Cases 2 and 3, the patients' ability to tolerate a relationship, despite its superficial nature, indicates some movement toward healthy resolution of the conflict.

Inability to tolerate closeness underlies the pattern of avoidance. By using this behavior pattern, the patient diminishes the threat inherent in any interpersonal relationship. Time, patience, tolerance, and acceptance of the patient's need to reduce his anxiety to a productive working level appear to be adequate solutions to the problem. However, unless positive intervention is initiated, the problem becomes a double bind for both patient and nurse, since they are participating in an avoid-avoid relationship which strengthens the pathology of the patient. The conflict is solved by mutual withdrawal.[3]

Therapeutically, then, the nurse assists the patient in resolving the conflict by helping him to learn a new pattern of relatedness to others. This is implemented at the earliest possible time in the nurse-patient relationship. The following principles and excerpts from the Case 3 nurse-patient data illustrate methods of dealing with the problem of avoidance.

Mr. R. was extremely anxious during early nurse-patient interviews. His speech was rapid and pressured. Gross hand tremors were observable, and the patient frequently wrung his hands. He had a facial tic. Despite the

[2] Peplau, H. E., *Interpersonal Relations in Nursing*, p. 106.
[3] See Tudor, G. E., "A Sociopsychiatric Nursing Approach to Intervention in a Problem of Mutual Withdrawal on a Mental Hospital Ward", pp. 193–217.

high anxiety level which was inferred from the patient's observable behavior, he was able to remain with the nurse for the entire interview.

The orientation at the first meeting included a specification of the
purpose of the interviews: "The interview time is for you to talk with me
about your problems."

The patient began the first interview with a discussion of the weather.
His next topic concerned the thoughts and feelings of hospitalized patients,
discussed in the second and third persons. The nurse interjected the questions, "What do you think?" and "What do you feel?" when they applied.
The patient did not answer the questions appropriately at this time. However, a positive intervention was ongoing from the first interview. Later
in the interview, the following intervention was used:

> *Patient:* The Communists have an entirely different system. And, ah, of
> course it is not correct, but they believe that the individual is not im-
> portant. That is the problem with the world at the present time.
> *Nurse:* And how does this relate to you?

Again, the patient did not answer the question appropriately. Rather, he
moved to a discussion of world problems.

On the basis of the data, it appeared that Mr. R. had heard at least
part of the orientation, for his content concerned "problems." Later in the
interview the nurse stated, "Mr. R., this is your hour, and I am interested
in your problems."

The nurse continued to orient the patient to the purpose of the interview during the initial sessions. She assumed that the patient's avoidance
might be based upon a lack of clarity about purpose. During session four,
the patient stopped in mid-sentence to ask, "Say, what is the reason for
this meeting, anyway?" The nurse repeated the purpose of the interviews.

The nurse continued to frame questions that related the patient's impersonal data to himself—his thoughts, feelings, and actions in the situations, he described. By the tenth session, the patient found it easier to talk
about himself and his problems.

After this time the patient was usually able to spend the greater part of
the interview discussing data relating to himself. He continued to use avoidance when his anxiety level became high. The nurse then focused on this
behavior when it occurred. She used a matter-of-fact approach, avoiding
verbal or nonverbal indications of disapproval.

During interviews ten through thirteen, the patient discussed his hallucinations and gave brief data relating to his homosexual experiences. During
interview fourteen, the patient spent most of his time discussing superficial personal data. During interview fifteen, he touched briefly on the

topic of his hallucinations. He then abruptly changed the topic to the environment. The nurse asked:

*Nurse:* Mr. R., are you avoiding talking about yourself?
*Patient:* Oh, no. (Continues discussing the environment for several minutes.)
*Nurse:* Mr. R., are you avoiding talking about yourself?
*Patient:* Yes, I am evading the issue. (He then discussed his hallucinations for the remainder of the interview.)

The nurse continued to point out the possibility that the patient was using avoidance when this behavior pattern was evident. By the twentieth interview, the patient identified this behavior in himself when it occurred and offered the following explanation for the behavior:

I'd like to mention that I'm uneasy. Sometimes I get so uneasy when I talk about myself that I have to talk about something else for a little while.

While the patient appeared to use avoidance less often, the nurse questioned whether or not the patient continued to use a more subtle method of avoidance. In analyzing the data of interviews fourteen through sixteen, the nurse found clues which indicated that when the patient appeared to be approaching a further discussion of homosexuality, he changed the topic to an impersonal one. Terms such as "odd" and "queer" began to come up in the data. Whenever this occurred, the patient's anxiety increased and he changed the subject.

During interviews seventeen and eighteen, the patient found a new method of avoidance. He arrived for the interview laden with written schedules of daily activities. He plunged into a recital of the material as soon as the interview began. The nurse did not record any of the data he read from notes. When the patient gave spontaneous data, the nurse recorded these data as she had previously done. During the recital of the notes, the nurse maintained a politely disinterested expression. The patient appeared to pay no attention to the nurse during interview seventeen and ignored the nurse's request that he tell her about the written material.

During interview eighteen, the patient continued to read the notes. After ten minutes the nurse said:

*Nurse:* Tell me about reading the notes.
*Patient:* It gives me something to do. (The patient continues reading.)
*Nurse:* Are you avoiding talking about yourself when you read the notes?
*Patient:* In a way, yes. (The patient takes out a new sheaf of notes to read.)
*Nurse:* Mr. R., is this the best use of your time?
*Patient:* No, it isn't. (The patient continues to read for two minutes, then puts the notes into his pocket.) There must be something else I'd like to tell you. Actually, there are lots of things I'd like to tell you.

The patient then began to discuss his homosexual experiences. After this meeting, the patient no longer brought notes with him to the meeting. For the next three sessions, the patient discussed with the nurse thoughts, feelings, and actions relating to his homosexual experiences. Avoidance was used minimally and briefly by the patient as a method of reducing anxiety.

Nursing intervention in avoidance with this patient was achieved in two ways. During the orientation phase, the nurse assumed that the patient, because of his high level of anxiety, might not have heard the purpose of the interviews. She stated the purpose of the interviews at each of the initial meetings. When the patient gave impersonal data, the nurse focused upon the thoughts, feelings, and actions of the patient, and how the data given related to the patient. She did not insist, however, that the patient change his behavior immediately. Change was gradual, but continual, during the early meetings.

During the working relationship phase, the nurse became more direct in pointing out to the patient her observations of the patient's behavior. The patient was soon able to recognize this behavior in himself, stated the purpose it served, and used it selectively.

Content analysis of the data gave clues to the nurse about the purpose of the behavior at different phases of counseling, enabling her to institute intervention to reduce the avoidance behavior and to facilitate discussion of problem areas for the patient.

# BIBLIOGRAPHY

JACKSON, DON D., The Etiology of Schizophrenia, Basic Books, New York: 1960.

PEPLAU, HILDEGARD E., Interpersonal Relations in Nursing, G. P. Putnam's Sons, New York: 1952.

SCHWARTZ, M. S., and SHOCKLEY, E. L., The Nurse and the Mental Patient, Russell Sage Foundation, New York: 1956.

SULLIVAN, HARRY S., Clinical Studies in Psychiatry, W. W. Norton & Co., New York: 1956.

TUDOR, GWEN E., "A Sociopsychiatric Nursing Approach to Intervention in a Problem on Mutual Withdrawal on a Mental Hospital Ward," Psychiatry: J. Study Interpersonal Processes, Vol. 15, May, 1952.

WOLBERG, LEWIS R., The Technique of Psychotherapy, Grune and Stratton, New York: 1954.

# 19 ANGER: A CLINICAL PROBLEM [1]

*Dorothea R. Hays*

Most people feel and express anger at one time or another. The nurse, and particularly the psychiatric nurse, is in a position where she has opportunity to recognize and deal with angry feelings and angry behavior. If she knows the concept related to anger and learns to make inferences from her observations, she can understand and control her own behavior and help patients to gain some insight into what is happening.

In the literature, major emphasis seems to be given to the problems related to anger in children, especially in relation to parents and teachers. There seems to be a need to examine the subject of anger with special reference to nursing.

Using selected literature and examples from two intensive nurse-patient studies, I will explore in this chapter the concept of anger and concepts related to anger and show how these can be applied to patients' experiences, and how the nurse can operate in situations where anger is present.

Anger serves a very useful purpose, if it can be felt and expressed freely, because it usually promotes a pleasant, powerful feeling, which is quite the opposite of the feeling of anxiety for which it is substituted. But it also veils the original threat which gave rise to the anxiety.

The concept of anger can be spelled out in four steps: (1) there is an experience of frustration, unmet expectations, or lost self-respect; (2) anxiety occurs; (3) the anxiety is changed immediately and usually without recognition into feelings and/or actions of power; (4) relief is felt.

[1] Originally published in *Nursing World*, 132:22–44, 1958.

Anger seems to follow three different experiences—frustration, a blow to the self-view, and unmet expectations.

Peplau [2] has defined frustration as "any interference with, blocking of, or barrier to a need, drive, or desired goal before satisfaction of these urges has been felt. . . ."

The steps in the concept of frustration which can be observed and/or obtained from the patient by questioning include: (1) the setting of a goal; (2) movement toward this goal; (3) an intervening obstacle; (4) anger. For instance, a hospitalized patient told the nurse, "I think about home, getting out of here, and going to work. I am mad at the whole place for being here." Her goal is to go home. The only way she has moved toward it so far is by wishing. The intervening obstacle, that she is not well enough, is not yet recognized by the patient. She freely expresses her angry feelings.

A blow to the self-view occurs when a person suddenly sees himself more fully, when he grasps the meaning of some dissociated or selectively unattended aspects of experience that are threatening his self-respect. Sullivan [3] says that a direct attack on the processes inhibiting awareness of these aspects would yield severe anxiety, anger, or resentment. Anger would be most pleasant of the three, because it is a powerful feeling and moves attention away from the threatened picture of the self. A patient, after telling the nurse about some experience in her past that was not socially accepted and that she could not accept as having happened to her, said: "I don't want to talk about that, it is past and forgotten; you make me sick." The patient recognized a difference in feeling, probably due to anxiety, and then became angry with the nurse.

Patients may expect a nurse to act a certain way, for instance, the way their mothers used to respond or the way a teacher or another person acted in an earlier experience. If the nurse then says or does differently, the patient may feel anxious and, in turn, become angry. A patient accustomed to a mother on whom she could not always depend found that the nurse was always there at the appointed time, even when the patient was late or ignored her. This patient expressed anger by saying: "You never do any work; just sit there and write, you and your pencil. . . . It seems you could find something better to do with your time."

According to Richardson,[4] the purpose of anger is to give a feeling of

[2] Peplau, H. E., *Interpersonal Relations in Nursing*, p. 86.
[3] Sullivan, H. S., *Conceptions of Modern Psychiatry*, p. 185.
[4] Richardson, R. F., *The Psychology and Pedagogy of Anger*, p. 53.

power which serves to enhance the lowered self-respect and stimulates the person to fight any obstacle between himself and his goal.

Anger may be expressed in various ways and change into several other feelings. A frequent response to the feeling of anger is in terms of oral or physical aggression, which may be more or less directed at the object causing discomfort or anxiety.

Peplau [5] classified aggression in four categories: (1) direct, (2) that directed against an object which resembles the original obstacle, (3) aggression against an object with decreasing resemblance, and (4) aggression directed toward the self. Direct aggression was expressed by one of the patients against a social worker who did not meet her expectations. The patient said, "She told me I would be out in a year. She is a liar and a thief. . . ." Aggresssion directed against a nurse who somehow reminds the patient of someone else whom he has a reason to be angry with is an example of the second category. A patient who felt angry and did not want to direct her aggression against any person suggested: "I wish I were out of here; I wish there was a kicking machine around to use some energy up." An example of aggression directed toward the self, but indirectly pointed at the obstacle interfering with a goal, is expressed in this statement of a patient: "I'll kill myself, then people will be sorry they did not help me to get out."

Feelings related to anger are hate and hostility. Both are, like anger, substitutes for anxiety.

Horney [6] defines hostility as a response to subjectively experienced humiliation. A person finds or thinks that another person does not have the expected respect for him. Rather than feel anxiety, he feels and/or expresses hostility. If we adopt unfriendliness as a synonym for hostility, the term "extreme unfriendliness" would be appropriate for hate.

Sullivan [7] sees hate as a mutual process between people evoking anxiety through humiliating each other in a relationship in which some conjunctive forces prevent a breaking up of the relationship.

The ability to feel and act out anger is learned rather early in life. Responses to frustration or anxiety-provoking situations change from diffuse rage to more and specific patterns of anger, aggression, hostility, and hate, as well as resentment and apathy.

According to Sullivan,[8] the child learns rage behavior from angry, punishing parents. If he then finds that an exhibition of rage aggravates the

[5] Peplau, H. E., op. cit., pp. 92, 95.
[6] Horney, K., New Ways in Psychoanalysis, pp. 66–67.
[7] Sullivan, H. S., The Interpersonal Theory of Psychiatry, p. 375.
[8] Ibid., pp. 211–13.

situation in terms of more punishment, he uses anger. If this, too, is not tolerated by the punishing parent, the child feels and exhibits resentment, which can be defined as feeling wronged. If this is not acceptable, the child must conceal his resentment, first from others, and later from himself. He then may become apathetic, or without feeling, and exhibit the dissociated feelings as a psychosomatic complaint only.

Patients use different ways of acting out anger, and from these the nurse can hypothesize about the attitude important adults might have had about anger when the patient was a child.

One patient told the nurse: "I have a pain in the head. I wish I were out of here!" Finding her goal impossible to reach, the patient might have felt and acted out of anger; instead she felt a pain in her head.

Patterns of anger are related to the particular development of the child, as well as to the general cultural frame in which he grows up. Richardson [9] describes the three different patterns of attributive, contrary, and indifferent reaction to frustration or anxiety-provoking situations. The attributive reaction pattern includes sarcastic or ironic remarks as well as imaginary attacks against the intervening obstacle. Contrary behavior has its roots in the Christian doctrine of "Offering the other cheek." Excessive kindness and politeness are shown where the situation calls for anger. The indifferent or "I don't care" reaction may be the result of repeated experiences of frustration coupled with the inability to do anything about it.

The nurse, in order to deal effectively with feelings of anger in her relationships with patients, has to understand the concept of anger, concepts related to anger, her own patterns of reacting to and dealing with anger-provoking situations, and how to recognize anger in patients and help them to cope with this experience in a meaningful way. This last skill includes three operations: (1) helping the patient to accept himself as feeling angry; (2) helping the patient to find out why he feels angry; (3) assisting the patient in using the energy inherent in anger in a constructive way.

In working with a patient who freely expressed anger, a pattern in nurse-patient interaction developed and was recognized. In the first phase of the pattern, the patient acted out her feelings of anger. For instance, she would pace back and forth and scream out her feelings of anger and hate. The nurse during this phase sat it out with the patient, asking short, non-directed questions aimed at clarification whenever she could get a word in, and showing no disapproval.

The next phase was one of reassurance. The nurse helped the patient to

[9] Richardson, R. F., *op. cit.*, p. 251.

explore what she had felt. The patient at one time described her feelings of anger as "a hateful feeling, and the body feels stronger." Often the patient felt guilty about having expressed anger. She wanted to know how the nurse felt about this. This patient once, when asked how she felt about her anger, remarked to the nurse, "You should be able to take it." But then she brought up a conflict in her own values toward anger and hate. She said, "I felt good yesterday [when she acted out anger], but I don't feel good today. I can't be hateful too long; the Lord said not to be hateful. When you are angry, it would be best to walk away."

Another patient, after showing anger with the nurse for several days, suddenly developed a stiff neck which disappeared when she felt more comfortable about expressing anger. At this stage, patients need some reassurance that anger is a common feeling and acceptable to the nurse.

The last phase in the pattern is an exploration of what brought on the anger, what other situations evoke the same reaction, and what alternate ways there are of dealing with them. Take for instance the patient who got angry because she felt frustrated in reaching her goal of going home. By using the concept of frustration, the patient and nurse together explored what the goal was, and what steps the patient had taken toward it. These consisted of defining her goal as wanting to get out of the hospital. Next, they found out what the obstacle was and what could be done about the situation. For this patient, it seemed to be best to change her goal temporarily from going home to getting well.

This patient had recognized her own anger and was able to talk about it. Some patients, on the other hand, may react with silence or apathy to feeling angry. Here the first step is for the patient to become aware of his feelings, to describe them, and to accept them.

Anger, like anxiety, evokes in the body physiological reactions which liberate energy. This energy should be used, if possible, to deal with the problem at hand, to learn about and/or dissolve the difficulty, or, if this is not possible, to work on some other constructive project. The nurse can help the patient with this by exploring with him whether the obstacle can be removed, whether there are other ways to reach the goal, circumventing the obstacle, or whether the goal needs to be changed, and then by assisting the patient in developing the necessary skills to deal with this and similar problems.

Anger is a concept which can be helpful to nurses in understanding and controlling their own behavior and in assisting patients in learning about the meaning of their anger reaction patterns.

The dynamics of the concept of anger used in this chapter include the following steps: (1) a blocked goal, reduced self-respect, or unmet expectations; (2) an unpleasant, uncanny, powerless feeling, which is part of the concept of anxiety; (3) a change of feelings, sometimes without recognition of the anxiety, into feelings or actions of power directed against the blocking object, a substitute, or the self; and (4) the feeling of relief.

This and related concepts have been explored with the help of literature and examples from two patients.

Patterns of experiencing, accepting, and expressing anger differ widely and are related to the cultural background and individual upbringing. Understanding and using one's anger constructively are learning tasks.

## BIBLIOGRAPHY

HORNEY, K., *New Ways in Psychoanalysis*, W. W. Norton & Co., New York: 1939.

PEPLAU, HILDEGARD E., *Interpersonal Relations in Nursing*, G. P. Putnam's Sons, New York: 1952.

RICHARDSON, ROY F., *The Psychology and Pedagogy of Anger*, Warwick & York, Baltimore: 1918.

SULLIVAN, HARRY STACK, *Conceptions of Modern Psychiatry*, W. W. Norton & Co., New York: 1953.

——— *The Interpersonal Theory of Psychiatry*, W. W. Norton & Co., New York: 1953.

# 20 AN INTERPERSONAL INTERPRETATION OF MANIPULATION

*Fern R. Kumler*

Manipulation is a term frequently used and infrequently defined in the literature and language of nursing. The need for a precise definition and operational clarification to guide nursing intervention is revealed by the following quotation: "One of the countertransference difficulties . . . is the fact that the therapist unconsciously frequently falls into a variety of ways of meeting the patient's demands without being fully aware that he has been manipulated." [1] What, then, is manipulation? What is its purpose? And what are the implications for nurse-patient relationships?

Manipulation is a process by which one individual influences another to function in accord with his needs without regard for the other's needs or goals. This definition clearly places the process in an interpersonal context and implies that at least one person in the interpersonal situation is not functioning at an adult level of respect for others.

Before clarifying the operations of manipulation, it might be well to review some aspects of growth and development that will help bring to light the full implications of the concept for nurses in their relationships with patients. It might be well also to clarify the terms this writer uses.

## CLARIFICATION OF TERMS

### RATIONAL AUTHORITY

This is authority based on knowledge and competence which is used to encourage and guide those subject to it to realize their potentialities. These potentialities involve the growth of the awareness of the integrity of the

[1] Fromm-Reichmann, F., *Psychoanalysis and Psychotherapy*, p. 264.

self as a separate and independent entity. The role of rational authority is temporary and requires constant self-evaluation. When the functions assigned to it are completed, it is dissolved.[2]

### THERAPEUTIC NURSE-PATIENT RELATIONSHIP

This is a relationship based upon the nurse's role as a rational authority. It requires the nurse's respect for the patient's potential for growth and provides for the stimulation of this potential. In the therapeutic relationship, there is mutual participation in the task of utilizing the relationship as a learning experience directing maturation. The therapeutic relationship is not an end but, rather, a means to an end.

### ADAPTIVE MANEUVERS

These are automatic behavior patterns which one adopts to reduce anxiety without experiencing learning through use of reflective thought.

## DEVELOPMENTAL ASPECTS

Every child begins his interpersonal experiences by using automatic behavior patterns to call attention to his needs and to gain love from the mothering one. In the first year of life, the infant is confined to the use of crying and prespeech verbalizations to manipulate the mother. However, as the child grows older and learns to identify others in the environment who will satisfy his needs, he tests and uses a variety of adaptive maneuvers to manipulate others in accord with his needs. These adaptive maneuvers are used to satisfy his needs and maintain his security without regard for the needs or goals of others.

How and when does the child learn to separate himself and his needs from those of others? How and when does he learn to respect the needs and goals of others? In other words, what is the process by which the child learns more mature patterns of interpersonal behavior? It is the experience of the integrity of the self as a separate and independent entity that permits the child to participate in a relationship based upon mutual respect and consideration. Unless the child is provided with the healthy and stimulating experiences of "freedom within limits," [3] he will not develop the personality structure or learn the use of the tools necessary for such

[2] For more complete definition and explanation, see Mullahy, P., *Oedipus: Myth and Complex*, pp. 267–68.
[3] Settlage, C. F., "The Values of Limits in Child Rearing."

a relationship. An examination of the meaning of healthy experiences of "freedom within limits" will clarify the value and effects of these limits.

When a mother lets the child know what she expects, she has set a limit. The wise mother does not expect complete and immediate conformity. She is consistent and firm in her expectations of the child's behavior, but realizes that the child's cooperation is necessary in the achievement of *self-control*. She is aware that children need to explore and experiment with new behaviors in conforming to expectations and at the same time striving for independence. The child's achievement of self-control is based upon the rudiments of cooperation—the patience of the mother and the readiness of the child to respond—not upon any condition or obligation that the child must fulfill to gain or maintain the mother's love.

Freedom within limits permits the child to explore and experiment with new behaviors and test his roles but offers guidance in achieving self-control. When a child achieves self-control rather than control by parents, there is a healthy identification with the firm but loving parents. He develops trust in others and trust in himself. He gains a sense of the integrity of the self as a separate and independent being. This includes a sense of love, worthiness, self-respect, self-esteem, and an ability to use cooperation, compromise, and finally collaboration as tools for learning mature levels of need gratifications in interpersonal relationships.[4] When the basic freedom to experiment within a consistent frame of reference is a continuous process, adaptive maneuvers in the service of manipulation are replaced by the increasing use of self-evaluation in relation to others. There is a minimum of anxiety experienced in this process of increasing independence from others and increasing dependence on the self. Interpersonal relations are increasingly based upon mutual respect and the ability to both give and receive love.

In contrast to the experiences of learning by experimentation and exploration under guidance, other forms of limit-setting predispose the child to the continuation of manipulative interpersonal behavior. Conformity to limits enforced by conditional love—conformity based upon fear of love and/or punitive retaliation—represents submission to control and not the achievement of self-control. Demands for strict and complete conformity based upon conditional love may also stimulate rebellion and a continual power struggle between parent and child. If limits are set inconsistently or

---

[4] Cooperation, compromise, and collaboration used as effective interpersonal tools mean the ability to give and take and to delay personal satisfaction out of consideration for and sensitivity to another's needs. For further explanation, see Sullivan, H. S., *The Interpersonal Theory of Psychiatry*, pp. 227–62.

if the child is caught in a "double-bind," [5] he cannot develop a frame of reference within which to identify himself and evaluate his expected roles with any degree of reasonable accuracy. The child is forced to continue manipulative maneuvers and must test adaptive patterns in each new situation. Lack of limitations and overindulgence deprive the child of an opportunity to achieve self-control. In such a situation the child is controlled by his complete dependency upon his parents. For this child the world exists to satisfy his needs. Lack of limitations by rejecting parents who demand too early independence of the child may result in a rigid system of attempted self-control by the child. The child's control then represents an adaptation to what he thinks the parents expect of him. Actually, it is control by fictional expectations.[6]

Limits set under the circumstances of conditional love, inconsistency, the double-bind, or the lack of limitations deprives the child of the development of the basic personality characteristics and the ability to use the tools needed to participate in mutually respectful, mature relationships. His sense of love, worthiness, self-respect, and self-esteem are dependent upon the response of others to his adaptive maneuvers. He has no sense of the integrity of the self as a separate and independent being. The child comes to view himself as a person whose needs are gratified by dependence on or submission to others or by dominance of or demanding from others. Cooperation is interpreted as submission to or dominance of others. Compromise and collaboration are used conditionally and not in learning more mature patterns of interpersonal behavior. The child has no concept of mutual respect, trust, or the ability to give and receive love. The question for this person becomes one of how to manipulate in order to get what one wants.[7] In other words, what adaptive maneuver will elicit the desired response from others?

## AN OPERATIONAL EXAMINATION
## OF MANIPULATION

Manipulation may be defined by the following interpersonal operations: (1) One person has needs that are not met by the other person. These needs may or not be in conscious awareness. (2) The anxiety level of the person with unmet needs rises. (3) The other person's needs or goals

[5] "In a double-bind situation, a person is faced with a significant communication involving a pair of messages, of different levels or logical type, which are related but incongruent with each other." Weakland, John H., "The Double-Bind Hypothesis of Schizophrenia and Three-Party Interaction," in *The Etiology of Schizophrenia*, D. Jackson (ed.), p. 376.

[6] English, O. S., and Pearson, G. H. J., *Emotional Problems in Living*, pp. 138–40.

[7] Fromm, E., *Escape From Freedom*, pp. 176–79.

are disregarded, consciously or unconsciously. (4) Adaptive maneuver(s) is (are) tried. (5) If the adaptive maneuver(s) elicits (elicit) the desired response, the needs are met, anxiety is reduced, and the automatic behavior pattern continues.

Steps 1 and 2 occur in every interpersonal relationship. However, Step 3 may occur for one of four reasons: (a) It occurs unconsciously. (b) It occurs in prolonged periods of extreme anxiety. (c) It occurs because the individual has never learned, as reviewed above, to participate in a mutually respectful relationship. (d) It occurs because of any combination of the above.

Steps 3 and 4 are of special importance for nursing intervention. When one individual disregards the needs of another in interpersonal behavior, the other individual is being used. For what is the other individual being used? Obviously, in this case, the other individual is being used to satisfy a need. At this point, the nurse must evaluate the adaptive maneuvers of Step 4 in terms of her knowledge of the patient's growth and development pattern and in terms of his current patterns of interpersonal behavior. She must be able to evaluate the patient's needs and evaluate to what extent her response will stimulate the patient's growth toward more mature patterns of interpersonal behavior and, thus, more mature levels of need gratification.

In nurse-patient relationships, manipulation is complete to the extent that behavior of the nurse is influenced to respond to the adaptive maneuver of the patient by adaptive maneuvers which meet the patient's needs but do not stimulate the growth of the patient. This implies that in successful manipulation, there is no learning experience, but, rather, a mutually adaptive relationship.

Successful manipulation may occur because of unconscious distortions of the nurse. This means that the nurse's response to the patient's behavior may be a result of her own anxiety and needs. She may be consciously aware of the patient's needs, but her response may be such that she unwittingly perpetuates the patient's behavior to relieve her anxiety or meet her needs. Therefore, the nurse must be reasonably aware of the feelings that the patient's behavior arouses in her and evaluate her response to these feelings in terms of the patient's behavior and needs.

## IMPLICATIONS FOR NURSING INTERVENTION

Nursing intervention is determined by the definitions of rational authority, therapeutic nurse-patient relationships, and freedom within limits. The definition of rational authority provides guidance to intervention by requiring that the nurse constantly evaluate and scrutinize her role in the relationship. The nurse's role is to use her knowledge and competence to guide the patient's growth toward self-awareness and independence. Her knowledge of growth and development and of the patient's present patterns of interpersonal behavior is her most valuable tool for the evaluation of the patient's needs and growth. It is a relationship in which mutual participation in the task of learning requires the use of cooperation, compromise, and collaboration. The relationship provides the patient with consistent and firm expectations. When the nurse defines her expectations, she is setting the limits. She must expect that the patient will test and explore the extent and consistency of these limits. The patient will attempt to re-establish previous patterns of interpersonal relationships to obtain need gratification. When the nurse provides a learning experience, she and the patient proceed to examine his behavior and its meaning according to the context within which it occurs. The patient is given the opportunity to become aware of himself in relation to others and to explore more appropriate forms of behavior.

Clinical examples will illustrate many of the foregoing statements. The following example illustrates some of the adaptive maneuvers used by one patient to establish and maintain a dependent relationship with the nurse.

*Patient:* If I tell you all about myself, what will you do?

(Then at a later date, quite angrily:)
If you're not going to do anything for me, I don't want to see you any more.

(At a still later date:)
You ought to be ashamed of yourself. You're a nurse. You're supposed to help me. What are you doing? I can't do anything. What can I do?

Each time the patient made reference to the nurse doing for her, the nurse set the expectation that the purpose of the interviews was to explore what the patient could do for herself. The patient tried many adaptive patterns in an effort to influence the nurse. She tried bargaining, demanding, derogation, and she tried to find the nurse's weakness. In the seventh interview, the following happened:

*Patient:* The social worker doesn't take care of me any more. I got a tutor who doesn't come to see me. . . . (Patient continued talking about others not taking care of her.)
*Nurse:* What's the connection between me and your social worker and tutor?
*Patient:* You're all the same. You don't do nothing for me. (The patient became very anxious and began crying.)

The patient gave every appearance of a helpless child, and the nurse became aware of her wish to respond and comfort in a mothering way the patient she viewed as a child. Being aware of her feelings in response to the patient's behavior and being aware of the patient's desire for dependency, the nurse evaluated to what extent her response would aid the patient's growth from dependency to independency. In this case, the nurse did not respond as a comforting mother. Instead, she waited until the patient was less anxious and provided for a learning experience. In reference to limits, the nurse had previously set the expectation that the patient was not helpless and that the relationship would be a collaborative effort in which the patient could learn by achieving self-control. In other words, the nurse had set a limit on excessive dependency in the relationship. Her response maintained that limit.

In using the model of freedom within limits, the nurse must remember that the patient will test behaviors in the process of learning self-control. If there is a lack of testing, the nurse must evaluate whether she has been manipulated into a dominance-submission relationship. In such a relationship, the patient may be doing everything to please the nurse. This means that learning and, thus, growth are not occurring. The patient is not gaining self-awareness and independence. The patient is using cooperation as submission. In such a case, the nurse must provide the patient with experiences in which the patient is encouraged to examine his behavior. For example: After many interviews in which the patient responded obediently to the nurse's questions and suggestions, the nurse said, "Did you say that because you thought I wanted you to?"

*Patient:* No.
*Nurse:* (Doubtfully.) Oh? Is that what you really think?
*Patient:* I don't know. I'm not sure.

At this point, the nurse asked the patient to express more of her thoughts. She also set the expectation that the patient would not be doing so to please her (the nurse), but that she would be doing so to learn about herself. Gradually, the patient began to express herself more and more as the nurse furnished encouragement and guidance.

The nurse is frequently viewed as mother-surrogate, and to gain the nurse's approval, the patient may use many of the maneuvers used in childhood. Nurses are familiar with the many maneuvers patients use. For example, the patient may be the nurse's helper, a tale carrier, a gift bearer, or a flatterer. To the extent that the nurse responds to the patterns with approval and to the extent that the pattern continues, the nurse has been manipulated.

The previous examples have shown the more subtle forms of manipulation. The following example demonstrates one of the more obvious forms. In this example, the patient attempts intimidation:

*Patient:* I'm mean, nurse.
*Nurse:* Oh?
*Patient:* I hit people.
*Nurse:* Tell me about it.

In this case, the nurse set the expectation that the patient would talk about her aggression. In other words, she set a limit on the form of aggression to be used in the relationship. Another way of setting the same limit is to inform the patient that she (the nurse) is not a punching bag and simply say, "You and I can talk about when you hit people." When the nurse responds to such patients by reassurance, avoidance, or clamping down to show who is boss and the pattern continues, she may very well find that she has been manipulated. Knowledge of the feelings the patient's behavior evokes in her and knowledge of the patient's patterns of behavior are her most valuable tools to assess the meaning of the patient's behavior. Giving the patient the opportunity to talk about and examine his behavior also provides the nurse with information to guide her responses to the patient in the later phases of the relationship.

Regardless of the form of the manipulative attempt, the forms described in this chapter or the more obvious forms of demanding or playing one person against another, the nurse's most valuable insurance against participation in a mutually adaptive relationship is her conscious knowledge of the goals of her response in relation to the patient's needs. In setting limits, she must know what she is limiting. Generally speaking, she is limiting excessive dependency in its varied forms and she is limiting aggression in its destructive forms. The purpose of her limit-setting is not to control the patient. Her purpose is to provide a consistent set of expectations for the patient and to provide guidance toward *self-control.*

## SUMMARY

Manipulation is a process by which one individual influences another to function in accord with his needs without regard for the other's needs or goals. It is an interpersonal process which may take many forms and which occurs unconsciously to some extent in all interpersonal behavior. It is of special interest in therapeutic nurse-patient relationships because it is incongruent with the goals of growth toward self-awareness and the use of cooperation, compromise, and collaboration in a mutually respectful relationship. The nurse's most valuable insurance against a mutually adaptive relationship is her own self-awareness, conscious knowledge of the goals of her response in relation to the patient's needs, and her skill in providing guidance for the patient to learn self-control.

# BIBLIOGRAPHY

ENGLISH, O. SPURGEON, and PEARSON, GERALD H. J., *Emotional Problems of Living*, W. W. Norton & Co., New York: 1945.

FROMM, ERIC, *Escape From Freedom*, Rinehart & Co., New York: 1941.

FROMM-REICHMANN, FRIEDA, *Psychoanalysis and Psychotherapy*, University of Chicago Press, Chicago: 1959.

JACKSON, DON D. (ed.), *The Etiology of Schizophrenia*, Basic Books, New York: 1960.

MASLOW, A. H., *Motivation and Personality*, Harper & Bros., New York: 1954.

MULLAHY, PATRICK, *Oedipus: Myth and Complex*, Grove Press, New York: 1948.

SETTLAGE, CALVIN F., "The Values of Limits in Child Rearing," unpublished paper given at the Conference on Family Living, Family Service of Philadelphia, February, 1958.

SULLIVAN, HARRY STACK, *The Interpersonal Theory of Psychiatry*, W. W. Norton & Co., New York: 1953.

# 21 NURSING INTERVENTION WHEN THE PATIENT SAYS "SHOULD"

*Ura A. L. Lazaroff*

In the nurse-patient relationship, the nurse must be alert to the patient's use of the word "should" as he talks about his past experiences. When the patient is speaking about his past in terms of "I should have felt," "I should have said," and/or "I should have done," he has used some of the intervening time to reconstruct the actual situation and to program his own participation in the event to his advantage. Most people have had the experience of being able to formulate and articulate "a perfect squelch" five to ten minutes after a conversation is terminated. The factor of importance in the nurse-patient relationship is the "what I did feel," "what I did say," and "what I did do" of the patient's experiences rather than the "shoulds," which are invariably different, if not polar opposites.

Everyone, through aculturation, has some idea of what he should do and what he should not do in relationships with his fellow men. The writer calls this complex integration of ideas the "should-system" of the individual. During the developmental years, each person evolves a self-system of which the should-system is a part. Sullivan[1] describes the self-system as a dynamic part of the personality that explains the personification of the self or the "I" to which an individual refers when he speaks about himself. In his writings, Sullivan states that there is a concept of a "good-me," "bad-me," and a "not-me" in the rudiments of the self. The good-me is a personification encompassing the organization of experiences that have been enhanced by reward or tenderness from significant other

[1] Sullivan, H. S., *The Interpersonal Theory of Psychiatry*, p. 167.

people. The bad-me includes the organization of experiences in which anxiety has been increased and experiences in which there have been forbidding gestures from the significant other people, usually the mother or mothering one. The not-me develops from experiences of intense anxiety, such as markedly forbidding gestures from the mother, and cannot be clearly organized or communicated by the individual because of the accompanying uncanny emotion. Also, there is an inability to connect the cause-and-effect factors of the experiences. This not-me of the self-system remains as a private part of the self.

The purpose of the self-system is to avoid or minimize incidents of anxiety in the process of education that is necessary for living in a society as a human being. Sullivan states, "The self-system is the principal stumbling block to favorable changes in personality . . ." and "is also the principal influence that stands in the way of unfavorable changes in the personality." [2]

As the human progresses from the infant stage of development into childhood, the personifications of the good-me and the bad-me merge—that is, in awareness the child thinks of himself as "I" being one person with one body. This fusion of the personifications is necessary for the purposes of communication when the child learns language. However, the less prominent view of the self remains with the individual, though not in awareness. If the self-system learns to postpone gratifications until a later time, the good-me emerges as the central part. If, in analysis of the situation, the realization of gratifications is not forthcoming, then the bad-me emerges as the central part of the self-system.

The child learns that he must cooperate with the parent. Training is necessary. In this training the child is taught what he ought to do and what he ought not to do in social living. In our complex culture, many of the ought's and ought-not's are at times contradictory. At other times the anxiety level of the child is such that learning cannot readily take place, and the meanings of situations in which the child finds himself are distorted or remain outside of awareness.

In the juvenile era of development, the child learns to accommodate himself to the social demands of others as he tries out the earlier learned patterns of behavior and compares his experiences with the experiences of others. At this time, what Sullivan calls "supervisory patterns" [3] become a part of the self-system. Supervisory patterns are censors of the various areas of behavior that an individual shows to other people,

[2] *Ibid.*, p. 169.
[3] *Ibid.*, pp. 238–40.

of what is the "right" thing to say or do. Editing of behavior is done in anticipation of the reactions of others.

The self-system is unstable—it changes through experience. However, there is resistance to change. Anxiety accompanies any behavioral change. The therapeutic situation is set-up wherein the patient may have interpersonal experiences in which he will have the opportunity to broaden his self-system.

The nurse facilitates this broadening by helping the patient to be comfortable enough that anxiety-producing experiences of the past can be brought back into awareness. Then the nurse helps the patient to take a look at what is happening in the situation in which he finds himself.

## NURSING INTERVENTION

Nursing intervention with the patient who expresses a self-system in which the should's have taken precedence over the real events is focused primarily in three areas: (1) The nurse elicits observation and description by the patient of his experience as to what action did take place in the situation and what were the patient's thoughts and feeling at the time. (2) The nurse casts doubt as to the real importance of the should's in relation to the actual happenings. (3) The nurse uses attenuating remarks for the purpose of weakening the should-system and facilitating the patient's looking at reality again.

For example, a female patient who was not married expressed the conflict between her thoughts and actions in her situation in the following nurse-patient interaction.

> *Patient:* Father has a feeling that I should be married.
> *Nurse:* Did he say this?

The patient's statement shows the ideas of the person who is significant to her. The nurse asked for the facts of the situation in order to help the patient clarify what actually occurred in the experience. This intervention is directed toward relieving the patient of distortions or projected fantasies in relationships with other persons.

At another time the patient described a relationship with a male friend in which they had spent time playing checkers. The patient's brother then asked the male friend not to see the patient any more. The patient argued with her brother following the incident.

> *Patient:* I just told him he shouldn't have said that to R. I didn't see R. after that. So, that friendship just ceased, that's all. I just was annoyed that my brother had spoken to him without saying something to me.

Maybe I should have left checker games and everything to someone else.
*Nurse:* What did you do when you got angry?

Here the should's have taken precedence over the real thoughts, feelings, and actions of the patient. The nurse elicited description of the actions of the patient. She asked the patient to describe what did happen rather than focusing on what might have been. The nurse encourages the patient to describe reality situations so that relationships between the cause-and-effect elements of the situation can then be looked at by the patient.

An additional example of the above is as follows:

*Patient:* The Bible says I should honor my father and mother that their days may be long upon the land. I think that's a Commandment, isn't it?
*Nurse:* Yes. What was your experience with your parents?
*Patient:* How can I honor them? My father deserted us when I was three weeks old. I can't honor a man I don't even know. If my honoring him determines how long he'll live, he must be dead by now. Yet I'm supposed to follow the teachings of the Bible.
*Nurse:* What about your mother?
*Patient:* I don't know. Sometimes I think I hate her. Sometimes not. I learned, as I grew up, that sex belongs to marriage. Not with my mother —her parade of men came first before me or anyone else. Honor her? At times I don't even know her. She tells me what I should do with words and contradicts the words with her own actions. Can I honor or even respect her? She has an appeal to me because I can't go home unless she takes me—but honor her and respect her? The Bible says I should.
*Nurse:* But you find the Commandment difficult at times?
*Patient:* Not difficult—impossible. I suppose if she dies young, I'll be to blame somehow.
*Nurse:* Blame?
*Patient:* Because I should honor her, but I can't always. It's really crazy you know—all that baloney that mothers know best. If I were her, I would practice what I preach.

One patient demonstrated low self-esteem and a desire for a more adequate should-system when he made an inquiry of the nurse. In this interaction, the nurse refocused on the patient's thoughts about the situation.

*Patient:* Do you believe if a sister bites you, you shouldn't bite back?
*Nurse:* What do you think?

By focusing on the patient, the nurse emphasized the importance of the patient's thoughts and showed acceptance of the patient no matter what he did or said.

One patient said that he had "bad thoughts" and indicated that he "shouldn't have these 'bad thoughts'."

*Nurse:* You say the thoughts are bad. Do other people say that the thoughts are bad?

*Patient:* I guess they would—they are so bad I can't say them.
*Nurse:* You don't know for sure?
*Patient:* I'm quite sure they would say they are bad.
*Nurse:* I don't know if your thoughts are bad or not, until you tell me what your thoughts are.
*Patient:* They are just so bad I can't.
*Nurse:* What basis do you have for saying your thoughts are bad?
*Patient:* Well, I know they are bad. (Moving restlessly in chair.)
*Nurse:* Are you uncomfortable? You are moving about.
*Patient:* (Nodding.) I feel nervous and everything.

This illustrates the inability of the patient to analyze or even describe the "bad thoughts" because of the unpleasantness of the anxiety that is produced when he talks about these thoughts that he thinks he shouldn't have. The nurse is instilling doubt about the actual severity of the unacceptableness of the patient's thoughts. Then the nurse points out to the patient the cues of behavior related to the patient's feelings. The doubt is subtle, since a wholesale doubt would threaten the patient's defense to the extent that the increase in anxiety might be devastating to the patient. Then the defense of verbalizing in terms of "should" would be reinforced.

In summary, the self-system develops to include a part which can be termed a "should-system." The should-system helps censor an individual's behavior in relationship with others. Sometimes the should-system is organized as a defense against anxiety when the person is unable to look at the reality situation clearly. The nurse facilitates the patient's return to reality by providing a comfortable interpersonal relationship, by eliciting the patient's observation and description of the full experience, by casting doubt as to the importance of the should's, and by using attenuating remarks in relation to the should-system.

# BIBLIOGRAPHY

SULLIVAN, HARRY S., *The Interpersonal Theory of Psychiatry*, W. W. Norton & Co., New York: 1953.

# 22

## THE CLINICAL PROBLEM OF "NOT-ME"

*Joan B. Baker*

"I would never say or do anything like that. It couldn't have been me. You must be mistaken." This remark could have been made by any one of us who had just been modified by another person of something we had said or done, of which we were entirely unaware. This mechanism is a highly complicated one termed "dissociation."

This word has many connotations to different people. The usual definition is similar to the one given by English and Pearson [1] in which dissociation is described as the walling-off of certain areas of the mind from consciousness in order to deal with conflict. Some typical examples of dissociative reactions in the usual sense are hysterical amnesia, sleep-walking, and multiple personalities such as illustrated in Stevenson's classic, *Dr. Jekyll and Mr. Hyde.*

In this chapter, the concept of dissociation is used in a slightly different sense. Dissociation is viewed dynamically as a clinical problem, as described by Sullivan.[2] The personality is made up of three personifications of the self (me). First, there is the *good-me* which consists of experiences and actions that have gained approval throughout the person's development. In ordinary conversation, this is "I." Second, there is the *bad-me* which is organized from anxiety-producing experiences and actions due to disapproval throughout the person's development. This part of the personality, as well as the good-me, is within the person's self-awareness, and this is the part of the individual that forces him to admit he is not infallible. The third personification is the *not-me*, which evolves due to the experience of intense anxiety over thoughts and actions that have been

[1] English, O. S., and Pearson, G., *Emotional Problems of Living*, p. 468.
[2] Sullivan, H. S., *The Interpersonal Theory of Psychiatry*, pp. 161–62.

130—

intensely forbidden by the mother or some other very significant figure. The intense anxiety aroused by the mother was poorly grasped and not formulated as belonging to the self.

Dissociation, as defined by Sullivan, occurs when the self (the part of the personality within awareness—good- and bad-me) does not notice or accept impulses, desires, and needs which are expressed from the part of the self that is not within awareness (not-me).[3] This limitation of noticing our own behavior extends to behavior of other persons. It is maintained by our experience of anxiety. In other words, there is a conflict between powerful needs and the restrictions the self imposes on the satisfaction of these needs.[4] Dissociated tendencies manifest themselves, but their satisfaction is incomplete or only found in sleep. The individual is not aware of these tendencies and has difficulty in the recognition of them. According to Peplau, a dissociated tendency can distort a person's enjoyment of life and his ability to relate satisfactorily with others.[5] Sullivan further illustrates this by pointing out that a person with a powerful dissociated system, when put at a task that requires all or most of his abilities within awareness, will when something or someone threatens to bring this system into awareness, neglect his task to fight off awareness of the dissociated system.[6]

If the nurse identifies a dissociative tendency or system in a patient, how can she handle the situation so as to help the patient and turn the experience into a useful and meaningful one? As a guide, the nurse might select her maneuvers using the principle *when feelings are not permitted expression and identified, feelings connected with the experience may be dissociated and operate outside the awareness and control.*[7] If a nurse or any other therapeutic person recognizes that a patient is not aware of his feelings and she does not investigate this with the patent, he or she may be aiding the dissociative process.

The case of Mr. A. illustrates the application of the foregoing principle. He was a 52-year-old, highly successful lawyer who was admitted to the medical ward with the diagnosis of myocardial infraction. When Mr. A. was growing up, some significant person in his development aroused the feeling of intense anxiety in him whenever he showed signs of fear or apprehension which were labeled "unmanly." Mr. A.'s self-picture, in this area, might then look something like this

---

[3] Sullivan, H. S., *Conceptions of Modern Psychiatry*, p. 22.
[4] *Ibid.*, *Clinical Studies in Psychiatry*, p. 61.
[5] Peplau, H. E., *Interpersonal Relations in Nursing*, p. 63.
[6] Sullivan. H. S., *Clinical Studies in Psychiatry*, p. 179.
[7] Peplau, Hildegard E., *op. cit.*, p. 125.

| Me | Not-me |
|---|---|
| Fearless | Fearful and apprehensive |
| Manly | Not manly |

When he entered the hospital, the nurse noticed that Mr. A., through-out all the tests and examinations, seemed to act as if this was routine for him. He did not appear to notice that he was seriously ill. From this small amount of quite significant data, the nurse might infer that Mr. A. had dissociated his feelings of uncertainty and fear. With this hypothesis in mind, she will then be alert to signs that support the validity of the hy-pothesis.

One day, when the nurse entered the room, Mr. A. was startled; how-ever, he quickly regained his composure and began a conversation. This startle response may be an indication that Mr. A.'s anxiety level is not as low as it appears on the surface. It may be an important nonverbal clue that something is bothering him.

Then Mr. A. proceeded to carry on a fearless conversation with the nurse. She may notice a cue to dissociation is inherent in "The doctor is coming to see me today to tell me whether or not I can sit up." (Pause.) "If I sit up too soon, it might be too bad." Thereupon, Mr. A. added quickly, "But the doctor knows his business and he knows what he is doing, so whatever he says is fine with me." Mr. A. may or may not be aware of what he said. However, if fear is in Mr. A.'s dissociated system, the meaning of it probably lies outside his awareness, since he quickly covers up his apprehension by expressing his complete confidence in the doctor and the lack of fear on his part to do what the doctor says. In other words, Mr. A. is quite busy keeping his feelings of fear out of his aware-ness.

What types of responses could the nurse make? "Yes, that's right, Mr. A., your doctor knows what he is doing." This reply could help Mr. A. to further dissociate his apprehension. The nurse is, in effect, saying, "Don't be afraid."

Another response might be, "You're afraid that the doctor will tell you to sit up too soon and that will be too bad?" This direct interpreta-tion or "frontal attack," as Sullivan [8] calls it, tends to bring into play processes in the individual that will blunt the interpretation or brush it off entirely. Mr. A. might respond thus, "Of course, I'm not afraid. I just said that the doctor knows what he is doing."

A third response might be, "You have confidence in your doctor, and you're wondering when *he* will tell you that it will be safe for you to sit

[8] Sullivan, H. S., *Clinical Studies in Psychiatry*, p. 181.

up." The nurse has restated to Mr. A. the meaning of what he has just said, without directly attacking his dissociated feelings or labeling these feelings, thus giving Mr. A. an opportunity to explore them further. It's not probable that Mr. A. will recognize his fear and apprehension with the initial maneuver of the nurse, but this is the first step in the integration of a dissociated system into self-awareness.

This case was given to illustrate two ways in which cues might be picked up by the nurse through observation and listening, and how these can then be used in making an inference as to the meaning of the behavior. In this case, using the inference that fear was in Mr. A.'s dissociated system, it was then shown how the nurse might test her hypothesis, or how she could close off communication with the patient, depending on her approach in the nurse-patient relationship. The nurse's investigative procedure is carried further in the subsequent clinical example.

In applying the concept of dissociation to psychiatric nursing, it is important to be even more acutely aware of its implications. According to Sullivan,[9] in schizophrenia there is a failure of the mechanism of dissociation. A schizophrenic patient becomes aware of the activity of the dissociated system. However, due to the previous processes which were built up to maintain the system in dissociation, the meaning of the behavior of which he is now aware eludes him. An analogy to this is the person who knows his multiplication tables and the alphabet and is suddenly presented with a complicated algebraic equation. He is aware of the numbers and letters, but what their meaning is or what to do with them completely perplexes him. In the schizophrenic, due to the stress from this inability to maintain a complete system of dissociation, control of the conscious contents is lost. Thus, the behavior within awareness and that which has previously been dissociated by the individual now all operate within the awareness, and the incomplete dissociation is manifest in the behavior of the schizophrenic. This incomplete dissociation is well illustrated by the hallucinations and delusions commonly experienced by schizophrenic patients.

Hallucinations are personifications of the not-me. The individual is aware of certain impulses or desires, but he is unable to accept these and integrate them into the self. Delusions are false beliefs, false interpretations, or exaggerations of facts which are the unrecognized expression of dissociated material.[10]

Because these dissociating tendencies are now operating in a very dis-

[9] *Ibid.*, p. 187.
[10] Fromm-Reichman, F., *Principles in Intensive Psychotherapy*, p. 174.

organized system of awareness, the individual needs help in reorganizing his self-system, since he cannot accomplish this by himself in his chaotic state. In other words, he cannot solve the algebraic equation without help in understanding the meanings of the problem. The schizophrenic patient needs help in learning to conceptualize.

The core of conceptual thinking lies in the ability to categorize or, to put it differently, to view an object as a bearer of certain general characteristics. For example, if someone says to us, "I live in a house," most of us have the concept of house pretty well in mind, so that the person doesn't have to describe what he means when he says house. This ability to categorize is what enables us to understand meaningful connections.[11] In schizophrenia, the patient's ability to do this is markedly disorganized.

The nurse's role in the psychiatric situation can operate with the same principle as discussed in the case of Mr. A. Thus, the opportunity to assist the patient to integrate his feelings and see meaningful connections (conceptualize) is used. To help observe this principle in action, the following case of Mr. X., a 23-year-old patient with the diagnosis of schizophrenia, is presented.

A nurse was working with Mr. X. in a nurse-patient relationship, which occurred for one hour, twice a week. After working with this patient for two months, his nurse developed the hypothesis from Mr. X.'s conversation that with this patient, feelings of anger were dissociated, i.e., being angry was in the not-me. The nurse decided to test her hypothesis and set up a quick exchange between herself and the patient to get the patient angry. After questioning the validity of what the patient was saying for a brief period during the interview, the following occurred:

(Long pause.)
*Patient:* Certain voices within me are telling me to do the craziest things.
*Nurse:* What are they saying?
*Patient:* Insane things.
*Nurse:* Tell me about them.
*Patient:* Well, a voice right now is telling me to slap you.
*Nurse:* Me?
*Patient:* Yes; the *voices*, of course, not me. I'm not angry at you. That's my sickness.

The patient was quite concerned that the nurse know and realize the voices were angry, not him. At this point the nurse tried to connect the things that had happened in the past in anger-producing situations to help Mr. X see the meaning and validity of this feeling. Initially, Mr. X. denied

---

[11] Hanfmann, E., and Kasanin, J., *J. Psychol.*, p. 525.

that he ever felt angry, but that the voices were angry and told him to do things he did not want to do.

During the following two months, Mr. X. and the nurse talked about other people who got angry and why they did, and why Mr. X. felt anger was "very bad." It became evident throughout the interviews that when Mr. X.'s father became angry, Mr. X. felt helpless and without control. To avoid the emerging anxiety, Mr. X. dissociated anger from his self-system. The conflict, then, appeared to be between the powerful need to express anger and the restrictions of the self imposed upon becoming angry.

Since much of Mr. X's time was being spent in controlling his feelings of anger, his enjoyment of other activities and relationships had been altered. He would stay away from certain people "because I don't like them." When the nurse explored the reasons for not liking certain people, he described feelings of anger. In other words, these people were doing things that Mr. X. found anxiety-provoking, so he avoided them rather than explore the reason these people made him angry.

Together, the nurse and the patient worked at interpreting the meaning of his feelings, validating with each other.

It is well to keep in mind that the purpose of interpretation and interpretative questions is to bring dissociated material into awareness and to show a patient how this material is expressed in verbal and nonverbal behavior.[12] This is done when the patient is ready to accept this material within his awareness. After analyzing several anger-producing situations, Mr. X. was able to formulate this uncomfortable feeling as anger. This was illustrated by the following which occurred three and one-half months after the relationship began.

When the nurse came to visit Mr. X., she discovered that he had been transferred to another ward. The reason was that Mr. X. had hit another patient. When the nurse arrived on the other ward, the conversation went as follows:

*Nurse:* I see you were transferred.
*Patient:* I struck another patient.
*Nurse:* How come?
*Patient:* I—Mr. X.—was angry.
*Nurse:* How did it feel to be angry?
*Patient:* It was a good feeling, but the loss of control I felt was frightening, and I was glad to have someone stop me.

The first step of integrating anger into self-awareness had been accomplished. Mr. X. was able to admit that he felt anger. The learning

[12] Fromm Reichman, F., *op. cit.*, p. 70.

process cannot stop here, if the feeling is to become useful and meaningful for the patient. Now the nurse must help the patient identify why he becomes angry and how he can use his anger constructively before the integration is complete.

In summary, dissociation occurs when a person experiences intense anxiety over certain experiences or actions. Dissociated impulses are not within the person's awareness. When something occurs that threatens to bring the dissociative system into awareness, anxiety is felt, and the individual develops processes to avoid the anxiety and thus avoids allowing the dissociative system into awareness.

When a person must keep busy at these processes to keep material dissociated, he misses an opportunity of forming relationships with other people and experiencing enjoyment in other forms of activity. Thus, when the nurse recognizes that a patient is dissociating, the therapeutic role is to help the patient integrate his dissociated tendencies into his awareness, which brings them under his control so that he is not always besing distracted from more enjoyable activities by anxiety. The nurse can help the patient integrate a dissociative system through the process of learning.

The steps of learning as outlined in this article involve observation of what is occurring, describing it, analyzing what has occurred and relating it to past events, and formulating the meaning of what has gone on. When this has been validated with another person, it can be used as foresight, and conceptualization has taken place. If the nurse in all her relationships with patients operates on the principle that the patient's experience is meaningful to the patient only if he is helped to integrate the experience into his awareness, she will be able to help the patient lead a useful, more meaningful life.

# BIBLIOGRAPHY

ENGLISH, OLIVER SPURGEON, and PEARSON, G. H. J., *Emotional Problems of Living*, W. W. Norton & Co., New York: 1955.
FROMM-REICHMANN, FRIEDA, *Principles of Intensive Psychotherapy*, University of Chicago Press, Chicago: 1950.
HANFMANN, EUGENIA, and KASANIN, JACOB, "A Method for the Study of Concept Formation," *J. Psychol.*, 3:521–42, 1937.
PEPLAU, HILDEGARD E., *Interpersonal Relations in Nursing*, G. P. Putnam's Sons, New York: 1952.
SULLIVAN, HARRY STACK, *Clinical Studies in Psychiatry*, W. W. Norton & Co., New York: 1956.
——— *Conceptions of Modern Psychiatry*, W. W. Norton & Co., New York: 1953.
——— *The Interpersonal Theory of Psychiatry*, W. W. Norton & Co., New York: 1953.

# 23 DISSOCIATION AND MEMORY GAPS

*Jane De Augustinis*

In the early twentieth century, Janet[1] described a phenomenon he had observed in certain of his patients, which consisted of a "strange absent-mindedness." He said there occurred a retraction of the field of consciousness, which could isolate and emancipate one function and suppress another from consciousness, producing blanks in memory and giving too much power to certain ideas. This process he termed "dissociation." This concept was more thoroughly developed and extended by those who followed Janet in the study of human behavior, particularly by Sullivan and Fromm-Reichmann.

Sullivan[2,3] believed that the expression of some things in personality was not recognized by significant other persons and so were never integrated in the self-system. He viewed dissociation as an anxiety-reducing phenomena which operates by restricting awareness. When the limitations of awareness are overstepped, anxiety is experienced. The person is extraordinarily sensitive to anything touching on dissociated material and, therefore, it is very difficult for him to recall anything significant about the actual situation that evoked the anxiety.

Fromm-Reichmann[4] also stated that the selection of subject matter for dissociation is determined by the cultural standards governing life, that is, those standards accepted by significant other persons. She further pointed out that experience of contrasting standards is highly threatening because it is connected with expected disapproval, and a very high degree

[1] Janet, P., *The Major Symptoms of Hysteria*, p. 331.
[2] Sullivan, H. S., *Conceptions of Modern Psychiatry*, p. 22.
[3] Sullivan, H. S., *Interpersonal Theory of Psychiatry*, p. 379.
[4] Fromm-Reichmann, F., *Principles of Intensive Psychotherapy*, pp. 80–83.

of anxiety ensues. Therefore, the individual attempts to bar them from awareness. She and Peplau [5] indicate that it is frequently not the events that happened that are dissociated, but the feelings accompanying them or engendered by them.

Dissociation may be defined as the separation from awareness of certain aspects (thoughts, feelings, and/or actions) of the individual's behavior, due to an experience of severe anxiety. Operationally, these steps occur:

1. In early life, certain thoughts, feelings, and/or actions of an individual are disapproved by significant other persons;
2. These standards are incorporated as the individual's own.
3. Later in life the individual experiences one of the disapproved thoughts, feelings, or actions.
4. Anxiety increases to a severe level.
5. The disapproved occurrence, frequently the feeling, is barred from awareness.
6. Anxiety decreases.
7. Dissociated content continues to appear in disguised form in thoughts, feelings, and actions of the individual.

The dissociated content is evidenced in many forms—dreams, fantasies, obsessive substitutions, parataxic distortions, or denial, among others. In psychosis, hallucinations and delusions are evidences of dissociated material that has partially entered awareness. However, one of the most common and certainly most obvious indications of dissociated material is the memory gap. In such a case the individual may forget an episode entirely or forget one or more aspects of the situation. For example, the actions and thoughts of the event may be remembered, while the feeling that occurred along with them are completely forgotten. The split may also be thoughts/feelings and actions or actions/thoughts and feelings. An extreme instance of memory loss is amnesia.

Memory consists of four general steps. First, there is assimilation of an experience, followed by formulation, integration, and recall.[6] When an event or some aspect of it is productive of a severe amount of anxiety, the individual will not notice the anxiety-inducer and bar it from awareness, so that it is not formulated and integrated and is unavailable to recall. Fromm-Reichmann [7] pointed out that early dissociated experiences, not being integrated, do not grow and mature with the rest of the personality. The individual's increased ability for judgment and evaluation does not

[5] Peplau, H. E., *Interpersonal Relations in Nursing,* p. 63.
[6] Piaget, J., "Principal Factors Determining Intellectual Evolution from Childhood to Adult Life," in *Organization and Pathology of Thought,* Rapaport, D. (ed.), pp. 154–75.
[7] Fromm-Reichman, F., *op. cit.,* p. 98.

affect the dissociated material, leading to parataxic distortions and mis-judgments of present-day interpersonal situations. Peplau [8] mentions that when material is dissociated, it operates outside awareness and outside the control of the individual.

Periods of high anxiety often have aspects that are not amenable to recall because of the dissociative process. In talking with psychiatric patients, particularly in attempts to elicit description, memory gaps involving actions, thoughts, and feelings are often very evident. The following clinical examples demonstrate the three aspects of experience that may be dissociated.

### ACTIONS

The patient was describing a typical day spent with her daughter in a period just prior to her hospitalization.

*Nurse:* Then what did you do?
*Patient:* Then we'd come home. I don't remember anything else. I don't remember much of what I did. It seems like so long ago. Then she was three—only a year and I can hardly remember anything.

### THOUGHTS

The patient was describing a period shortly after her husband had left her.

*Nurse:* What did you think?
*Patient:* I didn't know what I thought at the time. I missed the other two children. I never cried. I never talked to anyone, so I don't know what I thought myself. I knew I missed my children and was a little unhappy. That's all.
(After a period of silence, the patient changed the subject.)

### FEELINGS

*Patient:* The other day when it snowed, it reminded me of the time I got sick. The first time I noticed I was sick—it was the first snowfall of the year. The first time I was afraid. I felt like—I don't know—I didn't expect it, and I thought something unexpected was happening. But last week when it was snowing, I was happy.

## NURSING INTERVENTION

Fromm-Reichmann [9] stated, "The therapeutic process is aimed at bringing a sufficient amount of dissociated material into awareness so that

[8] Peplau, Hildegard E., *op. cit.*, p. 125.
[9] Fromm-Reichmann, F., *op. cit.*, p. 58.

understanding of it may follow." Verbalization facilitates recall of the facts of the experience which may then be formulated and integrated in light of the individual's increased ability for judgment and evaluation. This growing awareness and understanding of contents, history, and dynamics of his interpersonal processes can help him to understand and cope with problem areas in his life.[10] Sullivan [11] pointed out that, in general, the schizophrenic episode is due to inability to maintain dissociation. He believed that the schizophrenic is aware of the activity of the dissociative system, but cannot get it into clear personal focus.

The job of the nurse is, therefore, to aid the patient in a growing awareness and clarification of his past and present experiences, so that they may be analyzed, formulated, validated, integrated, tested, and used in future experiences. The following principles may be utilized to guide the nurse in carrying out this necessary, though difficult function.

*The nurse encourages description of the events surrounding the period of the memory gap, starting with the aspects the patient does remember.* Peplau [12] points out, "The process is largely one of expanding experiences dimly intelligible to the patient at first, so that they become better understood by patient and nurse."

> *Patient:* I remember going, but I don't remember who I saw or anything. I remember seeing the kids, but I don't remember seeing him or the girl there.
> *Nurse:* What do you remember?
> *Patient:* I just remember going and getting the ride home.
> (More description followed.)

*The nurse encourages repetitive description of events involving dissociated material.* With each repetition, more aspects will be recalled. The dissociated material will come into awareness when the individual is able to handle the anxiety associated with it.

> (Patient was describing a childhood experience.)
> *Nurse:* Go on.
> *Patient:* I don't remember any more.
> *Nurse:* As you repeat things, more and more will come back.
> *Patient:* I do. . . . As I tell things to you now I don't always remember. But later I remember. And as I think about it more and talk about it, things come back.

*When more material comes into awareness, the nurse aids the patient to examine the situation in the framework of the learning process.* The

[10] *Ibid.*, p. 59.
[11] Sullivan, H S., *Clinical Studies in Psychiatry*, p. 187.
[12] Peplau, H. E., *op. cit.*, p. 63.

nurse may use restatement, reflection, and interpretations to aid the patient in description, analysis, formulation, validation, integration, testing, and use of the conclusions derived. In this way the nurse helps the patient to clear up distortions and to test reality at his present level of development. Fromm-Reichmann [13] believed that dissociated material revealed under treatment must be tied together and worked through repeatedly in the frame of reference of the patient's interpersonal processes. The formulations from the various situations discussed can often be tied together in light of various concepts and themes noted by the nurse.

*Since a high degree of anxiety is associated with dissociated material, the nurse allows and aids the patient to utilize measures to reduce and control his anxiety.* Sullivan [14] explained that anxiety occurs when a person experiences anything that tends to enlarge the margins of awareness. He stated, "in dissociation any juggling of external events which would necessitate acceptance of the dissociative system by the self would probably lead to panic." Therefore, the nurse assists the patient in keeping anxiety at a low level and works through dissociated material only when the patient is able to accept it without severe anxiety.

(Patient was describing a period of great anxiety in which much material was dissociated.)
*Patient:* I remember the house had stairs, the kitchen was big, with a lot of windows. The bedrooms were upstairs. There was a big living room and kitchen. That's all I remember.
(While talking, patient shifted a great deal, started humming, breathing deeply. Anxiety becoming quite high.)
*Patient:* Now what would you like to talk about?
*Nurse:* That's up to you.
*Patient:* I'm tired of talking. I wish somebody else would talk.

When the patient's anxiety increased, the nurse allowed her to change the subject as a means of reducing the anxiety. Later in the relationship, the patient was able to discuss the episode and to recall more information that she hadn't remembered previously.

## PREVENTION

The nurse can play a significant role in the prevention of dissociation. Since the dissociative process functions in periods of very high anxiety, the nurse who is alert to this fact can talk with the patient, encouraging verbalization of thoughts, feelings, and actions following a threatening

[13] Fromm-Reichmann, F., *op. cit.*, p. 81.
[14] Sullivan, H. S., *Clinical Studies in Psychiatry*, p. 217.

situation. Because feelings, particularly, are dissociated, the focus may often be on this aspect.

Peplau [15] states:

> Counseling in nursing has to do with helping the patient to remember and to understand fully what is happening to him in the present situation, so that the experience can be integrated with rather than dissociated from other experiences in life.

The psychiatric patient, who is prone to periods of high anxiety because of the partial eruption of dissociated content into awareness, can be particularly helped by the nurse to utilize these experiences to enlarge his field of awareness and integrate them as part of his self-system.

# BIBLIOGRAPHY

FROMM-REICHMANN, FRIEDA, *Principles of Intensive Psychotherapy,* University of Chicago Press, Chicago: 1950.

JANET, PIERRE, *The Major Symptoms of Hysteria,* The Macmillan Company, New York: 1913.

MULLAHY, PATRICK, *Oedipus: Myth and Complex,* Grove Press, New York: 1948.

PEPLAU, HILDEGARD E., *Interpersonal Relations in Nursing,* G. P. Putnam's Sons, New York: 1952.

RAPAPORT, DAVID (ed.), *Organization and Pathology of Thought,* Columbia University Press, New York: 1951.

SULLIVAN, HARRY STACK, *Clinical Studies in Psychiatry,* W. W. Norton & Co., New York: 1956.

—— *Conceptions of Modern Psychiatry,* W. W. Norton & Co., New York: 1953.

—— *Interpersonal Theory of Psychiatry,* W. W. Norton & Co., New York: 1953.

WOLBERG, LEWIS R., *The Technique of Psychotherapy,* Grune and Stratton, New York: 1954.

---

[15] Peplau, H. E., *op. cit.,* p. 64.

# 24

## THE NURSE STAFF,
## THE NURSE–CLINICIAN,
## AND A HYPERACTIVE PATIENT

*Margaret A. Marshall*

The subroles which, when considered together, comprise the work role of the staff nurse have been delineated by Peplau.[1] Subroles can be delineated as well for the practicing nurse-clinician. The focus of the expert psychiatric nurse-clinician is direct psychotherapeutic intervention with individual patients and groups of patients. Within the clinical setting, such nurses have additional nursing subroles which include consultant, membership on the interdisciplinary team, nursing researcher and research assistant, and resource person to staff. It is the resource-person role and functions that are the focus of this chapter.

An instance of the clinician's utilization of the role and functions of the resource person began with the following exchange between a clinician and a head nurse. Data are reconstructed from notes taken during the conference.

(*H.N.*—Head Nurse; *P.N.-C.*—Psychiatric Nurse-Clinician.)
*H.N.:* I have on my ward a difficult patient. She is so impossible. If you have the time, perhaps you'd be willing to give me some help with her.
*P.N.-C.:* I have about twenty minutes. Tell me about the difficulty.
*H.N.:* Anna A. was admitted to an acute admission service 58 days ago. Since then, she has made two trips to the infirmary service, and I have had her on my ward (also an admission service) for about a month. Staff can't stand her. I'm now past the point of staff hostility toward both the patient, for her behavior, and myself, for assigning personnel to take care of her. I now have what could best be termed "open mutiny." Personnel flatly refuse to take care of her. Just before I came to lunch, one of the staff came out of Anna's room, slammed the door with sufficient

[1] Peplau, H. E., *Interpersonal Relations in Nursing*, pp. 43–70.

force that the unit rocked and stated that no amount of money would induce her to go into that room again. The staff member was upset to the point that, had the superintendent, chief nurse, Pope, and President of the United States has been making a tour, she would have said the same thing. Perhaps even more.

P.N.-C.: You said the patient came in 58 days ago?

H.N.: Yes—though maybe by now it's 59 days. It seems a nightmarish eternity. I'm at my wit's ends. It is an effort to come to work and face this day after endless day. I get up, sit on my bed, and have to convince myself that I should come to work. It's getting harder every day to talk myself into it though. On top of that, I've had a rash of vague complaints from staff which leads to an increased absenteeism, so that we are working short-staffed. Not that I blame them—I'd like to be absent myself.

P.N.-C.: Tell me something about the patient.

H.N.: Anna? This is her third admission to a hospital, but her first here. She was treated elsewhere before. She's 37, slight, and attractive. The thing we are all reacting against is her hyperactivity. She has not slept more than two hours in any twenty-four since she came in. On top of that, she has developed hyperemesis. Her medications have been altered frequently. She vomits about twenty minutes after oral medications are given and has developed an acute esophagitis. She was transferred to the infirmary for treatment, but created such a disturbance that they were unable, in fairness to the other patients, to keep her. She is dehydrated, since fluids are not retained. Her weight loss has been about twenty pounds, I'd guess. Due to her hyperactivity, we have been unable to weigh her. Her clothes hang on her, though, compared with the fit at the time of her admission. For the past two or three days now, her temperature has ranged between 102.6 and 103.2 degrees Fahrenheit. I'm just up to here (placing hands across her face at the brow line).

P.N.-C.: What seems to evoke the negative or hostile feelings in staff?

H.N.: Five minutes in the room with Anna! Staff now interpret my assigning her to their care as punishment. I have tried to take on her care myself, but I only work eight hours a day, so I must have their aid. Anna is on a high-protein fluid feeding by mouth every hour. I just must have staff cooperation to carry out the orders, and I can't get it.

P.N.-C.: Do you notice unfavorable patient reaction toward Anna A., also?

H.N.: Yes. I should tell you—one aide was overheard talking with a patient group. What she asked the patients to do was to report to the ward doctor that they couldn't stand Anna any longer and attempt to induce the doctor to transfer her. The aide said to them that, if enough patients complained, the doctor would have to do something. You know—transfer one to satisfy many. That didn't work, because infirmary wouldn't accept her, and she isn't ready for a continuous treatment service.

P.N.-C.: Is the patient unusually anxious?

H.N.: I think she is.

P.N.-C.: Then it is possible that staff reacts to the anxiety she generates, communicates to them, and that they observe in themselves?

H.N.: Yes—that's probably what it is.

P.N.-C.: The same thing might be true, then, of the other patients?

H.N.: Perhaps so. If she'd just go to sleep for eight or ten hours, so the rest of the group could get some rest, the situation might be more tolerable. But she doesn't. Fifty-eight days of this! If it isn't stopped I may have real problems with the patient group generally—you can feel the tension in the air as soon as you step into the ward—and the staff group specifically.

P.N.-C.: Suppose I arrange to see the patient later today or early tomorrow. After a visit we may be able, together, to work out a program which will be helpful to both the patient and the staff.

H.N.: The sooner, the better; you are welcome to her. Anything that anyone can do will be better than what I now have.

The patient was visited by the clinician. Anna was isolated in a seclusion room at the front of the unit in which an overhead light burned. Due to the location of the room, all traffic entering the ward, with frequent opening and closing of the doors, passed by her door. Similarly, all patient traffic was concentrated at that particular point, since patients had to move past the patient's room going to and from activities. The patient moved constantly about in her room, which had been stripped of all furnishings with the exception of the bed. She carried on a rapid, endless monologue which was shot through with profane and obscene words. The patient seemed oblivious of the presence of the clinician. Her clothing hung loosely on a slight, gaunt frame.

The initial change in the situation occurred in the nurse, who experienced a sharp increase in anxiety. Appraisal resulted in the judgment that the anxiety was being emphatically communicated by the patient and observed by the nurse. This nonverbal transmission of the feeling of anxiety has been described as a common occurrence between mother and infant: ". . . the emotional contagion by which the infant may become aware of the emotional state of his mother without the mediation of any of the known sense organs." [2] The capacity for recognition and accurate appraisal of empathically observed feelings in the interpersonal situation is acquired with experience and is a tool useful to the clinician in identifying the emotional aspects of the experiences of her patients.

The patient failed to respond to the greeting of the nurse. Repeated efforts to engage the patient in conversation were likewise fruitless. The nurse took steps to reduce her own anxiety by doing a concrete, routine task—recording her observations in a notebook. The almost instantaneous increase in the clinician's anxiety in the presence of the patient, when considered with the hyperactivity, verbosity, and scatter in language content, was indicative of a severe anxiety state in the patient (see p. 326).[3]

[2] Witenberg, E. G., Rioch, J. M., and Mazer, M., "The Interpersonal and Cultured Approaches," p. 1419.

See also, Sullivan, H. S., The Interpersonal Theory of Psychiatry, pp. 41–45; Conceptions of Modern Psychiatry, p. 17.

[3] See also, Hays, D. R., "Teaching a Concept of Anxiety," 1957, pp. 4–8.

It was evident that one of the first goals of the nursing staff would be to interrupt and then reduce the anxiety of the patient.

Immediately following this contact with the patient, the clinician arranged to confer with the head nurse to attempt to work out a comprehensive nursing-care plan for Anna A. It was important to work out a program with realistic goals, so that the staff members could begin to have small successes in working with this very anxious, overactive patient.

In the conference between the clinician and the head nurse, two factors received major consideration. The first is the cardinal principle of nursing: *The nurse will support the healthy aspects of the patient while moving the pathological in the direction of health.* The second is comprised of the three major categories of care, which, when taken together, constitute the care plan. These three categories are: (1) alleviation of the acute symptoms of the patient; (2) a general supportive care program; and (3) specific intervention into, and correction of, the underlying causes of the manifested pathology.[4]

Of greatest importance was planning a program of care to intervene in the high anxiety level of Anna so that her physiological needs could be met. The punishment to her physiological equilibrium was immeasurable. Her chart bore evidence that Anna was sleeping no more than two hours in any day, and that her failure to maintain a sleeping state had existed since prior to her admission. In spite of her temperature elevation, which would tend to produce drowsiness and subsequent sleep, the patient's high anxiety state kept her in almost perpetual motion. Best and Taylor [5] state that there is a point of continuous wakefulness that is lethal to humans. Laboratory experiments demonstrate that lesser animals, including dogs, may expire in as few as 14 days of continued sleep deprivation. In humans, the power to maintain equilibrium is grossly impaired during long periods of sleeplessness due to neuromuscular fatigue and the consequent loss of muscle tone. Medications, both oral and intramuscular, had proved ineffectual in slowing down the patient's body processes sufficiently to encourage and then support a sleeping state. Personnel expressed disbelief that the patient could "walk around with half of the unit's barbiturate supply in her buttocks and still not sleep." Such, however, was the case. The self-perpetuation of insomnia in high anxiety states, and in the classical "nervous" type of insomnia, is noted by McGraw and Oliven.[6]

[4] Ebaugh, F. G., and Tiffany, W. J., Jr., "Infective-Exhaustive Psychoses," pp. 1244–46.

[5] Best, C. H., and Taylor, N. B., *The Physiological Basis of Medical Practice*, p. 1487.

[6] McGraw, R. B., and Oliven, J. F., "Miscellaneous Therapies," pp. 1564–65.

In the era of the widespread use of hydrotherapy, two procedures were used to induce sleep. One was continuous warm tub baths which, by relaxing the patient, lowered muscle tonus and induced sleep.[7] The other, which was considered a method to abate the excitement in this case, was cold wet packs, which serve to stimulate cutaneous circulation, lessen the body temperature, and then act as a sedative.[8] The latter is accomplished by the initial vasoconstriction with a concurrent reduction of the blood supply to the skin. As soon as body heat is produced by this activity, the blood flow through the skin is at once augmented through the action of the heat-loss centers in the hypothalamus. An alteration in the blood flow follows which serves to bring deeper warm blood to the surface of the skin with vasodilation.[9] The warmer blood, from a deeper circulatory source, loses temperature by the process of evaporation when it is brought to the skin level, which is in contact with the cold packs. The body temperature is lowered by this artificial means which would normally occur when the body is at rest. Since the agency in which Anna A. was a patient had discontinued hydrotherapy, the cold wet pack, also called the sedative pack,[10] would be the alternative to the treatment of choice for the purpose of inducing sleep in this patient in the event anxiety was not reduced sufficiently in an interpersonal relationship that normal sleep would follow.[11]

The major purpose served by inducing sleep, regardless of the technique employed, is to allow restoration of the normal body equilibrium. This was particularly important for Anna A. One alteration achieved in sleep is a reduction of the pulse rate, the blood pressure, and the respiratory rate.[12] Cardiac decompensation is one of the major complications of prolonged hyperactivity. The general body processes are reduced with sleep, which might also serve to alleviate the hyperemesis Anna had manifested for several weeks. Sleep seemed to be the route by which progress toward achieving the first two of the three categories of total care could be established. The third category of care would be dealt with later.

The general, over-all plan, formulated in accordance with the cardinal principle of nursing care and in keeping with the three broad categories of care, was as follows:

First, the head nurse, functioning in the team-leader role, and the

[7] Wolberg, L. R., *The Technique of Psychotherapy*, p. 31.

[8] *Ibid.*, p. 31.

[9] Fulton, J. F., *A Textbook of Physiology*, pp. 779–80.

[10] Harmer, B., and Henderson, V., *Textbook of Principles and Practice of Nursing*, pp. 626–32.

[11] The author gratefully acknowledges the assistance of Isabelle Dutcher, R.N., M.A., in the preparation of the physiological aspects of this paper.

[12] Best, C. H., and Taylor, N. B., *op. cit.*, p. 1486.

clinician, functioning in the resource-person role, would meet with the total nursing staff to discuss the patient's symptoms, feelings, and physical status and would encourage the personnel to express their feelings toward the patient. When such feelings are explored openly, there is greater opportunity for resolving the difficulties that are noted in the interpersonal situation. It was deemed essential to use this procedure as a first step in eliciting staff cooperation for the improved care of the patient, and in aiding staff to gain a measure of control over the excessive anxiety they experienced in the presence of the patient.

Second, the patient would be moved to a room at the far end of the hall rather than being isolated at the front of the unit where she could be stimulated by the opening and closing of the doors and the incessant traffic of patients and staff. Further, her room was to be kept ventilated and darkened to cut down the external stimuli as much as possible.

Third, a volunteer from the staff group would be sought to care for Anna with some consistency. If no one volunteered, the head nurse would assume responsibility for most of the care of the patient. Because of the frequency of feedings and the hyperemesis, with the subsequent esophagitis, the staff volunteer would spend at least five or ten minutes with Anna immediately prior to each feeding. She was to encourage the patient to lie quietly in bed. She was also to speak quietly with the patient in short, direct sentences. When the patient began to relax, she was to be given her high-protein liquid feeding. The staff member would then remain with the patient for a short time, again encouraging the patient to rest. The goal of this procedure was to temporarily interrupt the anxiety and, at the same time, to provide the patient with both rest and nourishment. In addition to the foregoing, it seemed probable that the stability of the contact would further aid in anxiety reduction by providing the patient with a familiar person who would tend to be consistent in her approach to the patient. The patient had previously been exposed to numerous staff members, each of whom reacted toward, and interacted with, the patient in individual ways. What was desired has been labeled by Peplau [13] as the "sustaining thereness" as a way of establishing for the patient a realistic expectation which would then be met throughout the eight-hour day. The staff member would also serve to interrupt, by her interaction with Anna, the ruminative and circular thinking patterns which only perpetuated the energy of anxiety, and would aid the patient in thinking along a linear route which could be expected to minimize the energy force of the anxiety. Theoretically, the meeting of the need for re-

[13] Peplau, H. E., *Interpersonal Relations in Nursing*, p. 129.

duction of anxiety is an interpersonal process,[14] and the high anxiety level of the patient would not be lessened by the patient in isolation. The "sustaining thereness," provided by consistent contact with the same person, would serve to minimize the patient's anxiety sufficiently so that feedings would be retained. Fluid retention would aid in restoration of the patient's fluid balance, thereby alleviating her dehydration and reducing her fever. Further, retention of fluids would curb the persistent hyperemesis and assuage the symptoms and discomfort of the esophagitis.

Fourth, a nurse-patient counseling schedule would be started as soon as the patient had rested more than four hours on two successive days. One major goal was to maintain an anxiety level sufficiently low to allow the patient to explore, with the nurse, the genesis of the anxiety and the situation which immediately preceded her hospitalization. A two-day delay was deemed essential to achieve initial control over the presenting symptoms and to prevent a recurrence of uncontrolled anxiety, since some anxiety usually occurs with establishment of such an interpersonal relationship.

Fifth, the clinician would meet with the staff for brief periods each day in order to keep current with progress made by implementation of the plan. She would also assist staff to work through problems encountered from day to day as personnel worked with the patient. The goal was to encourage, receive, and sustain staff interest and cooperation.

In addition to the above, the clinician was to meet with the ward doctor to relay the care plan for Anna. In the event that sedative packs were used as a vehicle for inducing sleep, a medical order for the treatment would be required. Further, the medical officer might have data that would lead to additions to, or modifications of, the formulated plan. The clinician would also arrange with a colleague a time that could be made available to the patient for a psychotherapeutic nurse-patient relationship. The colleague would be the nurse who worked with Anna A. when the third category of care was initiated.

This, then, was the general plan. With its implementation, the anxiety of Anna A. began to decrease. On the first night, her sleep was interrupted after two hours, at which time the patient was "noisy." She fell asleep for a second time in the early morning hours with sedation and slept another hour and a half in what was charted as "fitful and restless naps." On the second night, the patient slept for nearly three hours. Upon awakening, she was "quiet and cooperative," and requested that she be escorted to the bathroom. Upon returning to her room, the night nurse remained with her. The patient subsequently slept an additional three hours. The third

[14] Witenberg et al., op. cit., p. 1420.

night, sleep was maintained for nearly five hours. Anna was quiet upon awakening, expressed surprise that "I am not in my room at home," and requested that the night nurse stay with her between rounds of the unit "because I feel too alone and nervous in here by myself." The nurse remained with the patient for brief intervals. Thus, by the third day of the planned program, it was evident that the alternative method of sleep induction would not be necessary, since sleep was forthcoming after the sustained relationship was begun.

On the fourth morning, a clinician began to orient the patient to the nurse-patient relationship. Within five days, presenting symptoms were alleviated to the extent that the patient was afebrile, retained all day feedings of high-protein liquids, and experienced minimal distress from the subsiding esophagitis. The experiences and status of the patient which precipitated a third hospitalization were explored during the working relationship with the nurse-clinician. During the second week, the ward doctor ordered soft, bland foods which were retained. Anna began a slow, progressive weight gain.

There were times during the nurse-patient relationship when anxiety was increased. When the clinician was with the patient, the causes of the anxiety were explored. At other times, Anna sought the company of her "day nurse" or night personnel. Usual sleep pattern of six to seven hours of restful sleep was restored during the third week. Sleep was then normally induced and maintained without sedation.

Within eight weeks, Anna was sufficiently improved that she was transferred to a continuous treatment service. Her nurse-patient counseling hours were gradually reduced as the patient began a predischarge program. The relationship was terminated after twenty-seven sessions. At the time of termination, the patient was asymptomatic, had regained her admission weight, had an awareness of the situations that provoked excessive anxiety in her, and was subsequently discharged as "recovered."

In summary then, the cardinal principle of all nursing care, particularly as that principle underlies psychotherapeutic counseling, guided the planning of the over-all nursing-care program for this hyperactive patient. That principle, to restate it, is that the nurse will support the healthy aspects of the patient while moving the pathological in the direction of health.

The clinician, in the role of resource person to the head nurse and the nursing staff, considered the three broad categories of care that must be included in all comprehensive patient-care plans. These are—

1. Alleviate the acute symptoms. In this particular instance, prime importance was given to a nursing program that would reduce the patient's

temperature; reduce the patient's anxiety sufficiently so that her usual sleep pattern would be restored; and work with the nursing and medical staff to provide a "sustained thereness" for this hyperactive patient.

2. Provide a supportive care plan so that the healthy aspects of the patient's status will be preserved. This was accomplished by soliciting the cooperation of the personnel who worked with this patient, and providing her with the same staff member throughout the eight-hour workday. By so doing, Anna was provided with a consistent relationship in which she could formulate realistic expectations concerning the actions and reactions of one person. Previously she had had to adjust to numerous stranger-to-stranger interludes. Active participation of staff in the nursing-care plan served to enhance the possibility that the members of the staff would form future interpersonal relationships with their patients. Further, it was demonstrated to staff that resources are available to give aid and guidance when needed.

3. Intervene and correct the underlying causes. The patient was provided with a nurse-patient counseling relationship in which the underlying causes of her behavior could be explored. Behavioral modifications along socially acceptable lines were tested by the patient with the nurse. This was accomplished during the twenty-seven interaction hours with the psychiatric nurse-clinician.

The clinician was functioning primarily in the resource-person role in this experience. She also used other subroles during the process of programming a care plan for Anna A. Among these nursing subroles were resource person to the staff, objective observer with the patient, and interdisciplinary team member. Some functions of the consultant role were also performed. A second clinician, a colleague of the resource person's, functioned in the counseling role almost exclusively since she worked directly with Anna A.

Throughout this therapeutic intervention into the hyperactivity of Anna, and during the planning and implementing of the over-all nursing program, the total staff, both nursing and medical, worked together for the benefit of one patient in particular—Anna A. This clinical experience, however, will serve as a basis for the formulation of care plans for hyperactive patients in general. The considerations made in preparation for the total care of this patient are basic to all of nursing and have application regardless of the illness or the behavioral manifestation of the energy of anxiety. The prime considerations, to reiterate, are the cardinal principle of nursing, and the three categories of care, which, when considered together, comprise the program of professional nursing care which can be provided to all patients.

## BIBLIOGRAPHY

BEST, CHARLES H., and TAYLOR, NORMAN BURKE, The Physiological Basis of Medical Practice, 2nd ed. Williams & Wilkins, Baltimore, Md.: 1939.

EBAUGH, FRANKLIN G., and TIFFANY, WILLIAM J., JR., "Infective-Exhaustive Psychosis" in *American Handbook of Psychiatry*, Silvano Arieti (ed.), Basic Books, New York: 1959.

FULTON, JOHN F., *A Textbook of Physiology*, 17th ed., W. B. Saunders Co., Philadelphia: 1955.

HARMER, BERTHA, and HENDERSON, VIRGINIA, *Textbook of Principles and Practice of Nursing*, 5th ed., The Macmillan Co., New York: 1955.

HAYS, DOROTHEA RICHTER, "Teaching a Concept of Anxiety," master's thesis, Graduate School, Rutgers, The State University of New Jersey, 1957.

MC GRAW, ROBERT B., and OLIVEN, JOHN F., "Miscellaneous Therapies," in *American Handbook of Psychiatry*, Silvano Arieti (ed.), Basic Books, New York: 1959.

PEPLAU, HILDEGARD E., *Interpersonal Relations in Nursing*, G. P. Putnam's Sons, New York: 1952.

——— "Principles of Psychiatric Nursing," in *American Handbook of Psychiatry*, Silvano Arieti (ed.), Basic Books, New York: 1959.

SULLIVAN, HARRY STACK, *The Interpersonal Theory of Psychiatry*, W. W. Norton & Co., New York: 1953.

——— *Conceptions of Modern Psychiatry*, W. W. Norton & Co., New York: 1953.

WITENBERG, EARL G., RIOCH, JANET MC KENZIE, and MAZER, MILTON, "The Interpersonal and Cultural Approaches" in *American Handbook of Psychiatry*, Silvano Arieti (ed.), Basic Books, New York: 1959.

WOLBERG, LEWIS R., *The Technique of Psychotherapy*, Grune and Stratton, New York: 1954.

# 25 SELF-CONCEPT AND THE SCHIZOPHRENIC PATIENT

*Shirley A. Smoyak*

Two factors in parental behavior, nondirectness and the switch phenomenon, contributed to the development of schizophrenia in John, a young patient in a mental hospital.

When this boy was dealing with the task of constructing his self-concept, his parents' attitudes and actions interfered seriously with his arriving at a healthy picture of himself. These factors operated to disturb John so seriously that, at the age of 14, he tried to commit suicide. Verbatim data from the psychiatric interview will be used in this chapter. At the time this chapter was written, John had been visited by the author for two one-hour sessions each week over a period of seven months.

The child develops his concept of self from reflected appraisals of his parents and other people in his environment. The parental appraisals of the child are of primary importance in the construction of the self-concept. From the rewards and punishments his parents give, the child begins to see himself as a person who at times is good and at other times, bad. Sullivan [1] describes the good-me as

> . . . the beginning personification which organizes experience in which satisfactions have been advanced by rewarding increments of tenderness, which come to the infant because the mothering one is pleased with the way things are going. . . .

Bad-me, on the other hand, states Sullivan,[2] is

[1] Sullivan, H. S., *The Interpersonal Theory of Psychiatry*, pp. 161–62.
[2] *Ibid.*, p. 162.

. . . beginning personification which organizes experience in which increasing degrees of anxiety are associated with behavior involving the mothering me. . . .

John, now 24 years old, has been a patient in a state mental hospital for the past ten years. He describes his childhood this way:

I wasn't ever punished; I was gently, subtly, verbally criticized. My mother babied me—she would always smile that way. I don't know if I'm a babied brat or just human nature. I never knew if that smile meant "You're a nice baby." Maybe she meant it just as a pleasant normal reaction. Maybe not. Maybe it was an appreciative smile, but it could have been a babying smile.

The outstanding characteristics of John's mother were vagueness and subtlety. Her responses to the child could not be categorized as meaning good or bad. As the boy puts it: "I never knew just where I stood." He recalls an incident with his mother which further illustrates this nondirectness:

I can remember the park where she used to take me. It was nice and we used to play cards. I would win every time, and she would smile as if I were a very good player. But I never knew if I were really good or if she was letting me win. There's a scientific reason for card winning—the other person, wittingly or unwittingly, lets you win. I don't know what the case was with her.

This situation of never knowing, or not being able to formulate a self-concept, is extremely anxiety-provoking. It is a terrifying panic-producing experience not to know who or what you are. In discussing the subject of playing cards, the nurse said, "John, what would happen if you lost?" His anxiety rose rapidly, and he shouted, "I'd go to pieces! I wouldn't know who I was!"

John's father also participated in this nondirect, vague pattern of relating to his son. The patient describes how he used to play checkers with his father, again winning every time, and again not knowing exactly how good or bad he was at the game.

In addition to this nondirectness, however, the patient's father used another, more confusing pattern: the switch phenomenon. At one time he would make one appraisal or take one course of action; but another time he switched to the opposite side. For example, his father would tell John that he was intelligent, a good scholar, and possessed brains. A few minutes later, he might tell John he was "a stupid boy and just a good-for-nothing." The father would tell the boy that to succeed he had to work hard and long, and do what he was told. On the other hand, he would also tell

John that all he needed was to be intelligent and outsmart others in order to succeed.

At times John's father became openly angry, using harsh, loud speech in his rage. When John tried this outlet for anger, he was told to shut up, that such behavior was insolent. The patient remembers his father having strict rules about what was manly and what was not. Yet the father participated in such unmanly actions as rubbing the patient's back when he was ill and using "very kind, syrupy-soft words."

Smoking was considered manly or masculine, but John's smoking was frowned upon. He describes the smoking this way:

> My father never said, "Don't smoke," but on the other hand, he never said I should. He doesn't smoke at all, and I have the feeling that he doesn't want me to. I've asked him to bring me cigarettes and he always says he will bring them, but never does. I can't figure it out.

This switch phenomenon has prevented John from developing a clear concept of self. As soon as he had categorized some trait or behavior under good-me, the switch occurred and the trait or behavior was characterized as belonging under bad-me. Possessing brains and being intelligent were at one moment desirable, at the next moment, undesirable.

He was not permitted to validate his actions, gestures, and words. In the absence of validation, John used autistic invention to explain what was going on. Being an alert and bright boy, he had to use his mental capacity to explain the situations in which he found himself. When he attempted from time to time to explain what he meant, his father would cut him off and his mother would give him no answer. Not being able to validate would leave him helpless. Rather than be helpless, John employed autism to make himself comfortable and provide explanations.

During one visit, the nurse remarked, "It seems as though you had to do a lot of figuring out by yourself as to what was meant." John's reply was:

> Either that, or take it for granted. He told me not to give him any of my "lip." My reaction was to be quiet, as if I knew I was wrong. I would become more wrong if I questioned his statement. To be honest, I didn't know what to reply. He had the upper hand.

During a previous discussion, the patient had stated:

> If I couldn't figure out something, I would make up an explanation. Then I would say it over and over and over until I really believed it thoroughly. Like I told myself that my mother loved me and that's why she smiled. The trouble is, when I talk to you, I wonder if it's that easy.

When John's efforts to seek explanations by means of consensual validation failed, he turned to autistic invention as a tool in finding answers. The nurse, in talking with this patient, is trying to reverse the process. Over the months, more and more autistic thinking has been replaced by validation. At present, John is confronting his father with the request that he make a definite stand on smoking. So far, his father has not done so and still is evading the issue. John's comment about this is, "I'm beginning to wonder who's sick around here."

## BIBLIOGRAPHY

SULLIVAN, HARRY STACK, *The Interpersonal Theory of Psychiatry*, W. W. Norton & Co., New York: 1953.

# 26 THE CHANGE FROM INSTITUTIONAL LIVING TO COMMUNITY LIVING [1]

*Shirley F. Burd*

Short-term home visits and discharge of a patient from a psychiatric fa-
cility represent movement from institutional living to community living.
Cruze [2] defines change as "movement from one type or another. It may
be movement from one place to another, or from one type of stimulation
to lack of stimulation, or vice versa." The writer has often taken part in
nurse-child interviews in a variety of institutional and community settings.
These children had been or were currently diagnosed as schizophrenic and
represented a variety of institutions.

Analysis of data obtained during these interviews suggested answers
to two of three vital questions about the change from institutional to community living. These questions are: What is the common process utilized
to effect the child's change in living from the institution to the community?
How can the nurse assist the child in making the change in living? What
are the other areas to be considered in the nurse-child relationship when
the child is diagnosed as schizophrenic?

Answering the initial question about the process used to effect change
in living seems simple when asked. However, the commonly held view of
the child differs from that of the nurse. Furthermore, assumptions may
prove to be anxiety-producing when one discovers that his view is not the
right view. Analysis of nurse-patient data with adults further validates the
process described by the children. Nursing colleagues validated the author's
experience, for each nurse had experienced some increase in anxiety when

---

[1] Originally published in *Nursing World*, Vol. 133, No. 10, October, 1959.
[2] Cruze, W. W., *Psychology in Nursing*, p. 354.

she first became aware that her thinking regarding the process of change in living was erroneous. Similarly, those reading this chapter may experience an increase in anxiety by reading about the possible erroneous nature of his or her thinking on the question.

The process of the change in living is related in a step-by-step manner by the children who take part in the working relationship phase of the nurse-patient studies or interviews. In this process the anxiety-producing factor is twofold, involving the person who initiates the process and how it is initiated. It is the patient who initiates the process of change, rather than any member of the nonprofessional or professional personnel. The initial step is one of personal decision-making. The child observes that other persons are making a change in living or "going home." The learning process utilized may be accompanied by wishes and hopes. This step is terminated by the child's formulation of a decision that he will go home and his selection of a plan of action.

The second step is to manipulate the power figure by currying favor. The identity of this person varies with the staffing policies of the various institutions represented by the children. The child's references to this step involve "be good." Terms the child uses in describing this step are "keep the peace," "don't upset Miss X.," "don't get into Miss X.'s hair," and "work, that's what Miss X. expects everyone to do." The child attempts to conform to the expectations, values, and anxiety of the power figure and all persons who might communicate with the power figure. The problem for the child in this step involves the multiplicity of expectations to be met. He usually identifies the major values and functions accordingly, in order to prevent an increase of anxiety in the power figure. "If Miss X. isn't upset by you, she likes you," he states.

If the child believes that Miss X. likes him, he can ask her about his going home or whether the power figure would ask the physician this question. This request is the third step in the process. Direct communication between the child and the physician may be limited due to many reasons. The obvious and logical person to make the child's needs known to the physician is the power figure who "likes" Johnny and confers with his physician regularly.

The fourth step includes the thought process and actions of the physician and the child. The physician makes a decision for Johnny regarding change from institutional living to community living, and the child encourages his family to write the physician about this change. Children, like adults, need to know the decisions and the underlying reasons. Since the child must have a reason for action or lack of action, he will autistically invent a reason if none is given. In doing so, he may also incorporate some of the thought pathology of other patients with whom he has discussed his problem of "no news."

The fifth step is that Johnny's family writes the physician or the institution indicating its willingness to have the child at home for a short or extended period of time. Freedman [3] writes of a limitation of the residential school for children diagnosed as schizophrenic: "During his absence, the family may become so reorganized that it can no longer accept the schizophrenic child back into the household." The physician and Johnny may encourage the family to make the change possible. However, the family makes the final decision about the possibility of change in living.

The physician presents the child at the staff meeting as the sixth step. Patients gain information about staff meetings from other patients and/or personnel. Children are no exception; they request and receive this information from someone. The child encounters an experience at the staff meeting that is somewhat similar to his expectations. The child's problem areas during this step are (a) an increase in anxiety and autistic invention of the decision and its reasons, if the communication of this information is delayed, and (b) the information obtained from other patients prior to staff which may be distorted according to the patient's thought pathologies.

There's a missing step in this process. The previously enumerated steps omit any progress toward getting better, or getting well. This is because children may defer this initial step until time to summarize the description of the process. The child often exclaims: "I didn't include getting well! That comes first. We both know that." "Getting well" and "understanding the problem" are two of the phrases used to describe the first step. All other steps are renumbered accordingly.

The question remains of how the nurse can assist the child in making the change from institutional living to community living. Children need to experience a satisfactory interpersonal relationship with one individual prior to satisfactory interpersonal relationships with many persons. This one-to-one relationship is an initial step in the development of the child.

The nurse carefully selects her expectations regarding the child in the initial phase of the nurse-child relationship. Children and adults tend to live up to the expectations of other persons. A useful and hopeful expectation of the nurse is that the child will return to his family.

In the initial description of the child's process of making the change, the child recognizes the need for a change in living, experiences the anx-

[3] Freedman, A. M., "Day Hospitals for Severely Disturbed Schizophrenic Children," p. 894.

iety, and converts the energy of the anxiety into a learning and/or problem-solving process in order to select a plan for action. In the nurse-child
relationship the nurse gives the child assistance, for he need not carry this
burden alone. The child becomes encouraged and hopeful about the future.

The theme of hopefulness extends to the family in the child-family relationships and the nurse-child-family relationships. Hopefulness acts as
intervention or prevention of possible reorganization of the family which
delays or prevents the child's return to community living.

The nurse-child relationship includes the major concept of anxiety.
This central concept is related to the child's problematic areas prior to
institutional living, as he views them, and his expectations of change in
the home and community at the time of his return. Experiential teaching
is used to discuss the concept of anxiety, the transfer of anxiety, the child's
usual energy-conversion patterns, and other energy-conversion patterns of
anxiety (see p. 325). The child now has a basis for investigating the "why"
of his behavior. He has an explanation and need not autistically invent
reasons for his behavior.

The child and the nurse investigate the problematic areas that led to
institutional living. What were the problematic areas? Was there any
similarity between areas? What were the child's behavior, thoughts, and
feelings? What made the situations a problem? What methods were used
to deal with the problem? What other methods could be used to solve
such a problem? What methods can be used when this and/or similar
problem situations are encountered in the future? Who might be of assistance to the child in the community setting? The child needs to know the
answers to these and other questions through his own learning process.

Time would be reduced considerably if the nurse made the above
formulations, but the usefulness of the nurse lecturing about her formulations of the child's behavior is questionable. This continues the child's
dependency on someone else to think for him. It is obvious that the nurse
will not be the child's constant lifetime companion. Therefore the nurse
assists the patient in reaching his own formulations. She is someone who
can and does validate the formulations of the child with him, and she
assists him in revising his formulations. The nurse's assistance in the child's
learning process decreases as the child gains the competencies of learning
and/or problem-solving.

As the child begins to make formulations regarding his own behavior
and that of other people, the discussions will focus increasingly on the
goal of making the expected change in living. The child needs to know
the administrative steps of the institution related to making the change

from institutional living to community living. He needs to know of possible and actual changes in the community; the family and the nurse share the function of providing him with such information. The expectation that the home and community will be the same as before can never be met. Change is a characteristic of urban societies. Anxiety is associated with change.

There are other problem areas which the nurse will consider in the care of children diagnosed as schizophrenic, and nurses must continue to look for the areas in which they might assist the children. This is done by studying the data obtained in a nurse-child relationship and the nurse-child-family relationship. How does the nurse care for the child other than in a custodial manner? What are the child's problems in the institution and upon return to the community? What are the parents' and/or family's interpersonal problems with the child?

The literature regarding children diagnosed as schizophrenic is extensive, as evidenced by the Kanner and Eisenberg reports.[4,5] But this literature does not include any reports made by nurses. By contacts with nurses throughout the country one becomes aware that nurses are involved both in nurse-child relationships and nurse-child-family relationships. These nurses know some of the problem areas experienced by the child. Two of the areas mentioned are the lack of educative facilities while in the institution and the inclusion of the child in an adult hospital population. Sharing the knowledge of these problems and the functions of the nurse through intradisciplinary and interdisciplinary conferences and the professional literature would expand the available information about how the nurse functions with these children living in an institution.

Children diagnosed as schizophrenic often make the change from institutional living to community living, but they need some assistance. Here the seven-step process answering the initial question of how some children effect this change in living has been described according to the view of the child. The question of method that the nurse can utilize in assisting the child to make the change in living has been described as a portion of the nurse-child and nurse-child-family relationships.

The child is assisted in his learning and problem-solving processes by a helpful conversion pattern for the energy of the anxiety-accompanying change. The other areas to be considered will depend on continuation of nurse-child and nurse-child-family relationships; use of the nurse's learning

[4] Kanner, L., and Eisenberg, L., "Review of Psychiatric Progress, 1957; Child Psychiatry," p. 7.
[5] *Ibid.*, 1958; Child Psychiatry and Mental Deficiency," p. 7.

process; and reports of the formulations in intradisciplinary conferences, interdisciplinary conferences, and professional literature.

## BIBLIOGRAPHY

CRUZE, W. W., *Psychology in Nursing*, McGraw-Hill Book Co., New York: 1955.
FREEDMAN, A. M., "Day Hospitals for Severely Disturbed Schizophrenic Children," *Am. J. Psychiat.*, 115:893–98, 1958.
KANNER, LEO, and EISENBERG, LEON, "Review of Psychiatric Progress, 1957; Child Psychiatry," *Am. J. Psychiat.*, 114:609–15, 1958.
——— "Review of Psychiatric Progress, 1958; Child Psychiatry and Mental Deficiency," *Am. J. Psychiat.*, 115:609–11, 1959.

# 27 AN ANTIDOTE FOR ALCOHOLISM

*Sheila Rouslin*

As the disguised language of the schizophrenic patient is symbolic and a symptom of an underlying thought disorder, so too is alcoholism a symbol for and symptom of an underlying psychological problem. Alcoholism, chronic compulsive drinking, can be viewed as the action that is representative of underlying unresolved thoughts and feelings. Operationally, the development of alcoholism as a repetitive pattern can be defined in the following way: A person has

1. A problem
2. Anxiety in relation to the problem
3. Conversion of the energy of anxiety to behavior—drinking
4. Withdrawal from problem through drinking
5. Anxiety relieved temporarily
6. Unsolved problem
7. Recall of problem
8. Anxiety in retrospect [1]
9. Repetition of drinking—unsolved problem—anxiety triangle

The problem still exists, the anxiety still exists, and the compulsive drinking causes secondary social difficulties which add more problems and concomitant anxiety.

Opinions differ concerning the generic roots of alcoholism. Generally, however, it is agreed that no single type of personality disorder is inherent in the alcoholic. The psychodynamics of alcohol addiction seem to have in common the finding of a low frustration tolerance and experiences that threaten security and consequently cause anxiety. These begin in the earliest stage of personality development. The pattern of seeking relief

[1] Sullivan, H. S., *The Interpersonal Theory of Psychiatry*, pp. 273–74.

—163

from anxiety and frustration by means of a fluid has its roots in this early stage of personality development.[2]

When a pattern of response is learned and practiced with a degree of success, there is little or no reason to change. In later years a person who has practiced appeasement of anxiety and frustration, rather than grappling with the sources, may experience some difficulty. As he becomes older, problems become more complex. Appeasement through a fluid, now alcohol, is the only way he knows to cope with his feelings about the problems. The way he deals with his current life experience is dependent on his earlier learning, which, when applied to later life, renders him unprepared and unable to cope successfully with his problems. The appeasement through a fluid is no longer a resolution, but it in itself becomes a secondary problem.

Thus, arrestation at an early stage of personality development and reinforcement throughout subsequent experiences of the pattern of response learned at that stage are the two components of the generic factors of alcoholism.

Two key concepts are relevant to the understanding of alcoholism; withdrawal and compulsion. Withdrawal is a behavioral reaction to anxiety, conflict, and frustration. A person—

1. Experiences anxiety or conflict or frustration
2. Acts, or wants to act, aggressively according to feelings
3. Perceives that actions are unacceptable by significant other persons
4. Experiences anxiety
5. Wants to please significant other person to ensure security
6. Withdraws, reducing anxiety

Compulsion refers to the tendency to repeat a certain kind of behavior without being able to inhibit it.[3] A person—

1. Has a thought or feeling that provokes discomfort
2. Is not aware of the discomfort
3. Feels a need to act or acts in a way that previously produced relief, usually opposite the original feeling or thought
4. Performs the action
5. Feels no more discomfort [4]

Both concepts have in common the experience of anxiety, the reduction of anxiety through action, and the final action opposite from the original desire.

[2] Zwerling, I., and Rosenbaum, M., "Alcoholic Addiction and Personality," pp. 623–39.
[3] English, H. B., and English, A. C., A Comprehensive Dictionary of Psychological and Psychoanalytical Terms, p. 104.
[4] Derived from Richter, D., "Operational Definition of Compulsion."

The theoretical application of the concepts to alcoholism is obvious. The alcoholic has a repetitive adaptive response to his problem that he has learned early in childhood. He withdraws from his problem by drinking. He does this automatically in order to relieve his discomfort. With constant performance of the act of drinking, the discomfort is relieved. Thus, the withdrawal-compulsive components of alcoholism. One thing remains, however—the initial problem, the particular cause for the withdrawal and compulsion.

In a nurse-patient interview, a patient whose central problem was an inability to cope with frustration described the vicious cycle of his use of alcohol:

> *Patient:* I'd have a problem, then become disappointed, then drink. Then there was catastrophe, plus I'd still have the problem I had in the first place.

He described the brevity of the relief of his discomfort and that although he knew, from past experience, the results of his drinking, he could not stop because he did not know what else to do.

Therapeutic intervention is possible with the alcoholic patient. One method that can be employed by the nurse is the problem-solving approach. This approach is particularly applicable to the pattern of the alcoholic, since no matter how you look at the maneuvers in the general pattern of the withdrawal-compulsive components of the pattern, the patient's initial problem still remains. If a patient cannot stop drinking because he does not know what else to do, why not help the patient learn the process of problem-solving, so that he *can* know what to do?

What is the problem-solving process? The process involves eight steps resulting in satisfaction.

1. Conscious awareness of the problem
2. Intention to deal with the problem
3. Pertinent evidence gathered to understand the problem
4. Consideration of means of action for solution
5. Implementation of one means of action
6. Observation of the implementation results
7. Evaluation of the implementation results
8. Revision in the light of Steps 1 through 7 [5]

A vignette from a nurse-patient interview is an example of the commencement of the problem-solving process.

> *Patient:* So what do we do—go back to the beginning when I first started to drink, or what?
> *Nurse:* Well, perhaps we can start this way. It is my understanding that

[5] Rouslin, S., "Operational Definition of Problem-Solving."

alcoholism is an unsuccessful attempt to solve a problem. In your opinion, what is the problem?

*Patient:* Well, I really don't know what the problem might be.

*Nurse:* You don't know?

*Patient:* Not unless it would be sort of a feeling of frustration I've had all along. I mean there were different things I wanted and couldn't get.

*Nurse:* Go on.

*Patient:* They go way back—suppose, I start.

The patient was aware of the problem (which, incidentally was substantiated in relating previous and living-through current experiences), intended to deal with the problem by having agreed to interviews with the nurse, and started gathering pertinent evidence to understand the problem. Later, in everyday frustrating problems that the patient faced during the course of the interviews, the patient went through the steps of problem-solving. One day the patient said:

*Patient:* If I were out [of the hospital] I'd go on a bender—I'm really getting the run-around with getting this new leg.

The patient did go out for the week end, but did not go on a "bender." Instead, he came back with a possible alternative solution in regard to replacing his amputated leg. When that alternative did not work, he tried another. He was learning to cope with his frustrating experiences by means of problem-solving, rather than appeasing the frustration by means of the withdrawal-compulsive pattern of alcoholism.

It is concluded that a destructive pattern can be replaced by a constructive one. If the mission of each pattern is to accomplish the same thing, viz., to solve the same problem, then there is no room for both patterns if they oppose each other. Therefore, the satisfying pattern is the victor. This can be called the "replacement phenomenon," since the destructive pattern is replaced by a constructive one.

The withdrawal-compulsive pattern of alcoholism fosters the problem, while the problem-solving pattern attacks the problem. The one pattern ends in a vicious cycle with the problem always unsolved; the other pattern culminates in a feeling of satisfaction with the problem being solved. Is there any doubt as to the pattern of choice?

In summary, alcoholism is an unsuccessful attempt to solve a problem. The use of alcohol has some generic roots in personality development and reinforcement during life experiences. The relevant key concepts to the understanding of alcoholism are withdrawal and compulsion. Therapeutic intervention is focused upon replacing the destructive withdrawal-compulsive pattern used in alcoholism with the constructive problem-solving pattern.

An implication for further clinical investigation is the use of the problem-solving approach for therapeutic intervention in other maneuvers involving the withdrawal-compulsive component, e.g., drug addiction.

## BIBLIOGRAPHY

ENGLISH, HORACE B., and ENGLISH, AVA C., *A Comprehensive Dictionary of Psychological and Psychoanalytical Terms*, Longmans, Green and Co., New York: 1958.

MARSHALL, MARGARET A., "Operational Definition of Problem-Solving," unpublished paper, College of Nursing, Rutgers, The State University of New Jersey, 1958.

NOYES, ARTHUR P., *Modern Clinical Psychiatry*, W. B. Saunders Co., Philadelphia: 1953.

RICHTER, DOROTHEA, "Operational Definition of Compulsion," unpublished paper, College of Nursing, Rutgers, The State University of New Jersey, 1956.

ROUSLIN, SHEILA, "Operationl Definition of Problem-Solving," unpublished paper, College of Nursing, Rutgers, The State University of New Jersey, 1959.

SULLIVAN, HARRY STACK, *Clinical Studies in Psychiatry*, W. W. Norton & Co., New York: 1956.

———— *Conceptions of Modern Psychiatry*, W. W. Norton & Co., New York: 1953.

———— *The Interpersonal Theory of Psychiatry*, W. W. Norton & Co., New York: 1953.

ZWERLING, ISRAEL, and ROSENBAUM, MILTON, "Alcoholic Addiction and Personality," in *American Handbook of Psychiatry*, Silvano Arieti (ed.), Basic Books, New York: 1959.

# 28 LISTENING FOR THEMES

*Alice A. H. Hadley*

The necessity for skills in listening was pointed out statistically in 1929 by Paul T. Rankin, supervising director of research and adjustment for the Detroit public schools. Rankin's study of the personal communication of 68 people in different occupations indicated that 75 per cent of his subjects' waking days were spent in verbal communication. Of this total, 9 per cent was spent in writing, 16 per cent in reading, 30 per cent in speaking, and 45 per cent in listening.[1] More recently, Nichols and Stevens [2] concluded that immediately after the average person has listened to someone talk, he remembers only half of what he heard, no matter how carefully he thought he had listened. However, Nichols and Stevens also found that in classes given in listening at the University of Minnesota, every group of students averaged better than a 25 per cent gain in listening skill.

Some general suggestions for improving listening skills are (1) reducing environmental distractions, (2) finding an area of interest in what is being said, (3) judging the content of the speech rather than the mode of delivery, (4) listening to the entire speech before planning a rebuttal, (5) working at listening by keeping an open mind in regard to emotionally charged words, and (6) developing flexible systems of note-taking. However, the most useful suggestion for improving listening skill seems to be looking for the central *idea* or *theme* of what is being said.

[1] Zelko, H. P., "The Art of Listening," p. 27.
[2] Nichols, R., and Stevens, L. A., *Are You Listening*, p. 5.

Peplau [3] defines a theme as, "a generalization, a summarizing characteristic, an abstraction of an event that actually consists of many details
best summarized by this theme." A theme can be considered in terms of a
single event, or in terms of a pattern that recurs throughout several events.
In a continuing nurse-patient relationship there may be several outstanding
themes for which the nurse can listen.

Various benefits accrue from this listening for themes. Peplau identifies
several. First, getting at the themes of interaction enables the nurse to
find out qualitatively what is going on between her and the patient. The
details of a situation are observed in such a way as to make inferences
about the situation. When the nurse validates her inferences with the
patient, the situation may become amenable to control. Awareness of
what is going on may lead the nurse and the patient toward shifts in the
way they interact in future situations.

Themes provide for economical communication of the total event.
When the theme is known, details can easily be recalled to expand and
clarify whatever needs to be remembered. If two situations are to be compared, the process is greatly facilitated by comparing total impressions
rather than details.

Themes can provide a frame of reference. That is, when past interpersonal themes are known, they can be used to study present relations.
The nurse can determine whether her present responses are reinforcing or
interfering with patterns laid down in the patient's previous experience.

Peplau also indicates that listening for themes gives the nurse an opportunity to use her reasoning capacities. She formulates concepts from
past and present observations, and from these infers the consequences of
present actions in the foreseeable future. She uses these inferences to foster
favorable changes.

A recurring theme abstracted by the nurse through listening to patient
J.P. in a psychiatric setting was in the nature of what he did not say. J.P.
vividly described his wife's actions as they figured in his hospitalization and
gave a blow-by-blow account of her behavior as an alcoholic. He omitted
any statements of his role in these situations.

Another theme discerned by listening was patient J.W.'s pattern of
giving. In the first interview, J.W. related to the nurse how he gave away
his occupational-therapy projects. In following interviews he mentioned
giving away cigarettes, although this was against the rules of the ward,
and giving away his mother's gifts of fruit and candy because he "just

[3] Peplau, H. E., "Themes in Nursing Situations," p. 1221.

didn't feel in the spirit of eating them." Thereupon, he attempted to give the nurse cookies and gum. The nurse discussed giving of gifts, both in terms of the nurse's giving of gifts and the patient's giving of gifts, with a nursing consultant. Several hypotheses were formulated:

(1) The giving of tokens by the nurse tends to anchor the relationship to a reward-punishment level of operation. It can prevent an investigative approach to the patient's problems from developing in the nurse.

(2) The giving of tokens by the nurse may invite interference in the interview by other patients when the interview is conducted on a ward.

(3) The demand for tokens by the patient may grow with succeeding interviews.

(4) The giving of tokens by the nurse may allow for autistic invention by the patient as to the reason(s) they are given.

(5) In the early phases of a nurse-patient relationship, gift-giving can create a social, rather than a therapeutic, atmosphere.

(6) If the patient has a pattern of giving, the nurse's acceptance of his gifts reinforces this pattern.

(7) In the early stages of the relationship, the giving of tokens can establish a pseudocloseness.

(8) If the patient has a pattern of giving, refusal of his gifts may cue nonautomatic behavior and permit investigation of the need for giving.

(9) The acceptance or refusal of patient's gifts by the nurse is an individual matter depending on the total content of the nurse-patient relationship.

Once a recurring theme such as giving is identified in listening to a patient, the next steps are discernment of the generic roots of the pattern, the purposes served by the pattern, and the relationship between the generic roots and the purposes.

Twenty-two-year-old J.W., whose father was dead, went out on a pass each week end with his mother. His mother spent the time talking with the neighbors at their homes; J.W. sat at home listening to the radio. J.W. related one of their infrequent conversations as, "She was polite to me and everything, but we ain't got no understanding. She talks about fixing up the place, drilling a new well, buying storm doors. She's always talking about the house." However, after each week end, J.W. returned from his visit with fruit, candy, cigarettes, and spending money which he promptly gave to other patients on his ward. The nurse speculated that J.W.'s giving might be an imitative pattern of his mother. The mother did not give of herself, but gave material things. J.W. developed this pattern for the purpose of winning approval or getting close to others.

In summary, a need exists to improve listening skills. Of the various methods for accomplishing the task, listening for themes in an event or series of events seems to be the most useful. Getting at themes in an interpersonal situation may enable the nurse to qualitatively find out what is going on between her and the patient. Themes can also provide for economical communication of a total event, facilitate comparison of two situations, and provide a frame of reference for studying present and future situations in terms of what went on in the past. Finally, the abstraction of themes gives the nurse an opportunity to exercise her reasoning and conceptualizing capacities. Two recurring themes, J.W.'s giving and J.P.'s leaving out his role, have been stated as they occurred in nurse-patient relationships.

## BIBLIOGRAPHY

BROWN, JAMES I., "The Measurement of Listening Ability," *School and Society*, 79:69–71, 1951.

"Can't Talk and Listen Both," *Science News Letter*, June 14, 1952.

GARRET, W. VAN, "Do You Ever Stop To Listen," *American Mercury*, Vol. 83, No. 394, November, 1956.

MERSAND, JOSEPH, "Why Teach Listening," English J., 40:260–65, 1951.

NICHOLS, RALPH G., and STEVENS, LEONARD A., *Are You Listening*, McGraw-Hill Book Co., New York: 1957.

PEPLAU, HILDEGARD E., *Interpersonal Relations in Nursing*, G. P. Putnam's Sons, New York: 1952.

———— "Themes in Nursing Situations," *Am. J. Nursing*, Vol. 53, No. 10, October, 1953.

REIK, THEODOR, *Listening With a Third Ear*, Grove Press, New York: 1948.

"Rules for Good Listening," *Science Digest*, 38:34, 1955.

STROMER, W. F., "Listening: How?" *English J.*, Vol. 41, June, 1952.

SULLIVAN, HARRY STACK, *The Psychiatric Interview*, W. W. Norton & Co., New York: 1954.

WYNN, D. R., "Good Listener," *J. Nat. Education*, Vol. 44, November, 1953.

ZELKO, H. P., "Art of Listening," *Rotarian*, 87:27, 1955.

# 29 HOPELESSNESS[1]

*Margaret A. Marshall*

What is hopelessness? What does it stem from? How can it be dealt with in the psychiatric hospital? The need to find answers to these questions arose during an educational experience in intensive nurse-patient relationships; it arose again during an experience in group work. Both experiences occurred in large mental hospitals.

What is hopelessness? Hopelessness has been variously defined in the very limited literature on this subject. Most definitions suggest that it is an absence of hope rather than the presence of a profoundly depressing feeling. Webster's *Dictionary* states that it is synonymous with despairing. Horney[2] states that hopelessness is the ultimate product of unresolved conflicts, with the deepest roots in the despair of ever being wholehearted and undivided. Gravenkemper[3] views hopelessness as "a looking forward to (an event or occurrence) with the deeply held belief that the anticipated will not occur."

What does hopelessness come from? There can be at least three, and undoubtedly more, origins of this feeling. The first origin occurs within the patient. Patients who are leaving the hospital after a first admission generally leave with a true feeling of lightheartedness and optimism. Subsequent readmissions, however, tend to alter the patient's attitude concerning his potential for survival in his family, his community, and his job

[1] This is a modification of an article of the same title which was published in *Nursing World*, Vol. 133, No. 8, August, 1959.
[2] Horney, K., *Our Inner Conflicts*, p. 183.
[3] Gravenkemper, K. H., "Two Instruments to Inventory and Classify Problems," p. 16.

situation. Rather than optimism, he leaves the hospital with what can best be termed "guarded pessimism"—guarded to the extent that the patient views his community stay as diminishing in length with each discharge. The patient leaves with the thought which can be summed: "Well here I go again. How long this time?" The thought is present at the time of departure that he will return for more care.

The second origin of hopelessness is within the family. Many people leave the hospital or a psychotherapeutic relationship with a private counselor before they are ready to sustain themselves in their interpersonal relationships with others without supportive care. The attitudinal changes in the family, then, are not notably different from those that occur within the patient. Many examples of this pessimistic attitude can be excerpted from nurse-patient data. Among these are the following:

Mrs. Jones has been hospitalized briefly following the birth of her second child, a girl, who was born less than a year after the birth of her first child. Within three weeks after the second delivery, she began to manifest symptoms of depression and stated that she neither could nor would care for these two infants without help. Mr. Jones tried to reassure her that she was capable of the task. He was obviously mistaken, for the following day he returned from work to find both infants howling and Mrs. Jones sitting in a chair, still in her nightgown and apparently oblivious of her crying babies. Her doctor was called. He advised hospitalization immediately, which was done.

Following an eight-week hospitalization, Mrs. Jones was "discharged as improved" and had no unsurmountable difficulties for over three years. During that time, she delivered her third child, after which she was cared for by a private counselor. With the advent of her fourth pregnancy, she became openly hostile toward her husband. She became so threatening toward him that she was hospitalized during the sixth month of the pregnancy. The child was born during the hospitalization.

When the infant was four months old, Mrs. Jones was sent home on an extendible pass, but reacted toward her family in such a way that her husband returned her to the hospital. Details of her behavior were not available, but she was retained for an additional period at the hospital. It was after this discharge that her husband began to comment, to her counselor and her family, in the presence of Mrs. Jones, "I just want her to stay well until the kids are in school, then I can manage the household while she is hospitalized, which, of course, she will be."

Attitude of another family was stated directly by a female patient as follows:

After the first time here all was okay but then I had an argument with Joe [the patient's huband] and I came back as a voluntary admission. While I was here, my mother-in-law moved in to the flat downstairs to take care of the children. Now when I'm home, if I raise my voice to the kids or to Joe, she runs upstairs with her "watch her Joe—she's slipping again" and I have troubles. Why is it that every wife can argue with her husband but me? Every couple has disagreements, but I'm not allowed because I've been a patient. This is unreasonable. I'm supposed to be a mat for everyone to walk on because one raised voice from me and my mother-in-law runs to tell Joe that I'm flipping my wig again. Isn't that crazy?

The third source of hopelessness is with personnel who provide care during hospitalization. It seems that this source is the one that must be corrected, since personnel do, wittingly or unwittingly, convey their personal attitude concerning the patient to both the patient and his family. It is possible that findings of research in this matter would highlight the fact that personnel are major contributors to the attitudinal changes in the family, which then have an impact on the patient's potential for community survival.

You can recognize the presence of a feeling of hopelessness at times when you go into a strange hospital. Hopelessness is looking forward to success, but anticipating failure. After about ten minutes of conversation with personnel, the hopelessness is communicated, either verbally or empathically. "These people never get well, so why try to do more than keep them happy, clean, and fed," the personnel seem to say. In other words, they would provide only custodial care.

On the other hand, you can enter another hospital and find a feeling of hope conveyed. The patients recover, go home, and stay at home with no problems with the family, community, or job. The goal of the personnel is to work together with the patient to expedite the therapeutic process and get the patient home. Could it possibly be true, then, that hopelessness is a problem, not only with the patient, but also with those who work with him?

In an individual nurse-patient relationship, hopelessness arose first after several weeks of work with the following patient, and in a unique way. To protect the identity of the patient involved, she will be called Anne.

Anne had been hospitalized about two and a half years when the relationship began. It was not her first admission to the hospital, she had been in and out of hospitals for about fifteen years. Anne had been on home visit for about one year of the two and a half years of the present admission and had been employed most of that time. The patient was unable to account for her return to the hospital after the leave, but thought it was the usual procedure to return and be examined thoroughly before being discharged permanently.

Anne had a mother who was living and a son who was married while she was hospitalized. The son, daughter-in-law, and mother lived together in a town about thirty miles from the hospital and visited the patient regularly once every month. The mother had been promising to take Anne home for a week end. No definite time had been set for the visit, but Anne expected that it would be at Thanksgiving. However, the family failed to visit during November and the week end was put off, by the patient, to Christmas. This was confirmed by the family when they came to visit early in December.

The patient was visited by the staff doctor, and during the course of the conversation, they discussed Anne's progress and the possibility of instituting week-end visits to her family and home. When the doctor proposed to present the patient to staff for approval of the visits, Anne said, "I am well enough to go home week ends, but not yet well enough for an indefinite stay. I do want to go, but I will come back and continue the process with the staff and 'my' nurse until I am completely well." Week-end visits were then approved by the staff.

In relating this conversation to the nurse, Anne verbalized the belief that her previous home visit had been unsuccessful because she had not completely recovered from her illness. She said that she was willing to remain for therapy this time in an attempt to ensure success when discharged from the hospital.

There had been no hint of hopelessness in the relationship up to this point. Then the precipitating event occurred. The mother wrote to Anne that the son and daughter-in-law had adopted a baby, and for that reason would be unable to have Anne at home for a week end. In her letter Anne's mother said that Anne should make up her mind that the hospital was the only home that she could ever expect to have. After all, Anne's mother wrote, she (the mother) was too old to cope with Anne and a new baby at the same time!

"This is a hopeless situation," Anne declared. "What do you do when the family breaks a promise? And when the staff has approved me for home visits? I've been replaced by an infant, a total stranger, in my own home! They'd rather have a baby than me."

All participation in activities ceased. Anne consistently failed to carry out her ward assignment—watering the plants—which would have taken about ten minutes each day. She then became physically ill and was transferred to a sick ward, where she remained for two weeks. After returning to her own ward, the relationship was weighed down with hopelessness. The patient moved backward rapidly to her psychotic state. "Why bother to get well," she reasoned. "I'm never going home anyway."

These problems were worked with for several weeks, with no obvious progress. The patient still failed to do her assignment or go to activities. The nurse then sought expert advice and guidance; she received both. It was then a matter of waiting for the subject to come up again in the next session. And it did.

"If you were in my place, what would you do? My family won't have me at home. My mother said so. The doctor should force them to take me as soon as I am well," Anne said. "What would you do?"

"I cannot put myself in your place, Anne," I answered. "I lack your experience; I can only speculate. I think, though, I'd get so well it would be perfectly obvious that I didn't need hospital care any longer. Then anyone could look at me and say, 'She doesn't belong here.' After that some arrangement could be made to send me either to my own home or to a foster home."

Anne considered this suggestion for about three weeks and finally decided that it would work. She started by carrying out her ward assignment faithfully; eventually she resumed all activities. Hopelessness did not come up for discussion again in the relationship, and good progress was made by the patient. Such good progress, in fact, that Anne was approved for home care three months later. The family had not yet called for the patient when the relationship terminated, but this patient was ready to go home. The problem had been worked through and solved.

It is not suggested that all hopelessness can be handled in the same way. The nurse should work under expert supervision and guidance. She should seek expert advice and follow it as long as she continues to work intensively with patients.

The relationship discussed above lasted for eight months. During that time the patient was seen regularly for one hour in the morning, three days a week, for five months; then two days a week for three months.

Interest in nurse-patient relationships has increased in recent years. Doctors have verbalized a willingness to supervise and guide those nurses who are willing to enter into a one-to-one relationship with patients or to work with groups of patients.

Supervision and guidance are illustrated in the National League for Nursing–Smith, Kline and French Company film, "Nurse-Patient Relationship." As long as mental illness remains a major health problem, the assistance of all the health professions should be utilized. The nurse is surely a member of the health team and might as well participate actively in helping all other members of the health team in the fight to prevent and to cure mental illness.

The hopelessness which arose during a group-work experience was similar, yet in some ways different. The hopelessness of Bill's situation was communicated to the group by the attendant, who said, "He's a hopeless case! Bill can't talk. He'll never go home. Do what you want, but after all, these patients are ten per cent mentally ill, and the other ninety per cent are just plain crazy. Bill is one of the 'just plain crazy' ones."

The nurses working with the group saw Bill for one hour each week. He was not verbal at the beginning, but was given support and encouragement. He was told repeatedly that he could talk when he felt safer and a little less anxious in the situation. The nurse sat quietly with Bill, speaking softly to him about the weather, the ward activities, and his fellow patients.

After three hours of this one-sided conversation, Bill was comfortable enough with the nurse to start talking with her about his fears, his problems, and his family. He related the conversations of the personnel about himself and other patients. He knew he was considered hopeless. They said he couldn't talk—so he didn't. He could, though, if he wanted to, he explained.

The attendants were, needless to say, impressed with this relationship and its outcome. When it terminated, the personnel showed signs of having learned, by demonstration, that it wasn't really true that 90 per cent of these patients are just plain crazy.

Perhaps nurses should all do more teaching by demonstration in order to clear up some of the misconceptions about mental illness. It may also be a good cure for some of the hopelessness, which is one of the most common problems in mental hospitals at the present time. Hopelessness, which comes from the patient, the family, and hospital personnel, is a heavy burden to the patient.

## BIBLIOGRAPHY

GRAVENKEMPER, KATHERINE HEPP, "Two Instruments to Inventory and Classify Problems," unpublished master's thesis, Graduate School, Rutgers, The State University of New Jersey, 1957.

HORNEY, KAREN, *Our Inner Conflicts*, W. W. Norton & Co., New York: 1945.

WOLBERG, LEWIS R., *The Technique of Psychotherapy*, Grune & Stratton, New York: 1954.

# 30 LONELINESS

*Claire G. Francel*

Of all the subjective states of mental illness, loneliness, perhaps, is the one most productive of psychic pain. Fortunately, relatively few people experience it during their lives. Some persons, unable to tolerate the continued presence of loneliness, choose suicide in preference to a lonely life. Others lessen its horror by the invention of a private fantasy world and the companionship of hallucinatory figures. All those unhappy people who pursue the neurotic way of life are acquainted with loneliness. By various defensive maneuvers, they handle its presence and are more or less miserable according to the success or failure of these psychic dynamisms of defense.

Loneliness is in essence the inability to love, combined with a negation of being; or to describe it otherwise, the lonely person has the terrifying experience of being unable to conceptualize himself as real, i.e. having existence. This is both a cognitive and affective unconscious dynamism; it is out of the person's awareness.

He literally does not know that he is. In order to love, one must first have knowledge of a beloved. This learning has never been accomplished by the lonely one. In examining the root of loneliness, one can trace in the childhood development the omission of this learning so basic to the foundation of a healthy personality. In infancy the human organism perceives through his senses a differentiation of objects in the environment and makes explorative attempts to investigate their essence, i.e., that which makes them what they are. Then, he can encounter opposition and punishment which cause the explorative activity to be experienced as dan-

178—

gerous and conducive to an unpleasant affective state that we call anxiety. If the child, in his attempts to examine his own body, again encounters the disapproving reaction from human beings in the immediate environment, he again experiences this drop in euphoria, anxiety. The child may then avoid further investigation. A sense of mystery remains about certain aspects of himself. Further, if interpersonal contacts impressed upon the child that in order to avoid anxiety he must act as others wish him to act, he again is denied the opportunity of learning what his own desires are. As a result, more aspects of his identity remain unknown. He becomes what others wish him to be, and unconsciously substitutes a drive for approval (unknown quantity) for love of self (unknown quantity). From such a dynamic pattern, one can understand how this child takes cues for behavior from the environment and knows himself only in the reflective appraisal of significant people.

Throughout the growing process, these people believe themselves to be unloved by others, even though they have been loved. They do not recognize love when given. Because of their own inability to love, tenderness on the part of others to them, often makes them intensely anxious. They experience a sense of unreality and deep loneliness.

As Peplau [1] has so well described it, these persons use many patterns of behavior to alleviate the anxiety and reduce the experience of loneliness: submission, imitation, worship of others, rebellion, anger, or lawbreaking produce responses of approval or disapproval from other people. The lonely one becomes familiar with handling such responses of others, and these may temporarily reduce the anxiety he experiences in interpersonal relationships. However, this never actually aids him in learning how to love himself, nor does it increase the awareness of his own existence (the sense of self).

When the above-described adaptive behavior fails, and it inevitably does, the intensely unpleasant experience of loneliness arises and reoccurs to haunt the person. He is truly faced with an existential crisis. As Shakespeare wrote, "To be or not to be. That is the question." Every year a certain number of people in society decide "not to be." These are the people who are successful in suicide attempts; they have resolved the dilemma of loneliness by taking positive action to end their lives. However, before the suicide attempt, the majority have indicated to society openly or subtly their intentions and the loneliness that motivates the destructive act. These attempts to communicate often trigger off anxiety in the listener, who reacts by withdrawal, ignoring, pretending the whole

[1] Peplau, H. E., "Loneliness."

situation does not exist—patterns of behavior that merely reinforce the sense of unreality in the lonely one.

If a suicide attempt has failed, the person may be jailed, hospitalized, or ostracized, according to the laws of the state. Whatever happens, he is usually blamed for wrongdoing, and his guilt and loneliness increase. Rarely does this dramatic cry for help procure skilled attention and understanding.

In this chapter, the writer examines ways in which loneliness is mishandled unwittingly and ways in which it can be eradicated through therapy.

The person committed to a mental hospital finds often that his loneliness is increased rather than relieved by being institutionalized. The basic dynamic of not knowing himself is often accentuated. One patient repeated over and over, "All I want is an understanding. What am I doing here? How did I get here?" Frequently, complaints voiced by patients in group work were: "No one tells you anything here. I ask a question; the nurse says 'ask the doctor.' I never see one. The last time I talked with one he said, 'What do you think?' . . . What did I do wrong? How does one get well? I try to cooperate, maybe if I do more work, I can get out."

The following excerpt from a group meeting describes the dilemma the lonely person encounters:

> *Patient:* I've been here five months. What is going to happen to me? I look around—these people are worse off than I am—I don't want to be here ten years and become like them. There is no one to talk with. The staff won't tell you anything. I have to figure out things for myself alone, and sometimes I get crazy thoughts, and what horrifies me is that I'm beginning to believe them.
> *Leader:* What are these thoughts like?
> *Patient:* That people are deliberately keeping me here; like even you two want to have me stay here for good.

This girl was attempting to resolve the not-knowing by means of autistic invention and, perhaps, developing the paranoid stage of schizophrenia.

In order to avoid the loneliness, she would substitute an unvalidated, erroneous conclusion that might reduce the anxiety, ease the terror of loneliness, but certainly prevented insight.

How hospital staff members unwittingly contribute to the sense of unreality in the patient is seen in the content of conversations between the staff and the patients. Pretending or ignoring are two patterns used by many staff nurses and attendants that add to patient's loneliness. Only "safe" topics are discussed, e.g., the weather, hobbies, movies, ward housekeeping, physical illness, the dances. These are preferred to discussions of problems in living which make the staff anxious. Subjects that are taboo in some wards are mental illness, mental health, anger, and anxiety. Thus, we see an air of mystery surrounds the whole area of mental health. Getting well, to many patients, is a magical process accompanying a resurgence of physical strength. Some patients interpret avoidance of the topic of mental health on the part of the ward staff as an indication that it is too terrible to mention: it is unspeakable and a disgrace.

In one of the group sessions, one patient emphasized that she had come to the hospital for treatment of a cold. It was a mistake, but she acted "good" here and did what she was told. In another group one patient said to another: "Confess, what did you do wrong that they put you here? Have you learned your lesson?" The patient saying this identified strongly with the staff and had been given ward responsibilities that allowed her to exercise power over other patients. To the patient who remembers no wrongdoing, the sense of unreality is magnified by what he perceives as mystery.

The idea that the mental hospital is a place of punishment like a jail is furthered by the "locked doors." One morning as this writer sat with a silent patient, one of the hospital aides walked by swinging in a wide arc a chain with about twenty keys attached. These keys jangled as he passed by. The reaction of patients was observed as the aide passed. Two patients shrank back into the chairs. A few patients stared in a fascinated manner at the keys. The silent patient turned and looked at me with a gaze of such despair that I turned away from those eyes until I could control my own anxiety.

Much emphasis is placed on cooperating, adjusting, getting along with others, conforming, and not making noise. Rewards are attached to "good" behavior on some wards. The "good" patients have coffee in the morning. The "workers" get extra food on one ward where the ward sociology was observed for four months. These controlling maneuvers of the staff are a repetition of approval-disapproval structured behavior that earlier in the life of the patient prevented learning and encouraged only adaptive living. This approval-disapproval pattern thwarts attempts to gain meaningful insight on the part of the patient; all it teaches the patient are the needs and wishes of the staff. Again, the individual's own desires are denied. In such a setting, one wonders if the lonely one will ever develop a sense of self?

Dramatic changes in behavior as a result of new learnings can replace loneliness with the states of peace and integrity of the personality. Group therapy seems especially conducive to this. Description of work that was done with a nonhospitalized group that met one hour a week for ten months follows: This period of time seemed to be a minimum amount needed for effective results. Establishment of skills and tools for continuance of the learning process after therapy was achieved in this time. Sixteen females participated. During the orientation phase, the leader outlined the rules or limitations that the group must abide by. They were three: (1) Each member is to speak in a spontaneous fashion, i.e., say immediately what comes into her thoughts without censoring it. (2) Each member who raises a problem is to discuss only her own behavior and refer to others only as they affect her behavior. The group will aid her only by questions; she does her own interpreting. (3) New behavior is to be tested between meetings and results reported to the group.

It took about two months to overcome resistance of the majority of group members, although resistance persisted in some members a couple of months longer. When the group entered the working phase, several stages in therapy became outlined.

1. The first stage of the group work was an examination of current and recurring behavior patterns by the group member; this involved a description of how she operated in interpersonal situations. Questions from other members, such as "Who gets you up in the morning?" "What do you dislike in other people?" "What situations make you most anxious?" proved advantageous to the person attempting to describe her own behavior. Often, the content discovered by the patient as she outlined the behavior was surprising and disconcerting. It was usually the first time that she had attempted to describe the type of life she lived.

2. The second stage was an attempt to discover the roots for present patterns. Childhood memories were re-examined and explored. Group members were often startled at the discovery that what had been thought a unique event in their lives had been undergone by other members.

3. The third stage was the expression of likes and dislikes toward key figures in the patient's life. Here, long-buried hostility and aggression toward relatives and friends were ventilated. Acceptance of the presence of hostility as it came into awareness allowed previously suppressed guilt feelings to emerge. While going through this stage, one girl, who had repressed anger at her mother for years, said that she had packed her bags and threatened to leave home when her mother asked her to mail a letter. Later, she laughed at the disproportion of her response to the little request. During this stage, the release of hostility in great amounts occurs. At this point, everyone is blamed by the patient for her unhappiness.

4. The fourth stage begins after the patient has tested new behavior, released hostility in small amounts, begun to assert her own wishes, and discontinued much of the approval-getting behavior. During this time, she receives support from group members and has begun to like herself. At this stage, the person takes a look at how the situations that resulted in loneliness came about. She now examines how she invited unhappiness; what her contributions to anxiety-producing relationships were. Alternative modes of behavior are examined and often the group member is able to point out what neurotic gains she achieved by acting in the chosen behavior. It is at this stage that insights are achieved. Remarks occurred such as, "Why didn't I ever see that before? It was needless. . . . I certainly acted as if I wanted to be rejected, didn't I?"

5. The fifth stage was the one in which appropriate love objects were chosen, and new behavior tried out in loving relationships with others. Once the group member had developed awareness and knowledge of self, and if support from the group had been adequate, a healthy love for self had developed. With the new learning, the person was now prepared to relate to others in respectful loving relationships. Needless to say, loneliness, an original learning defect, had been eliminated.

## BIBLIOGRAPHY

MERTON, THOMAS, *Seeds of Contemplation*, Dell Publishing Co., New York: 1948.
PEPLAU, HILDEGARD E., "Loneliness," *Am. J. Nursing*, 55(11):1426, 1955.
SULLIVAN, HARRY STACK, *The Interpersonal Theory of Psychiatry*, W. W. Norton & Co., New York: 1953.
————— *Clinical Studies in Psychiatry*, W. W. Norton & Co., New York: 1956.
ZILBOORG, GREGORY, "Loneliness," *Atlantic Monthly*, **161**:45-54, 1938.

# 31 HALLUCINATIONS[1]

*Katherine H. Gravenkemper*

> Another person's hallucinations may seem humorous to some people, but nurses cannot afford to deal so lightly with the problem.

Many jokes have been told about the psychiatric patient who thinks he is Napoleon, hears voices from God or talks to people who aren't there. Perhaps one of the reasons for these jokes is that the experience of a hallucination is so foreign to us; it is something we cannot understand and it makes us anxious. Perhaps joking about it alleviates the uncomfortable feeling that thinking about it causes.

While this may be an effective maneuver for most people, the professional person in a psychiatric setting cannot laugh at hallucinations and summarily dismiss them. The nurse must understand the why, when, and how of hallucinations and then find adequate means of handling them before she can expect to help the patient.

This chapter is written on the assumption that to know about a certain phenomenon reduces one's fear, dread, and anxiety when faced with the phenomenon, and that measures can then be taken to correct, remove, or change the phenomenon.

To understand hallucinations we must begin with the self-system of the individual. This self-concept is the way the individual sees himself and the way he believes other people see him. It has its roots in early childhood, where it is elaborated and maintained through the appraisals of significant people in the child's life. These appraisals become internalized. Sullivan[2] says the self-system is made up of these "reflected appraisals." It contains those things in his personality for which he received approval from adults

[1] Originally published in *Nursing World*, Vol. 132, No. 6, July, 1958.
[2] Sullivan, H. S., *The Interpersonal Theory of Psychiatry*, p. 161.

(the good-me), those for which he received disapproval (the bad-me), and all other things in the personality which, when expressed, were neither approved nor disapproved—the not-me. To these aspects of the self, the individual refuses awareness, does not notice. These impulses, desires, and needs become dissociated from the self.[3] This is the not-me. These dissociated impulses, desires, and needs are discharged in unnoticed acts when the self is functioning smoothly.[4] But during panic, this self-system receives a mortal blow and becomes disorganized. More correctly, the total personality is disorganized and must reorganize (reintegrate) as quickly as possible in any way that it can. Usually this is a state of terror. It is at this point that the individual comes to the reality of dissociated components in his personality—the not-me phase of the self-concept.

Sullivan states that since one of the complex functions of the self-system is to defend itself from the knowledge of these dissociated impulses, desires, and needs, this revelation of dissociated motivations is accompanied by feelings of revulsion and suspicion. He further states that the next step in this process is the "noticed activity of one of the zones of interaction (auditory, visual, oral, etc.) as the expression of a dissociated system." In other words, the individual hears voices, statements, or experiences other events, which seem foreign to him, but are actually the expression of the dissociated part of the self-system.[5]

This is the theoretical basis of hallucinations. But how do hallucinations operate? Every normal person can hear his own thoughts because thoughts are generally expressed internally by auditory verbal images. As one patient jokingly put it, "It's all right to hear voices, but not to answer them." This patient, of course, was referring to actual hallucinations, but his comment aptly illustrates our statement that we all hear our own thoughts but do not "answer them."

The individual whose dissociated motivations have been brought to the level of awareness has revealed to himself a hitherto dissociated part of himself over which he has no control. Because of the perceptual quality of his thoughts, he is afraid that people around him will hear his thoughts and his "real" self will be revealed to the world.

In the next phase, the individual still recognizes these thoughts as his own, but he also believes that others can read these thoughts. He begins to hear others repeat (steal) his thoughts verbally. This must produce an uncanny sensation. As one patient described the experience, "It's frighten-

---

[3] *Ibid., Conceptions of Modern Psychiatry,* p. 23.
[4] *Ibid.,* p. 138.
[5] *Ibid., The Interpersonal Theory of Psychiatry,* p. 360.

ing, I like my privacy. It seems rude to invade anyone's privacy. How did he know what I was thinking?"

Finally, the individual no longer recognizes the thoughts as his own and projects them completely to others. The individual projects everything that is painful or causes anxiety. In other words, he puts distance between himself and the unpleasant phenomenon.[6] One patient verbalized this very succinctly when he said, "I try to escape these thoughts that I receive, especially those that are the memory of bad language that you hear. I have a very strong feeling that these are not really my own thoughts."

How does the nurse deal with the patient who has hallucinations? How should she respond? How can she best make this a learning experience for herself and the patient?

First of all, she should realize hallucinations are real experiences of the patient. Whether anyone else can see or hear these figures is immaterial; the fact that they are experienced by the patient makes them real for him. It is, therefore, a problem within the realm of nursing care. It should also be remembered that the patient's first experience with an hallucination is deeply disturbing. The nurse will probably only meet this kind of hallucination on acute admission wards. Since I have had no experience with patients hallucinating for the first time, I cannot suggest any methods of dealing with them; undoubtedly, the patient at this time needs complete acceptance, a feeling of understanding and support, more than anything else.

Later in the illness, hallucinations may become commonplace to the patient and about as important as ordinary conversation. They fill a need the patient has been unable to fill in any other way. Various patients have described the needs in these ways: "There are patients on this ward who have actually gone out of their minds to communicate, so they manufacture little people. I think it must be loneliness." Or, "When I don't know what to say to you, I talk to them." (This patient had developed a pattern of talking with hallucinatory figures whenever she became anxious.) Another patient who used hallucinations in order not to feel lonely declared, "Don't say I'm lonely, how could I possibly be? I have all these children, and if they die off, I just make more."

From this, we can formulate the guiding principle that the patient who hallucinates has a strong need to believe in the reality of the hallucination. We also may hypothesize that the patient will not begin to doubt the reality of the hallucination until the need that the hallucination is fulfilling has begun to be met in some other way. To discover the purpose

[6] Arieti, S., *Interpretation of Schizophrenia*, pp. 243-53, 299.

of the hallucination and to satisfy the need in another way are the functions of the nurse.

But how does the nurse do this? And how can she control her own anxiety? More important, what can she say to the patient when she obviously can neither see nor hear the hallucination? Probably the first rule the nurse should keep in mind is to convey the idea to the patient that she cannot see or hear these things, but that she is willing to learn as much about them as the patient will tell her. When I arrived on the ward one morning, a patient very sociably pointed to her hallucinatory figures and said, "I think you know all these people." I answered, "No, I don't. I only know what you tell me about them. What are they doing?"

The patient went on to name them, describe them, and tell why they were there. By my action, I conveyed to the patient the fact that I accepted these figures as very real people to her, but at the same time I maintained my separate identity by admitting that I could not see them.

It should also be remembered that it is very unlikely that the patient distinguishes these hallucinatory voices from real voices. He may become angry with you for interrupting. This is easily handled, if the foregoing step has been well established, by simply stating you did not know that they were talking.

In the beginning, all the nurse's efforts should be directed toward getting the patient to describe his experiences and then gradually establishing the reason for the use of hallucinations. Once this is established, it leads to valuable clues in interpreting other data that the patient reveals.

A typical conversation may follow this pattern:

Nurse: How come you've spent so much time talking with your children [hallucinations] today?
Patient: Was I doing it much? I must be uncomfortable.
Nurse: Uncomfortable?
Patient: Yes, I didn't want to talk about Mrs. S., as we did yesterday.

Finally, when the patient's anxiety has been reduced enough, when he is comfortable with the nurse, and their relationship is well established, the day will come when the following conversation may be heard:

Patient: I've had enough! I don't want to hear any more!
Nurse: Hear any more?
Patient: Yes, voices. It's sort of hard to discuss with anyone because they're just voices, but I need them. How else am I going to manage alone?

This is the time for the nurse to move in and suggest and discuss other ways of handling the feelings that arouse the hallucinations. But, the events leading up to this point do not occur overnight; they take months of patient listening, acceptance, and description. And even when the patient has reached this point, he may temporarily backslide because the thought of living without these hallucinations is as frightening as the first experience of hallucination was. But if the relationship with the nurse has been one in which any problem can be discussed, this, too, can be gradually overcome.

The next step is taken when the patient begins to edit these experiences himself and starts to distinguish the real experiences from hallucinatory experiences. One patient in this phase said, "Write that down, it sounds right. The other, before, was a little ticklish. I thought that's what happened, but I'm not sure any more." The task of the nurse now is to help the patient distinguish for himself just what is reality and what is hallucination.

Finally, when the needs for the hallucination have been met in a non-hallucinatory manner, the hallucinations will gradually disappear altogether. One precaution: One of the major reasons for the disappearance of hallucinations is that the patient has found that he can communicate with someone. That someone, in this case, has been the nurse. Before terminating the relationship, the nurse should be sure that the patient's ability to communicate has been expanded to include others.

A hallucination is an inner experience expressed as though it were an outer event. It arises out of the dissociated motivations of the self-system and is an uncanny, yet real, experience for the person. Nursing procedure for these patients consists of accepting the hallucination as a real experience to the patient, while not participating in the pathology, and helping the patient to find the reasons, the need, for the hallucination.

## BIBLIOGRAPHY

ARIETI, SILVANO, *Interpretation of Schizophrenia*, Robert Brunner Publishers, New York: 1955.

SULLIVAN, HARRY STACK, *Conceptions of Modern Psychiatry*, W. W. Norton & Co., New York: 1953.

——— *The Interpersonal Theory of Psychiatry*, W. W. Norton & Co., New York: 1953.

# 32

## THE "VEIL" PHENOMENON IN AN HALLUCINATING SCHIZOPHRENIC

*Rebecca S. Isani*

This chapter is a clinical study of the "veil" phenomenon in the descriptions given by a hallucinating patient. It seeks to examine the gradual unfolding of this description against the background of certain interviewing techniques.

A search through major psychological and psychiatric sources reveals no previous report on the occurrence of the "veil" phenomenon. The author regarded it as a hallucinatory experience and in her contact with the patient followed the principles of interpersonal technique discussed in this chapter. Hallucination is effectively defined by Gravenkemper in the preceding chapter as "an inner experience expressed as though it were an outer event. It arises out of the dissociated [1] motivations of the self-system and is an uncanny, yet real, experience for the person." Hallucination differs from perception primarily in that the former is not the sensation of awareness caused by external stimuli, but by the person's own thoughts. The hallucination does, however, give the patient the sensation of hearing, smelling, tasting, or feeling, just as if it were an experience coming from external environment.

In defining the psychiatric interview, Sullivan [2] states, "The patient has at least some expectation of improvement or other personal gain from

---

[1] Harry Stack Sullivan, in his *Conceptions of Modern Psychiatry*, describes dissociation saying: "For the expression of all things in the personality other than those which were approved and disapproved by the parent and other significant persons, the self refuses awareness, so to speak. It does not accord awareness, it does not notice; and these impulses, desires, and needs come to exist disassociated from the self, or *dissociated*. When they are expressed, their expression is not noticed by the person." (Pp. 21–22.)

[2] Sullivan, H. S., *The Psychiatric Interview*, p. 16.

the interview." Whereas it is necessary that the patient be kept from acquiring exaggerated or false hopes, it is also essential that he be told that he can derive benefit from the interviews by developing a better understanding of himself through discussing his difficulties with the nurse. The nurse needs to understand the problems as viewed by the patient in order to formulate how she can be of assistance in his recovery. This approach motivates the patient and prepares him earlier for a rapport, which is essential if the interviewer is to succeed. It also maintains the goal of helping the patient. In the words of Sullivan, "That the patient will leave with some measure of increased clarity about himself and his living with other people is an essential goal of the psychiatric interview." [3]

Since the interview series is a learning experience for the patient, the steps of the learning process can be used as a conceptual framework for the nursing intervention. The nurse begins by helping the patient to develop his ability to observe and describe, then assists him in sequence through the other steps of the learning process that follow (i.e., analysis, formulation, validation, integration, testing, and application). This chapter discusses the nursing intervention during the descriptive phase of the "veil" phenomenon—the phase in which attention is directed toward further developing the patient's ability to recall and describe in detail a particular event(s) or experience(s).

Basic to the nursing intervention in the following series of interviews is that hallucinations are very real to the person who hallucinates. The information that can come from the patient's descriptions of hallucinatory phenomena is essential knowledge in the care based on the patient's increasing understanding of himself. A person's thought process uses many important symbols that can be followed up by a nurse to develop a greater understanding of the patient and to help the patient to understand himself. As Peplau [4] has stated, "Symbols are also representative of emotional ideas or desires; they may be interpreted in order to reveal underlying themes, wishes, or wants that cannot be expressed directly." This chapter is limited to one of these symbols, the "veil," as viewed by one patient.

## THE DESCRIPTIVE PROCESS:
## NURSING INTERVENTION AND EFFECTS

Over a four-month period, 22 fifty-minute interviews were held with a middle-aged schizophrenic patient who had been hospitalized for over 15

[3] *Ibid.*, pp. 18–19.
[4] Peplau, H. E., *Interpersonal Relations in Nursing*, p. 301.

years. The general technique followed was to invite the patient to talk about herself, explaining that this would aid her in understanding herself and help the nurse in understanding the patient. The interview series was initiated with a question wide enough to leave the choice of topic of conversation unrestricted for the patient, and in eliciting description, the principles indicated below were among those adhered to:

1. *In counseling, the nurse takes the direction in communication easiest for the patient to follow.* This allows the latter to select topics related to his own needs. The patient's needs are of primary importance to the nurse, and, as in the following example, the patient will discuss these if given an opportunity.

   *Patient:* Well, what do we talk about this morning?
   *Nurse:* Anything that will help you to better understand yourself.
   *Patient:* I was hearing voices again last night.
   *Nurse:* Tell me what the voices said to you last night. (The patient continued to talk about her hallucinations for the remainder of the interview.)

   If the nurse introduces the subject herself for the hallucinating patient, or in any other way shows too prominent an interest in the hallucination, he may exaggerate his descriptions to please her.

2. *In counseling, the nurse takes the patient's focus and elaborates it.* In this series, the writer focused on the topic brought up by the patient and elaborated by such statements as, "Describe this to me," "Tell me more about this," and a number of what, when, which, and where questions, as in the following instance:

   *Patient:* I would think of terrible things . . . outrageous things.
   *Nurse:* What; for instance?

   If the nurse focuses away from the topics brought up by the patient, he may interpret this as a lack of interest and understanding in his problems and withdraw even further into his hallucinations.

3. *In counseling, when the patient presents much content, the nurse has a choice in selecting the focus.* In these interviews, when what appeared to be a hallucination was mentioned, the nurse steered toward this as a focus and solicited detailed description. Under no circumstances was the subject pursued if the patient showed unwillingness or an uncomfortable stage of anxiety.

The first mention of the "veil" was made in the fifth interview. At first, this "veil" was vaguely referred to as "it." The nurse's questions elicited the information that the "it" was the "veil."

*Patient:* I get a moving in my head. . . . It was terrible.
*Nurse:* What is the "it"?
*Patient:* It is something in my head. Sort of a veil that moves.
*Nurse:* When does the veil move?
*Patient:* It moves all the time . . . .

Thereupon, the patient changed the topic, showing various signs of anxiety, and the nurse talked with her about topics that were more comfortable for her.

The "veil" was not mentioned again until the tenth interview, and then, too, it was only briefly referred to. Details began to emerge in the eleventh interview. When the patient has come to the point of feeling secure with the nurse, he may show a willingness to share his hallucinatory experiences with her. It is very important that the nurse does not show surprise or disbelief, and that she tells the patient that she does not share his pathological symptoms but is willing to explore them with him. *"The nurse points out simply that she does not see, hear, taste, smell, or feel the hallucination phenomenon."* [5] In this series, the nurse used the statement: "I don't see the veil. You need to describe it to me, so you and I can figure the veil out together." Arieti [6] writes that the "therapist should simply tell the patient that he does not hear these voices and will maintain an attitude of cordiality and relatedness." Fromm-Reichmann [7] suggests:

> . . . the psychiatrist should not argue about their hallucinatory, delusional, or illusionary character. He should state quite simply and clearly that he does not see or hear what the patient professes to see or hear, that he does not share the patient's hallucinatory, delusional, or illusional interpretation or evaluation of facts.

After that, continues Fromm-Reichmann, he should interest the patient in investigating why he hears or sees what the psychiatrist does not, when the hallucination first appeared, and ask the patient to account for any previous real experiences that preceded the present hallucinatory experience.

Gradually a description of the "veil" emerged. For some time the indefinite "it" was used by the patient, and the first descriptions were vague. Each mention, however, added to the picture, and for the nurse this experience was like fitting a puzzle together. The "veil" was described in interviews Nos. 5, 10, 11, 13, 14, 15, 16, 17, and 19. This indicates that once the initial rapport had been established, the descriptions were forthcoming in increasing detail.

Initially, the patient described one "veil," and this had "thoughts" writ-

[5] Clack, J., "An Interpersonal Technique for Handling Hallucinations," p. 14.
[6] Arieti, S., "Introductory Notes on the Psychoanalytic Therapy," p. 84.
[7] Fromm-Reichmann, F., *Principles of Intensive Psychotherapy*, p. 175.

ten on it. During the fifteenth interview, she mentioned a "veil" that was blank. She spoke of a third during the sixteenth interview. No description was given of the third "veil," though the patient drew it on paper as a fleecy cloud. The first "veil," however, was the one mentioned most frequently in the interviews. The following clinical data provide one example of the patient's description:

> *Patient:* It moves inside my head a lot. The "it" is a shadow that moves. It is a veil. I haven't any words to describe it with.
> *Nurse:* What are your thoughts when the shadow moves?
> *Patient:* I have thoughts inside the veil. I move the veil that has the thoughts.

At various times, the patient described it as black, brown, a combination of light gray and white, and neutral ("no color at all"). She said that the color of the "veil" changes. The only indication of the material composition of the "veil" was that "it is like a big ball of cotton." [8] In size, it was large enough to cover the eyes. It moved in four directions—forward, backward, up, and down. One example of movement and dynamics of the "veil" is in the following clinical data:

> *Patient:* I have thoughts inside the veil. The thoughts move in the veil. I move the veil that has the thoughts. . . . I push the thinking in my head.
> *Nurse:* Tell me about pushing the thinking.
> *Patient:* I push it—that is all.
> *Nurse:* What do you do when you push the thinking?
> *Patient:* . . . I stop the thinking sometimes too—I stop it. I press down on it.
> *Nurse:* You press down? Tell me how you press down?
> *Patient:* I press down on the part that moves.
> *Nurse:* What are you thinking when you press down?
> *Patient:* A lot of things. When I don't want to think, I press down and then I won't think of it.

An attempt was made to obtain an illustration of the "veil" on paper during the sixteenth interview. The nurse said: "I am trying to see the 'veil' the way you see it. I have to see it the way you tell me, so make me a picture." The patient drew the "veils" on the paper offered her (Figs. 1, 2, 3). Under the first and second figures, the patient wrote "no thinking." She pointed out the dark spots in Figure 3 as "thoughts." By the time the pictures were drawn, the patient had become very anxious.

"Whenever the patient is anxious, the nurse assists the patient in the

---

[8] Woodburn Hern, in an article on the experimental production of hallucinations, reports that one subject described his experience: "my mind seemed to be a ball of cotton wool floating above my body, or something seemed to be sucking my mind through my eyes." ("The Pathology of Boredom," p. 4.)

recognition and the naming of the anxiety in order to initiate the patient's learning and/or problem solving," writes Burd (see p. 311). In this case, the nurse got the patient to recognize her anxiety by asking her, "Are you nervous?" In addition, she permitted the patient's use of one of her patterns of reducing anxiety (choosing a more comfortable subject and walking to obtain a cigarette). When the anxiety had been reduced, the conversation was refocused on the "veil."

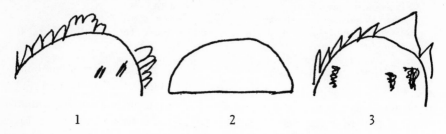

|    1    |    2    |    3    |

A hallucination of this nature is dissociated material, and its recall is painful to the patient. This may result in problems of communication. The self-system tends to keep the information dissociated, and the recall of this material results in anxiety which may make it difficult for the patient to communicate with the nurse.

## ROOTS AND PURPOSE OF THE "VEIL"

In this series of interviews, the nurse had insufficient data to ascertain when the "veil" phenomenon occurred initially. On each of three occasions a different answer was given by the patient when asked when she saw the "veil" for the first time. Her replies were—

Last May, around Mother's Day.
When I first heard the voices. No, a couple of months later.
After I took shock treatment, I started to hear the voices and see the veil—
    in February.

More data would be required to obtain understanding of the time that this patient had the initial experience with the "veil" phenomenon.

The function of the "veil" appears to be the prevention of anxiety-producing thought. The patient described the occasions during which she saw the "veil": "When I don't want to think, I press down and then I won't think of it." Further clarification of the time when the "veil" is noticed is inherent in these data:

*Nurse:* What are you thinking when the veil moves?
*Patient:* . . . Wild thoughts; thoughts that upset me.

*Nurse:* Give me an example of a wild thought.
*Patient:* They prove to me that I didn't believe in God; and prove to me that I was not a woman . . .

The "veil" had the additional purpose of aiding the patient in the production of thoughts that were comfortable to her. These replaced the undesirable thoughts temporarily. As already mentioned, one of the "veils" described had "thoughts" on it. "It makes thinking. . . . When I press down, it makes the voices come." The patient has made a connection between the "voices" and the "veil." She described terrorizing "voices," but also "voices" that were not unpleasant. During the nineteenth interview—the last time she referred to the "veil"—the patient offered and gave the nurse a demonstration of how she brought on the "voices." Her method was to press down on her eyelid with her finger. As previously indicated, the eye was the location of the "veil."

It seems reasonably apparent that the "veil" was selected because it could serve as a screen to maintain dissociation of unpleasant thought and feelings. In Western culture, the veil is generally accepted as a symbol of separation. The secular meaning of the word, according to *Webster's Dictionary* is "a fabric hung up, or spread out, to intercept the view, and hide an object; a curtain. . . . Hence, a cover, disguise, mask." "Assuming the veil," in the Catholic faith, refers to entering the cloistered life of a nun, entering a life of separation from many worldly things. Again, the central idea is one of separation. As a Catholic, the patient may have been particularly aware of this meaning.

Speculating further, one can also conceptualize the "veil" as an example of autistic thinking. Autistic thinking is largely a tool of childhood through which thoughts, feelings, and words have a magical power of fulfilling needs, wants, and wishes. Frequently, the "voices" are very terrorizing to schizophrenics. This patient could have invented the "veil" to have control over these voices.

Like other hallucinations, the "veil" is a thought disorder. In this series of interviews, the nurse, using interpersonal techniques, tried to aid the patient in uncovering the need(s) she attempted to satisfy through hallucination. The interviews were a step toward aiding the patient to differentiate between the real and the hallucinatory, that she may realize there are better ways to satisfy the same need(s). It is the role of the nurse to suggest these better means, including increased interpersonal relationships. Once they succeed, the hallucination will disappear. Progress may often be slow, but the positive approach discussed in this chapter appears best suited to aid the person diagnosed schizophrenic who hallucinates.

## BIBLIOGRAPHY

ARIETI, SILVANO, *Interpretation of Schizophrenia*, Robert Brunner Publishers, New York: 1955.

——— "Introductory Notes on the Psychoanalytic Therapy," in *Psychotherapy of the Psychoses*, Arthur Burton (ed.), Basic Books: New York: 1961.

CLACK, JANICE, "An Interpersonal Technique for Handling Hallucinations," in monograph No. 13, *Nursing Care of the Disoriented Patient*, pp. 16–26, American Nurses' Association, New York, 1962.

FROMM-REICHMANN, FRIEDA, *Principles of Intensive Psychotherapy*, Phoenix Books, Chicago, Ill., 1950.

HERN, WOODBURN, "The Pathology of Boredom," *Scientific American*, Vol. 196, January, 1957.

PEPLAU, HILDEGARD E., *Interpersonal Relations in Nursing*, G. P. Putnam's Sons, New York: 1952.

RENDER, HELENA, and WEISS, OLGA, *Nurse-Patient Relationships in Psychiatry*, McGraw-Hill Book Co., New York: 1959.

SCHWARTZ, MORRIS, and SHOCKLEY, EMMY, *The Nurse and the Mental Patient*, Russell Sage Foundation, New York: 1956.

SULLIVAN, HARRY STACK, *Conceptions of Modern Psychiatry*, W. W. Norton & Co., New York: 1953.

——— *The Psychiatric Interview*, W. W. Norton & Co., New York: 1954.

# SECTION

# III

## CLINICAL RESEARCH

# 33 NURSING INTERVENTION INTO THE AGGRESSIVE BEHAVIOR OF PATIENTS[1]

*Janice Clack*

What is the best nursing intervention that can be used by all nursing personnel to help the patient use aggression as a meaningful learning experience? When the patient acts out aggression, other patients and nurses react to him, often quickly and automatically, and without much benefit to anyone in the situation. This aggressive action and reaction, of patients and nurses, are common occurrences in the experience of most psychiatric nurses.

The author defines aggression as any verbal and/or nonverbal, actual or attempted, forceful abuse of the self, another person, or thing. There are observable behaviors antecedent to aggression. These antecedents defined operationally in order of their emergence yield the following explanation of aggressive behavior:

First, *the person holds expectations*. These include needs for prestige and status, wants, wishes, and drives. These expectations may be witting or unwitting; they are products of the patient's past experiences with other people significant in his living. In later interpersonal situations, the patient picks up cues that trigger these expectations into operation. He anticipates the fulfillment of these expectations, even though they may not be communicated clearly.

Second, *the expectations are not met*. Either wittingly or unwittingly, other people in the situation, perhaps even the nurse, do not recognize or meet or help the patient to meet his expectations.

Third, then, *the person experiences a higher level of anxiety*. He may

[1] Read at American Psychiatric Association Convention in Toronto, Ontario, May 11, 1962. Permission to publish this paper received from the *American Journal of Psychiatry*.

feel helpless, powerless. His previous ability to execute self-control is considerably minimized, if not lost, and this loss is felt at this point. This loss of self-control is a common occurrence as shown in clichés such as, "He makes me so mad I can't see straight," or "I was so mad I could have exploded."

In the fourth step, *aggression occurs.* Anxiety may have been previously so distressing to the patient that early he found ways to convert it into aggression in order to feel more comfortable, that is, to rid himself of the felt powerlessness. This impressive result—the utility of aggression—is then sought in similar situations of anxiety. Aggression may be called into operation so rapidly, when expectations are not met, that the patient has no recognition of the expectations or of feelings of anxiety that occur.

Then, a fifth step occurs, namely, *justification of the aggression.* The temporary feelings of relief obtained from the acted-out aggression are of short duration; in other words, "the calm after the storm" is not long-lasting. The needs or expectations are still present, though perhaps not uppermost in his mind. When these are called out again, as they will be, Steps 1 through 4 will recur and culminate again in aggressive behavior.

The patient will temporarily be bogged down in the aggression and attempts at justification. The nurse most often gets manipulated into participating in this pattern. The pattern becomes cyclic and, with each round, snowballs until finally the initial behavior is obscured and unrecognized by the patient. It is evident that some therapeutic intervention *by nurses* must halt this operation from continuing in the pattern just spelled out.

It is not the author's intention to advocate suppression of all acting-out of aggression, nor to advocate complete license so that a patient may vent fully his aggressive tendencies. It is the intention to explore ways that a patient can be aided in expressing aggression in a manner that leads to feelings of satisfaction and security in interpersonal relationships.

The crucial factor in regard to whether the patient's aggression is perpetuated or turned toward resolution is not the type of hospital physical environment, but the type of nursing care he receives. Two additional and important factors are the consistency of constructive intervention by the entire nursing staff toward that patient, and the reliability of the theory from which that intervention is derived.

Three types of interaction patterns that can or do go on between nurse and aggressive patient can be described:

1. The pattern of countertransference reaction or counteracted anxiety
2. The pattern of manifest anxiety reaction or free-floating anxiety

3. The pattern of therapeutic reaction requiring application of therapeutic nursing intervention wherein the nurse constructively uses the energy anxiety

## COUNTERTRANSFERENCE REACTION

In the countertransference reaction, or parataxic distortion, the nurse re-enacts and, in a sense, relives the mother-child relationships which she knew as a child. She, however, utilizes the mother role as her actual mother used it, placing the patient in the position and predicament which she, the nurse, knew as a child. The nurse acts inappropriately to the here-and-now situation, in light of theoretical explanation, but appropriately to her own unrecognized and unresolved difficulties.

Frequently, this inappropriate nurse action revolves around the nurse's attempts to set limits on the patient's freedom to act out aggression; however, this so-called limit-setting is usually acted out by the nurse as a form of countertransference in an attempt to stop the aggression of the patient. There is frequently an extreme lack of talking-through the behavioral situation with the patient. Therefore, the patient does not develop foresight to use when anxiety or aggression arises the next time. And, neither does the nurse learn about aggression and develop foresight to use in later instances of it in the work situation.

In making systematic observations of ten nurse-patient interactions wherein the patients were overtly aggressive, the nurses were found to be unable to observe their own behavior. Nor could they state an explanation of their behavior. Usually, these nurses explained the patient's behavior by saying, "Oh, he's just imitating another patient and wants attention." But, when observational data of the nurse-patient interactions were analyzed, the nurses were found more frequently to cut off communication with the patient through such means as making moral judgments, secluding the patient, being counteraggressive, intimidating, or angry. In every instance where the nurse stated that the patient wanted attention, the nurse, in action, deprived the patient of her attention. Why is there this incongruency between what these nurses stated as the needs or expectations of the patient and the nurses' action in regard to those needs?

## THE PATTERN OF MANIFEST REACTION
## TO ANXIETY

A second type of interaction was studied in which nurses were observed to manifest free-floating anxiety in attempting to cope with the aggressive patient. These nurses frequently met with repeated failures in their attempts; that is, they reported no change in patient behavior and manifested more anxiety themselves. Nurses seemed not to know what to do with and for the aggressive patient. Responses then noted in these nurses were helplessness, ingratiation, avoidance of aggressive patients, and a tendency toward changing the environment for the patient. Such nurse responses often do not allow the patient to express his actions and, more important, inhibit the patient from exploring his thoughts and feelings regarding his aggression experiences. The patient's pathology, though it be hidden temporarily, does not usually just go away. It must be brought out into the open, explored, and ultimately understood.

The following pattern of helpless inconsistency most often occurs in the anxious nurse as reaction to behavior of the aggressive patient: The patient's aggression works to give him power at the expense of rendering the nurse anxious, that is, powerless and helpless. The nurse is likely to feel intimidated and then respond momentarily with anger in a failing attempt to regain her status, self-control, and power. Subsequently, the nurse flounders helplessly, trying to think of something she can do that works. She tries different approaches which are inconsistent, and she feels even more anxious and helpless.

This pattern of helpless inconsistency is exactly reversed in the interaction of the aggressive patient and the nurse in countertransference. In this latter pattern, the nurse counteracts her anxiety and is initially mobilized with power, maybe in the form of anger. The aggression of the patient calls out the countertransference reactions and aggression in the nurse. The nurse maintains her power at the expense of rendering the patient powerless, helpless, more anxious, and eventually more aggressive and then more anxious. This pattern, in contrast to helpless inconsistency, might be called the pattern of consistent incongruency.

Both patterns are likely to be called out in the absence of clear theoretical knowledge to explain the patient's behavior. Both result from the lack of a reasonable model the nurse can use, either mechanically or with understanding, in instances of aggression. The nurse has no better way to explain the situation. If she did, she would use it, and her actions would more likely reflect understanding of what went on.

## THERAPEUTIC NURSING INTERVENTION

The author has classified nursing intervention into the aggressive behavior of patients into three areas.

## GENERAL CONSIDERATIONS OF NURSING CARE

It seems the cause of some inept nurse attempts lies in the expectations held and in an orientation of "good" versus "bad" behavior. The nurse has expectations about herself as a person and as a nurse; she also holds expectations wittingly or unwittingly about patients. These latter expectations of nurses seem to fall into two categories: (1) They expect the major pattern of acting out aggression to continue and to remain the same, or (2) once the patient is able to execute some self-control, over a period of time, and "act good," the nurse expects the self-control to be maintained continually. Both expectations get communicated to the patient, and both are more unrealistic than not.

One of the most important points to be communicated is that the practice of all nursing lies in three operational steps seen in order of their emergence. These are—

    1. The nurse observes the patient's behavior
    2. The nurse then interprets her observations
    3. The nurse then intervenes into the behavior on the basis of her observations and interpretations

Interpretation of observed behavior requires the nurse to use reliable theoretical frameworks that yield, in part, explanation of the patient's behavior. When the nurse acquires the habit of analysis of nurse-patient interactions, she will gradually become able to observe keenly and to analyze the actual ongoing situation between herself and the patient. The nurse validates her observations, her interpretations, and what she actually did, her intervention, with another person. The nurse knows how to and when to set limits on the patient's freedom to act out aggression. She refrains from making moral judgments regarding the patient's behavior, for such judgments only relinquish an atmosphere for exploration of behavior. The nurse refrains from cutting off communication with the patient. She aims for consistency of intervention into the patient's behavior. She assesses the level of her and of the patient's anxiety and aids him and herself in taking measures to reduce anxiety to the level where learning can take place.

In general, the nurse aims toward acting appropriately to the elements of the situation presented in her interaction with the patient—acting appropriately in light of reliable explanatory theory. Therapeutic intervention into the aggressive behavior of patients is built upon recognition of the dynamics of the situation and upon concepts explanatory of observed human behavior.

Research-tested patterns of nursing intervention specific to aggression have not yet been reported, but the need for even hypothesized approaches, such as the following, is clearly apparent.

## A COMMON APPROACH FOR ALL NURSING PERSONNEL

One concept explanatory of aggression, presented at the outset of this chapter, is useful to all nursing personnel. This simply stated concept of anxiety can be used as a guiding framework in intervening into aggressive behavior.

The approach suggested here calls for a talking-through of each aggressive episode of the patient's in an interpersonal situation between the patient and his nurse. One nurse could regularly be assigned to the care of a particular patient. Each time this patient acted out aggression, the nurse would use time with that patient in talking about his behavior that has just occurred. It is absolutely necessary to deal with each episode of aggression in order to steer the patient toward resolution of his problem in this regard.

The nurse must endure extreme testing by the patient, which occurs at the cyclic point of aggression-justification-aggression. To get out of this cycle, and to make the aggression a basis for learning something new for the patient, the nurse directs the patient over and over again to explore what went on or what led up to the aggression. She encourages the patient to observe and to describe what his expectations were, what happened instead of the anticipated fulfillment, and to describe his reactions, his thoughts, feelings, and his actions. It is at the initial clues of anxiety, before conversion to aggression, that the nursing intervention is most opportune. Even so, the nurse directs the patient to explore the antecedents of his aggression.

The author hypothesizes that when one nurse copes with each aggressive episode of a patient's, for a period of time, and directs that patient to talk-through the antecedents of his aggression, even on a superficial level, the patient will soon begin to steer his own efforts toward more understanding and resolution of his aggression.

## PSYCHOTHERAPEUTIC INTERVIEWING

These nursing interviews with the aggressive patient might occur on two levels: (1) the individual nurse-patient interview and (2) group therapy led by a nurse for aggressive patients.

This approach might be used by the psychiatric nurse–clinical specialist. These interviews occur at regularly specified intervals for the usual duration of fifty minutes. The nurse is qualified to talk-through any behavioral experience the patient might bring to the interview. The psychiatric nurse has a broad framework of concepts and processes that she uses in interviewing. In a therapeutic environment such as this type, an aggressive patient has a potential opportunity for greater depth in experiential learning than that provided in the general approach.

Through such learning, he may resolve some of those experiences that led up to the automatic use of aggression. The patient, through understanding of his thoughts, feelings, and actions, gains in self-control, his proclivity for anxiety is minimized, and his competencies for satisfying interpersonal relationships are enhanced.

## BIBLIOGRAPHY

DOLLARD, JOHN, and MILLER, NEAL E., *Personality and Psychotherapy*, McGraw-Hill Book Co., New York: 1950.

——— et al., *Frustration and Aggression*, Yale University Press, New Haven: 1939.

FERNANDEZ, THERESA M., "How to Deal with Overt Aggression," *Am. J. Nursing*, 53(17):113–21, 1953.

FROMM-REICHMANN, FRIEDA, *Principles of Intensive Psychotherapy*, University of Chicago Press, Chicago: 1950.

MAIER, NORMAN, *Frustration*, McGraw-Hill Book Co., New York: 1949.

MASSERMAN, JULES H., *The Practice of Dynamic Psychiatry*, W. B. Saunders Co., Philadelphia: 1955.

MENNINGER, KARL, *Man Against Himself*, Harcourt, Brace and Co., New York: 1938.

REDL, FRITZ, and WINERMAN, DAVID, *The Aggressive Child*, The Free Press of Glencoe, New York: 1957.

SEARS, ROBERT R., "Non-Aggressive Reaction to Frustration," *Psychol. Rev.*, 48:343–46, 1941.

SYMONDS, PERCIVAL M., *The Dynamics of Human Adjustment*, Appleton-Century-Crofts, New York: 1946.

WOLBERG, LEWIS, *The Technique of Psychotherapy*, Grune and Stratton, New York: 1954.

# 34 INDIVIDUAL PANIC: ELEMENTS AND PATTERNS[1]

## Gloria Oden

Frequently, the admission of a patient to a mental hospital is preceded immediately by a dramatic episode in which the patient appears to have lost control of his actions. Before the episode, the patient is often able to function in society at least to a minimal degree. Suddenly something happens to the patient which (1) causes him to lose control in large part over the contents of his awareness and (2) results in extremely hyperactive behavior.

The uncontrolled and uncontrollable behavior does not persist indefinitely. Such extreme behavior is incompatible with life, and if continued over a prolonged period of time, exhaustion and death would result.

Following this acute episode of apparently purposeless activity, another behavior change is frequently noted. Behavior becomes bizarre. From verbalizations and actions by the patient, it can be inferred that a less healthy personality organization is in operation. The patient often requires hospitalization.

Sometimes relatives and friends proffer explanations about the cause of the patient's acute episode. At other times, significant persons are at a complete loss to explain the patient's behavior.

For the purposes of this chapter, the temporary disorganization of the personality manifested in the behavior above is termed "panic." Its fuller description was the primary aim of this study.

What is panic? What happens during a panic episode? On these questions hinge the answers to still other questions for which this study pro-

[1] Adapted from Oden, G., *Panic, A Descriptive Study*, master's thesis, Graduate School, Rutgers, The State University of New Jersey, May 1962.

vides a basis. What therapeutic interventions can be developed that would assist the individual in panic to reorganize his personality along healthy lines?

There is a dearth of research in the area of panic. No definition of panic based upon systematic observation is generally accepted. No generally accepted interventions for panic are described in the literature, nor any generally accepted methods of prevention.

It is necessary to understand fully the phenomenon, panic, in order to prevent it or to use successful intervention when it occurs.

During a panic episode, the personality becomes disorganized. Following the panic, the personality reorganizes, frequently in the direction of increased psychopathology which requires institutionalized psychiatric care. Prevention of panic would reduce the incidence of mental illness. Intervention in panic would prevent or reduce the degree of increased psychopathology, thereby maintaining many individuals at a level of mental health that would permit them to function adequately in the community.

The initial step in clinical research is systematic observation of a problem area. Interpretations of observations are then made, using available concepts and generalizations already validated by the experience of experts in order to reach explanations of what is observed. From this, preventive measures and interventions are postulated, then tested, whereupon successful ones are validated, accepted, and standardized.

To date, no one has done a systematic observational study of individuals in panic as an initial effort toward a scientifically based solution to the problem. Instead, each individual—professional or layman—reacts in his own way when confronted by another person undergoing panic.

The word "panic" is derived from the name of the god Pan—half-man, half-animal—who inspired contagious fear and terror in travelers. *Webster's Dictionary* defines panic as "a sudden fright, especially a groundless fright; terror inspired by a trifling cause." Panic is conceptualized in various ways. According to Meerloo: [2]

It [panic] has gradually come to express different degrees of fear, alarm and perplexity. In the European languages (German, Dutch, French) it has a stronger meaning than in English. In Europe it is used primarily to express strong collective emotions of terror, perplexity, dread and horror. In English it is just as frequently used to express individual reactions to danger, dread, awe, the nightmare, and even more subtle anxieties, such as the "blue funk," the startle reaction, and so forth.

Panic, then, is used synonymously to describe two phenomena: group behavior and individual behavior. Implied in the concept are two modes

[2] Meerloo, J. A. M., *Patterns of Panic*, p. 10.

of human experience. They are emotion and action. A possible third mode of experience is intimated as well, that is, thought.

In reviewing the literature on panic, it was found that while the approach to the subject and the focus of interest differed in both types of panic, there were similarities of emotions, thoughts, and actions described in both. The intention of this research is to study individual panic. However, a review of the literature on both group panic and individual panic is deemed purposeful because of the approach used by many authors in discussing group panic. Attempts have been made to study group panic in a systematized manner. Several authors,[3] in writing about group panic, have attempted to collect data in an organized manner and to describe, analyze, and report their findings. Descriptions of individual panic are based most frequently upon generalizations culled from clinical experiences and described on a less-than-systematic basis. Analysis of panic behavior is usually made on the basis of theoretical concepts. Most often, studies of group panic are undertaken during wartime and during times of civilian disasters, such as fires, earthquakes, explosions, and tornadoes.

The works of authors describing the mass panic of wartime and disaster tend to view it as disorganized behavior based on fear. The focus of their interest is on the development of prophylactic measures to prevent panic. Emphasis is therefore placed on the causative and precipitating factors in panic, rather than upon panic as a complete entity including causation, precipitating factors, the panic episode itself, and the result of panic for the participants.

Writers on the subject of individual panic tend to view panic in its totality rather than to emphasize any one aspect of the experience. Because authors on this subject provide a theoretical framework for understanding the phenomenon of panic, the literature on individual panic was reviewed first.

Panic is not an experience separate from all other experiences. It evolves from other experiences. Moreover, it is generally agreed by writers in psychiatry, psychiatric nursing, and related disciplines that panic is related to

[3] Caldwell, J. M., Ranson, S. W., and Sachs, J. G., *Group Panic and Other Mass Disruptive Reactions*, pp. 541–67.
Foreman, P. B., "Panic Theory," pp. 295–304.
La Piere, R., *Collective Behavior*, pp. 437–62.
Meerloo, *op. cit.*, p. 116.
Quarantelli, Enrico, *The Behavior of Panic Participants*, pp. 187–94.
*Ibid., The Nature and Conditions of Panic*, pp. 267–75.
Schmidelberg, W., "The Treatment of Panic in Casualty Area and Clearing Station," pp. 162–69.

anxiety. Virtually every work published on the dynamics of human behavior discusses anxiety. The term "anxiety" is variously treated as a concept in relatively static terms or as a process. The majority of authors discuss panic briefly and in reference to the behavior of individuals in a state of panic.

The general consensus is as follows: that panic is a high degree of anxiety; that it is like fear, except that the origin is unknown or irrational; that it is probably the most extreme form of behavior disturbance; that there is lack of coordination in behavior; that rational thought is no longer in operation. Various authors classify panic behavior as an escape mechanism or as assaultiveness, with the preponderance stating that the behavior is predicated upon a wild desire to flee from the situation. Sullivan, for example, contrasts this flight response with the very different behavior seen in loneliness, an equally extreme emotional disturbance, but one which impels turning toward someone. In effect, it is a state in which an individual is no longer able to function as an organized human being and in which erratic, uncoordinated motor reactions can be observed.

Sullivan [4] defines panic as a high degree of anxiety in which there is "an acute failure of the dissociative power of the self. . . . All organized activity is lost. All thought is paralyzed. Panic is, in fact, disorganization of the personality." Sullivan conceptualizes panic as part of a polar construct of anxiety extending from pure euphoria on the one theoretical extreme to a state of pure anxiety on the other. Anxiety progresses from the euphoric state through mild anxiety, moderate anxiety, severe anxiety, panic and terror, to pure anxiety.[5] Panic is seen as a tentative state, a state wholly incompatible with life. The personality reintegrates as swiftly as possible, often in a state of terror in which every energy is directed toward flight. In describing panic, Sullivan [6] mentions circus movements, random activity, and incoordination of the skeletal muscles as well as changes in perception in which visual perception becomes extremely limited, and auditory perceptions become limited or distorted.

In discussing individual panic, its relationship to psychopathological reorganization of the personality is noted. Peplau [7] states:

> Personality is always organized along more or less productive lines. During panic, however, it disorganized quite rapidly and a new reorganization follows. The new organization may be an improvement; it is more likely that it will be along pathological lines.

[4] Sullivan, H. S., *Conceptions of Modern Psychiatry*, p. 134.

[5] Mullahy, P., *Oedipus: Myth and Complex*, p. 292 (citing an unpublished lecture by Harry Stack Sullivan).

[6] Sullivan, H. S., *op. cit.*, p. 137.

[7] Peplau, H. E., *Interpersonal Relations in Nursing*, pp. 132–33.

Individual panic is frequently discussed in terms of its relatedness to psychotic processes. Based upon clinical observations, Arieti [8] has outlined the sequence of events at the beginning of a psychosis. He states that there is—

> . . . a sequence of stages: first, a period of intense anxiety and panic; second, a period of confusion, when everything seems strange and crazy; and third, a period of psychotic insight. When this insight occurs, the external world is understood according to a new system of thinking, which, of course, follows the motivational trends of the patient.

If this is the sequence of frank psychosis, is it not possible to develop interventions for use during the period of intense anxiety that culminates in panic, in order to avert a psychotic reorganization of the personality? In another publication, Arieti [9] maintains that he believes this to be the case. He states that intervention in the early stages of panic can avoid progression to a full-fledged panic.

Spiegel,[10] in discussing panic which she claims precedes a changeover to schizophrenia, emphasizes the lack of ability to communicate with and relate to others. She states that there are changes in the usual mode of experiencing time and space. She describes individuals in this type of panic as clutching and clinging to a trusted person. This behavior is in direct contrast to the flight behavior described by other authors.

Spiegel's statement regarding the panic participant's inability to communicate suggests that intervention based upon verbal exchanges with another is not possible during a panic episode. Is this view valid, or is it possible that during the panic episode there is some degree of anxiety reduction which would make it possible to communicate verbally with the individual in panic? Would such communication further reduce anxiety rather than allow it to be maintained at a totally noncommunicative level?

Schwartz and Shockley [11] note a limitation placed upon those present with an individual in panic. They state that there is a profound effect upon other individuals in the panic situation, to whom the anxiety of the one who panics is communicated. They stress the importance of the roles of other individuals in maintaining, increasing, or reducing the anxiety of

[8] Arieti, S., "Interpretation of Schizophrenia," p. 331.

[9] Arieti, S., "Introductory Notes on the Psychoanalytic Therapy of Schizophrenics," pp. 72–74.

[10] Spiegel, R., "Specific Problems of Communication in Psychiatric Conditions," pp. 931–32.

[11] Schwartz, M.S., and Shockley, E. L., The Nurse and the Mental Patient, pp. 182–85.

the panic participant. Wolberg [12] stresses the need for the therapist to maintain calm in treating an individual in panic, in order to assist the patient in achieving stability.

The importance of maintaining a nonanxious or a controlled degree of anxiety as a therapist for the panic patient is complicated by the seemingly sudden onset of panic. Arieti [13] describes the sudden nature of panic. He notes also the decrease and distortion in visual and auditory perceptions, and the focus of thought on one, or a few related obsessive ideals.

The aspects of panic discussed thus far have pertained to the phenomenon of individual panic. What has been written in the area of group panic?

Strauss,[14] in his compilation of the literature on group panic, classifies panic conditions into three categories: physiological, caused by fatigue, toxic reactions, etc.; psychological, caused by feelings of anxiety and powerlessness; and sociological, caused by a lack of group solidarity. It appears that these categories, which are not mutually exclusive, could be applied also to the individual in panic. The appropriateness of the first two categories is obvious. The third could be applied to the individual in panic in terms of his perceptions of "not belonging."

Strauss [15] also found that writers on the subject of group panic tended to agree that there were characteristic descriptive features of mass panic (preponderantly military). These included collective surprise, shock, suggestion, mass imitation, mental contagion, shattering of group bonds, and wild flight. Writers agreed upon conditions that influenced panic episodes. Physical debilitation, which included fatigue, exhaustion, poor nourishment, bad health, and previous shock, was cited as an influencing factor in panic. The exact role of debilitation was unknown. It was frequently suggested, however, that this condition weakened the ability to think clearly. High emotional tension and heightened imagination were also generally argued to be preconditions of panic.

Other causative factors in panic agreed upon by various authors include lessened mental ability and the perception that one's life and body were in extreme danger.[16]

Brousseau [17] found that sharpened imagination, noises, distractions,

[12] Wolberg, L. R., *The Technique of Psychotherapy*, p. 589.
[13] Arieti, S., "Introductory Notes on the Psychoanalytic Therapy of Schizophrenics," pp. 72–74.
[14] Strauss, A., "The Literature on Panic," pp. 317–28.
[15] *Loc. cit.*
[16] *Loc. cit.*
[17] Brousseau, A., *Essai Sur La Peur Aux Armées 1914–1918*, pp. 19–30.

emotional tensions, and the feeling of isolation triggered panic episodes.

Kelland [18] believes that the causative factors in panic are consciousness of powerlessness and the futility of stemming the inevitable.

Munson [19] views panic as the result of unexpected events which result in a violent change in the current of thought. He also emphasizes certain psychological processes: illusion, hallucination, suggestion, and contagion.

Quarantelli,[20] in his study of the nature of group panic in civilian disasters, finds:

> Panic can be defined as an acute fear reaction marked by a loss of self-control which is followed by non-social and non-rational flight behavior. Covertly there is an acute fear reaction, i.e., an intense impulse to run from an impending danger. . . . Panic participants do not weigh the social consequences of their flight and are highly individualistic and self-centered in their actions in reference to one another. There is no consideration of alternative courses of action to flight.

In addition, Quarantelli [21] views the fears of panic participants as future-oriented, in terms of not being able to escape an impending threat. These feelings dominate from the first and prevail throughout the entire panic episode. Individuals in panic do not feel trapped; there is, rather, a feeling of possible entrapment.

Both Strauss [22] and Quarantelli [23] agree that the current conceptions of panic are inadequate because of their lack of empirical basis. Strauss [24] suggests studies based on direct objective observations of panic, and the use of documents, interviews, and published descriptions of panic as sources of information. He emphasizes the need for the development of new tools with which to study the phenomena of panic.

In panic episodes, whether of an individual or group nature:

1. Panic is a high degree of anxiety.
2. In panic, the ability to function as a human being is either absent or severely limited.
3. While varying phenomena of change are emphasized by different authors, it is agreed that during a panic episode there are abrupt and drastic changes in thoughts, feelings, and actions, as compared with usual behavior.
4. The anxiety of panic is contagous. It is empathically communicated to other persons present with the person in panic. The anxiety of others tends to increase markedly in degree.

[18] Kelland, C., "How Men and Women Act Facing Terror," pp. 44–45.
[19] Munson, E., The Management of Men, pp. 105–17, 242–44.
[20] Quarantelli, E., The Nature and Conditions of Panic, pp. 272–73.
[21] Ibid., p. 272.
[22] Strauss, A., op. cit., p. 326.
[23] Quarantelli, E., The Nature and Conditions of Panic, p. 268.
[24] Strauss, A., op. cit., p. 326.

With the foregoing as a theoretical background, an exploratory study was designed to seek answers to the study question: *What common elements and patterns of individual panic can be identified from observations and descriptions of the experiencer, the researcher, and other individuals present during a panic episode?*

The following definitions were employed for the purposes of this study:

1. *Panic* is a temporary disorganization of the personality manifested by hyperactive behavior and disorientation without a physiological basis.
2. *Individual panic* is panic experienced by a single person, as opposed to collective panic experienced by a group of persons.
3. *Experiencer of panic* designates the individual who undergoes the panic episode.
4. *Panic episode* designates a time interval extending from the time the experiencer of panic and/or other individuals note changes in thoughts, feelings, and/or actions which, in the opinion of these individuals, appear to have influence on the panic episode, until the time when the experiencer of panic falls asleep, or until two hours after admission to the hospital, whichever occurs first.
5. *Observations* are the perceptions of a panic episode by the experiencer of panic, the researcher, and other persons present during any part or all of a panic episode.
6. *Descriptions* are verbatim data given to the researcher or research assistant about observations of a panic episode. This includes the observations of the researcher and research assistant.
7. *Other individuals* are persons present during any part or all of a panic episode who are available and willing to describe their observations of the episode, excluding the experiencer of panic.

Data were collected at a 750-bed metropolitan city hospital where emergency psychiatric cases are admitted. Patients admitted are residents of and visitors to the city. Hospital stay for psychiatric patients is short-term. The mean length of hospitalization of the patients reported in this paper was 3.6 days. Admitted psychiatric patients are tentatively diagnosed, after which they are discharged, transferred to nonpsychiatric units of the hospital, transferred to jail, or transported to state, county, or private psychiatric facilities as indicated. There are two psychiatric receiving units, an 18-bed male unit and a 12-bed female unit. Upon admission to the hospital, all patients are taken first to the emergency room, examined by a staff physician, then transferred to a psychiatric unit if this is indicated.

The sample consisted of seven patients admitted to the psychiatric service who met the following criteria:

1. Any person who was hyperactive upon and/or before admission to the hospital.
2. Any person who was disoriented.

3. Any person who, in the judgment of the medical staff present in the emergency room, had no physiological basis for his hyperactivity and disorientation.

Every person in panic is not hyperactive. Some persons respond to panic with "freezing-on-the-spot" behavior. For the purposes of this study, only persons manifesting hyperactive responses to the panic situation were observed.

Disoriented verbalizations provided the indicant that the thoughts of the person were disorganized. Expressions of bewilderment as to time or place and inability to remember events immediately preceding hospital admission are examples of disorientation.

Data collected on any person subsequently diagnosed as organically damaged or as panic of physiological origin were discarded. In order to avoid data collection on patients whose symptoms were of physiological origin, data were not collected on the following cases:

1. Any patient transferred from a nonpsychiatric unit of any hospital to the psychiatric unit of this hospital.
2. Any person over 60 years of age.
3. Any person who presented clinical evidence of acute alcoholism, drug addiction, diabetes mellitus, severe mental retardation, or toxic reactions to disease processes or drugs.

If any of these conditions were found to exist, data were discarded.

Combined techniques of observation, interview, and questionnaire administration were utilized in data collection.[25]

# CASE STUDIES

## CASE 1

The patient was a 45-year-old Caucasian female. She was married, but had been separated from her husband for more than a year. She had four children. Prior to separation, the patient had spent one year in a mental hospital. Between the time of her separation and until two weeks before the panic episode, she had lived alone. For two weeks before the panic episode she had lived with her mother. Occupational history for the past year indicated that the patient had changed jobs four times. Her jobs included cook, waitress, saleswoman, and factory worker.

Respondents for this case included three sisters and two police officers. Biographical data were secured from the patient's siblings.

[25] Due to space limitation, description of data collection, processing, analyses, and tables are omitted. The case data, however, are presented in detail for each of the seven subjects who comprised the study sample.

For several months before the onset of the panic episode, family members report that they had noted behavioral changes. The patient had become increasingly argumentative, complained of ill health, and neglected her appearance.

The panic episode occurred in the early evening. Earlier that day, one of the sisters phoned the mother to inquire about the whereabouts of the sister's child. The phone call apparently upset the patient, who argued with the mother about the call. Later in the day, the three sisters visited the mother's house. The patient attacked the mother verbally, and an argument ensued between the patient and her sister. The patient became increasingly upset. At the onset of the altercation, the patient's verbal responses were appropriate. According to the sisters, she "threw up to us things that happened in the past." As the argument progressed, the patient's verbalizations became less appropriate, until "nothing she said made sense."

Finally, the patient assaulted the sisters physically. The sisters fought with her. Suddenly she ran out of the house, clad in pajamas, robe, and slippers, "screaming and yelling." During this time, one sister phoned for police assistance.

The patient remembered the argument and stated that her sisters had assaulted her. She had no memory of having left the house.

Her first memory following the reported assault was "standing on the porch and the police were coming in with me." When questioned repeatedly about the interval between the time of the assault and standing on the porch, the patient responded, "I don't know" and "nothing happened." She was able to describe events prior to leaving the house and following her return with the police. When questioned about her feelings during the panic episode, the patient stated, "I was afraid. I was mad. First I was afraid, then mad, back and forth." When asked what she thought of during this time, she stated, "I can remember that all I could think about was how they drink—my sisters, Henry my husband—evilness." When questioned about perceptions, the patient answered, "I saw their faces coming at me."

Police officers reported that they had received instructions to intervene in a family fight. On arrival at the house, they found the patient standing on the porch. The police officers assumed that the patient was the complainant, and questioned her about what had transpired. They reported that the patient talked in riddles and in circles. The police officers accompanied the patient into the house to assess the situation. On arrival, the police officers described the situation as "bedlam" and "a mess—everyone was shouting and screaming. The mother was hysterical." The police separated the protagonists, and, after interviewing them, attempted to persuade the patient to accompany the police to the hospital. The officers stated that the patient talked in circles. She talked about Henry and drinking, and "did not appear to hear anything we said a lot of the time."

Finally, after a "little while," the patient agreed to accompany the police officers to the hospital. Both officers reported that she was reluctant, but agreed to come. Family members stated that the police had succeeded in calming the patient. The patient reported that she was afraid to go, but that she thought she "would be away from her sisters and the police were nice."

On arrival at the hospital, the patient was quiet. She was oriented and answered questions appropriately.

She looked around the emergency room and occasionally smiled at the police officers who remained with her. The admission procedure was uneventful and no medications were given. The patient was interviewed shortly after her transfer to the psychiatric unit. The interview lasted approximately fifty minutes. The patient was able to remember events after the arrival of the police at her home as well as events before she ran out of the house. Descriptions of events of the panic episode were not given in order of occurrence by the patient. During the course of the interview, the patient pieced together what had occurred and was able to enlarge upon details of the episode. With assistance, she was able to describe events in order of sequence. When asked how she felt at present, the patient replied, "I feel better now—just a little afraid once in a while." The patient stated that she felt tired and fell asleep shortly after the interview was terminated.

The diagnosis of this patient was "psychotic reaction, undiagnosed." The patient remained in the hospital for eight days. The hospital chart described no episodes of hyperactive behavior during her hospital stay. On the eighth day, the patient was released to the custody of her mother.

In discussing their success in calming the patient, one of the police officers stated that, in his experience, "diversionary measures helped." He said that he had found that if the patient was talking about something, it was a good idea to ask questions about the topic and encourage the patient to talk. He specified that this patient had said that she worked every day and had a good job in a toy factory. The officer questioned the patient about the job, and the patient talked about her job during the entire trip to the hospital.

## Case 2

The patient was a 30-year-old, female Caucasian. She was single. The patient had a history of mental illness, having been hospitalized intermittently during the past three years. She was not gainfully employed at the time of her current admission to the hospital. However, she had been employed as a nurse in a general hospital for three months, up until two weeks before hospitalization.

Respondents for this case study were one staff nurse and two police officers. The patient was alone immediately before the panic episode, and no family members were available for interview. The initial account of the episode was the patient's. No validation was available. The first portion of the case study is the patient's verbatim account of the episode.

> I was in a private psychiatric hospital. The doctor wanted me to leave. I don't know why. My brother came for me and we left. I had brought my car to the hospital, so I went in my car. He went in his. I was supposed to follow him. I lost him. I was on a highway. I remember I got to a restaurant close to the tunnel. Last stop for gas, 17 miles—I remember that sign. I went in. I had a cup of coffee. Then I met two women who were psychologists and they insisted that I call my doctor. I didn't want to, but they said I was in no condition to drive, but they would take me anywhere I wanted to go. I called the doctor. He wanted me to go back to the hospital for the night.

The police officers stated that they had been alerted to investigate a disturbance at a highway restaurant. Upon arrival, one officer remained in the patrol car, the other entered the restaurant. The patient was in the phone booth telephoning. She was shouting. Two women were outside the booth, speaking to her. He went over and asked the patient what was wrong. She was shouting and yelling incoherently. Verbalizations concerned her brother and three hospitals which the patient named. The police officer was unable to convince the woman to leave with him. After about six minutes, the patient agreed to go to her car to speak with the police officer. They left the restaurant and entered the patient's car. The police officer unsuccessfully attempted to elicit information from the patient in order to notify her family. She was incoherent. Finally, she agreed to drive with the officer, in her car, to police headquarters. The officer left the car to inform the second police officer. The patient started the car and sped toward the parking lot exit. At the exit, the patient turned in the wrong direction, driving down the highway in the direction of oncoming traffic. To avoid a head-on collision, the patient drove the car onto a center island. She continued down it at high speed. The police car followed in pursuit. One of the officers shot out the tires of the patient's car, halting it. By this time other police cars had converged on the scene.

The police officers then broke into the patient's car. They found her cowering on the floor of the car. Her face was buried in her hands; she was crying and cursing. She attempted to escape. With the assistance of additional police, she was handcuffed and moved to a police car. A decision was made to take her to X Hospital. The patient cried and screamed that she did not want to be taken there. The police officers stated that they would take her to another hospital instead. The patient became calmer. She remained quiet until the police car was a short distance from X Hospital. At that point she recognized the area and realized that she was being taken to X Hospital. She became hyperactive again.

The patient arrived at the hospital shortly after midnight. On arrival at the hospital, she was screaming and assaultive. Assistance was needed to bring her into the emergency room. She was put into full restraints, and 100 mg. of Sparine were administered intramuscularly.

The patient recognized a staff nurse. She screamed at the nurse, cursing her. The patient alternated between hyperactive and quiet behavior, first screaming at and about the nurse and then begging not to be kept in the hospital. During that interval, she was transferred to the psychiatric ward. On arrival on the ward, she was moved into a bed and restrained. Her behavior was less overactive. She cried quietly. She was oriented as to place and within five minutes was able to be interviewed.

The patient was interviewed for a period of eighty minutes. At the start of the interview, she was unable to recall anything except her arrival at the hospital. As the interview progressed, the patient remembered scattered fragments of the episode, but not in order. With assistance, the patient remembered more and more of what happened. She would repeat details, gradually piecing the episode together in order of its emergence. There were, however, three gaps in the events which the patient was unable to recall.

The patient remembered being in the restaurant. She remembered that the police officer had been with her in the car. She could not remember the events between the time she was in the restaurant and when she was seated in the car talking with the police officer.

The second gap occurred between the time the police officer left the car and when she drove off.

The third gap in description occurred between the time that the police officers broke into her car, and when she was en route to X Hospital. She did, however, recall one detail—being handcuffed. She described this detail as "the handcuffs came toward me."

When asked what she had thought about at the beginning of the panic episode, the patient replied, "X Hospital, X Hospital, and here I am." When asked how she felt at the beginning of the panic episode, the patient stated that she could not remember.

While in the parking lot and afterward, the patient stated she was "scared like hell." Her thoughts were: "What can I do—jump out of the car—hide?"

The patient's perceptual attention focused on many insignificant details in the environment during the entire panic episode. These details appeared disproportionately large in her visual field, according to the patient. Examples of this are the road sign, when traveling to the restaurant, the red lights revolving on top of the police cars during the patient's attempted escape, and the handcuffs applied after the patient was caught. She also reported that all she could see when she arrived at the hospital was that "filthy pig of a nurse." She explained her total behavior with the comment, "I'm not mean. I was upset and scared."

The researcher remained with the patient for a total of two hours. The patient was awake when the researcher left the ward.

The patient remained in the hospital for one day. Her diagnosis was "psychotic reaction, undiagnosed." Notations on the chart designated the patient as homicidal and suicidal. She was transferred the following day to a mental hospital.

## CASE 3

The patient was a 29-year-old, female Negro. She was married and the mother of three children. The patient was unemployed; she was described as a housewife. She had no previous history of mental illness.

Respondents for this case included the patient's father, sister, and brother-in-law, and two police officers. Biographical data were secured from the patient's sister and brother-in-law who live in the same building as the patient. The patient's father was unable to answer questions about behavioral changes in the patient prior to the panic episode.

According to the sister and brother-in-law, the first behavioral change noted in the patient occurred two to three weeks before the panic episode. The patient appeared nervous and restless, stayed by herself more, and spoke less. For one to two weeks before the panic episode, the patient's daily routine changed. Meals were served at irregular hours, and the patient appeared less able to handle household routines, although she seemed busy. For four to five days before the panic episode, the patient slept less than usual. Her sister stated that she was up at night, walking. The patient stated that she was unable to sleep.

At the onset of the panic episode, no participants were present. The initial account of what occurred is a verbatim description by the patient.

> I remember I was in the kitchen, frying fish. I was alone. Just me and my little baby. She was playing. My four-year-old was in the living room, playing. Before I went to the bathroom, I was nervous. My bathroom and kitchen are attached. I went into the bathroom. When I came out, my nerves . . . The baby was crying and calling. Wait! Bathroom—kitchen— maybe there was a noise—the kids beating pans and spoons. The beating of the pans and spoons became louder and louder until I couldn't stand it. I came out of the bathroom to turn the fish. I turned or was turning the fish and something came up in my chest. Something—like—a-a fear. All I could see was the kitchen table. It looked long or something—long—long—noise —noise all around. My seven-year-old daughter—I grabbed her. She ran. I said, "I won't hurt you, Cookie." She said, "Turn me loose and I'll get Aunt Mabel." Then I turned her loose. She ran and kept going. Then my baby cried and I grabbed her. I was out on the street, laying on the sidewalk. How did I get on the street? I was on the street and my brother was trying to drag me back in the hall. Oh, I don't remember. On the street I was screaming and running. They caught me. They said I would hurt myself. I ran half a block. I was afraid.

The patient's brother-in-law ran after the patient when told by the patient's daughter what had occurred. With the help of two passers-by, the patient was forcibly returned to her apartment, screaming. She became hyperactive again. She screamed "Get away! No! No!", ran around the kitchen, knocking over the table and attempting to avoid persons in the apartment. By this time the noise had brought several persons to the scene. Someone phoned for police assistance. Persons present struggled with the patient, attempting to subdue her.

The police arrived within ten minutes, and with help, placed the patient in full restraints. She was removed by police ambulance to the hospital.

The patient remembered some of the events after returning to her apartment. She stated:

> I wanted to scream. Then, like a dog—like a fury, I was beating a stove, a table. I bit my tongue and my mouth like I was eating hard. I hit the table—tried to pick it up—like going crazy. I never did that before—picking it up, knocking it over. Then I was like out cold. I don't remember. I can't remember. I don't remember. Then they were looping me. Then they put a bag on me. I looked up at brass buttons. I said, "What are you folks

doing here?" They carried me somewhere—a long trip—sounded like a car with a motor. I was by myself. I was laying, tied up, looking up. I was laying on a floor. Then that's all. Then there were lights over me. They said, "You're in the hospital." Then I saw a lady I knew.

On arrival at the hospital, the patient was screaming and struggling in the body bag. She was transferred immediately to the psychiatric unit. En route she appeared to hear nothing that was said to her. Her verbalizations were screams, interspersed with "No! No! . . . Help! . . . Stop!" On arrival on the ward, she looked at the ward attendant and stated, "I know you. You live near me." The patient became less active. She was transferred to a bed, undressed, and hand and ankle restraints were applied. She appeared to become aware of her surroundings during this time. The researcher began to question the patient about fifteen minutes after her arrival on the psychiatric unit. Initially, the patient stated repeatedly that she could not remember what had occurred prior to admission to the hospital. With assistance, she was able to remember fragments of events, but not in the order of occurrence. When questioned further, she was able to enlarge upon details, and then to serialize almost all of what had occurred. There were three gaps in the account, the events of which the patient could not remember.

When asked what she had thought during the beginning of the panic episode, the patient stated that she had thought about escaping. When asked what she was escaping, the patient said she did not know, but that she had a fear, and that she had to escape it. When questioned about what she thought about later, when she was back in the apartment, she stated that she wondered why all the people were there and why the room was in disorder.

The patient remembered several perceptions during the panic episode which appeared out of proportion to their realistic size. Two were visual. These were the kitchen table and the brass buttons on the police officer's uniform. The other perceptual distortion was auditory, "The beating of the pans and spoons louder and louder until I couldn't stand it." The patient stated several times that she was tired and wanted to sleep. After seventy minutes of interviewing, the patient concluded the interview by stating that she wished to sleep. She fell asleep immediately. The researcher observed and interviewed the patient for a total of one hour and forty-five minutes.

The patient was diagnosed "hysteria." She remained in the hospital four days. At the end of that time she was released to her husband's custody.

## CASE 4

The patient was a 34-year-old, married, Negro female. She had six children. In February, 1960, her husband deserted the family. At that time the patient was hospitalized in a mental hospital. One of the respondents cared for the patient's children during the patient's hospitalization.

Respondents for this case included two friends of the patient and two police officers. The respondents stated that the patient had been hospitalized in a mental hospital until three weeks before the panic episode. On leaving the hospital, the patient returned to her home and resumed caring for her family.

According to the friends' statements, the first behavioral changes noted in the patient began about one week before the panic episode. The patient became "more nervous." During this time, the patient ate little and was unable to sleep. She spoke constantly of dying. The day before the panic episode the patient was no longer able to function in her own household. At this time the patient was taken to live at the home of one of the respondents.

On the evening of the panic episode, the patient was observed trembling. Following this, she had an involuntary bowel movement. She then began screaming, "Help me! Help me!" She did not appear to recognize the respondent. She began running around the house. Her movements were described as slow and weak. The single respondent present during this part of the panic episode reported that she ran after the patient and caught her. The patient struggled to escape, but was too weak to do so. The respondent stated that the patient was incoherent. The only words the respondent recognized concerned death. After a short interval, the patient appeared calmer. The respondent was able to communicate verbally with the patient. The respondent asked simple questions about the patient's children, and the patient was able to respond accurately to the questions.

For three hours the respondent stayed with the patient. During this time, the patient's behavior alternated between disoriented behavior, when the patient appeared unable to hear the respondent, and oriented behavior, when the patient spoke "intelligently." The patient was not hyperactive during this period.

At the end of three hours, the second respondent came into the house. The patient became hyperactive again, screaming, running, and struggling with both respondents. The patient appeared unable to hear the respondents when they spoke to her. One respondent phoned for police assistance. By the time police arrived, the patient was quiet again and recognized her friends.

All the respondents stated that the patient appeared nervous and afraid. The police decided to take the patient to the hospital. The patient agreed to come, then refused. She was described as so frightened that she could no longer move and practically had to be carried to the police car.

The patient was ambulatory on arrival at the hospital. She moved slowly. Her behavior was frozen-to-the-spot. She appeared terrified. She was moved from the emergency room to the psychiatric ward via wheelchair. She offered no resistance when she was undressed and put to bed. On the ward, 50 mg. of Sparine were administered intramuscularly. The patient lay rigidly in the bed. She was unable to communicate with others. She responded to the researcher's questions with "I'm afraid. I'm going to die." She did not speak with the researcher at any time. No description of the panic episode was obtained from the patient.

The patient was observed for one and one-half hours. At the end of that period she fell asleep.

The patient was diagnosed as "schizophrenic reaction, undifferentiated." She remained in the hospital four days. She then was transferred to a mental hospital.

## CASE 5

The patient was a 38-year-old, male Negro. He was married and the father of three children. He had no history of mental illness. He had been employed as a commissary helper for nineteen years and was gainfully employed at the time of his admission to the hospital.

Panic participants in this case were the patient's son and two hospital personnel, a doctor and a nurse. The patient's wife and sister supplied biographical data. Neither of them was present at any part of the panic episode.

The patient's family noted behavioral changes in the patient for approximately six days before the onset of the panic episode. The patient's usual behavior was described as very quiet. About six days before the panic episode, the patient became very talkative. His family stated that he talked constantly about art and painting (his hobby) and seeing-eye dogs. This behavior persisted for four days. On the fourth day, the patient stopped eating. He spent part of his time "marching around the house like a soldier." His behavior alternated between hostile verbal attacks and gift-giving. On the day before the panic episode, he stayed home from work. He called his employer, stating that he was ill. The patient explained his behavior to his family by saying that he was waiting for the delivery of a mirror he had purchased. He stayed home from work the following day as well. The following excerpts are from verbatim data given by the patient's son:

> At six A.M. on the day he got sick, Dad woke me up to go on a train ride. He kept talking about seeing-eye dogs. We went on the train. He talked, talked, talked. To make it worse, a seeing-eye dog and a blind man got on the train. My father talked louder and louder. The blind man got off the train and we followed him. He talked to the blind man and tried to take the man's arm. The man said no. Dad kept talking about seeing-eye dogs. From there we walked to the art league, then to the garment center, then to a church, then to a restaurant. All the way he kept stopping people to talk to them. He stopped traffic in cars and tried to talk to them. Then we went to a department store, and Dad bought me six pairs of pants, a coat, and a suit. After that we went to buy shoes. He made me buy combat boots. Then he changed from nice to cross and yelled at me. Then he changed back to nice. We left the store, and he made me run after him all the way to the train station. He ran real fast. I could hardly keep up. We got on the train and Dad went to buy me a soda. He gave me the train pass to show the conductor. He told me not to give it away—just show it. It turned out it was my mother's pass, and the conductor took it away from me, because it wasn't mine. Then my father came back, screaming and arguing. When we got to the next stop, Dad ran off the train and I ran after him. On the platform he made me sit on the floor, and he took off my shoes, coat, and shirt. Boy, I was freezing. Then a man came and said to bring me inside. Dad said I had heart failure and couldn't move. An ambulance came and we got into it. My father told me not to say anything. They thought I was sick. At the hospital he asked for information, then collapsed. He was talking and yelling.

The first indication the hospital personnel had that they were treating the wrong patient came when the patient suddenly started screaming and shouting in the emergency room. Personnel attempted to quiet him and a struggle ensued. The patient was restrained and put into a bed. He appeared to hear no one. His verbalizations consisted of screams and shouting such as "Get out! . . . Stop it! . . . I'll kill you!" Ideation included war, seeing-eye dogs, tanks, and God. He shouted, screamed, and struggled for forty minutes. During this time, he was transferred to the psychiatric unit. Occasionally, during the period of hyperactivity, he appeared to hear words and phrases used by other persons and included these in his verbalizations. After forty minutes of hyperactivity, he became quiet, looked around the ward, and asked what had happened. Hospital personnel spoke with him and told him where he was. At this time the patient was interviewed.

The patient was willing to speak with the researcher, but avoided answering questions about what had happened. He described a few of the events that had transpired after he had left home with his son. He stated that he had visited the art league and a department store, but would not or could not describe what had happened. He described having been on the train and going to buy a soda. He stated that he had argued with the conductor and that he had "tried to tear his head off like he learned in the army." (The patient's son stated that he had not hit the conductor.) He remembered getting off the train and said that after that he had "blanked out and woke up here on the ward."

The patient refused to enlarge on any of the details he had given. He stated:

> I don't remember what happened. Something rose—happened. I never told anyone about this. In Belgium a jeep turned over and hit me. If I let myself think about the war—the tanks, the ditches—I'd go crazy. I won't remember. I'd go crazy. I won't remember what happened today, just like I won't remember the war. I'll go crazier if I do.

The patient avoided discussion of thoughts, feelings, and perceptions connected with the panic episode. A total of two hours was spent in observation and interview of the patient. The interview lasted fifty minutes.

The patient remained in the hospital for six days. According to the patient's chart, his behavior was frequently bizarre, and his verbalizations were often incoherent. The patient was overactive during this time, but did not have to be restrained. He was diagnosed as "schizoprehnia, schizo-affective." After the sixth day, he was transferred to a mental hospital.

## Case 6

The patient was a 43-year-old, female Negro. The patient was unemployed; she was described as a housewife. She had no previous history of mental illness.

Respondents included two friends and two hospital personnel, a doctor and a nurse. Biographical data were secured from the patient's husband, who did not witness the panic episode.

According to the patient's husband, the patient had been worried about the health of her mother, who had been ill for three months. The mother had "become sicker" about two weeks before the onset of the panic episode. The husband noted that the patient appeared nervous for about two months before her panic episode. The patient had made plans to go to the hospital for a major operation at that time. The operation was scheduled for the day following her panic episode. One month before the panic episode, she was reported to have become forgetful. Examples of this behavior were that the patient would forget plans she had made and that, on two occasions, she had walked past her house and around the block several times without recognizing where she lived. Her husband stated that he had had to go outside and call to her to come in. For two weeks prior to the panic episode, the patient had slept little and had lost her appetite.

On the day of the panic episode, the patient had gone to a hairdresser. The beautician, who knew the patient, reported that the patient seemed a little dazed when the beautician spoke with her. While the patient's hair was being dressed, she spoke to the beauticians about going to the hospital for an operation on the following day. The beauticians stated that the patient "talked on and on about the operation she needed." Suddenly, the patient "got stunned and slumped a little. Then she started talking wild, loud, and fast about operations and fibroids. She didn't make sense." She vomited, then tried to run outside. The patient was so weak, however, that she was unable to leave. One beautician held the patient. She attempted to obtain the husband's telephone number from the patient by shouting to her. The patient appeared not to hear anything that was said. She was screaming about fibroids and operations. She continued trying to escape from the beautician's grasp to run out the door, but was unable to do so. After the beautician shouted at the patient "many times," the patient heard the question and supplied her home phone number.

One beautician attempted to phone the patient's husband. There was no answer. She then phoned for police assistance.

Within a few minutes, two police officers arrived. They asked the patient to accompany them to the hospital. The patient made feeble attempts to escape. The police assisted the patient to the police car, almost carrying her.

On arrival at the hospital, the patient entered the door, then began running around the emergency room. The police called hospital personnel for assistance. She was caught by two police officers, who held her. With the assistance of a nurse, the patient was taken to an examining room. During that time, the patient was shouting incoherently. The only word heard clearly was "fibroid."

A doctor entered and asked the patient her name and address several times. The patient stated she was "Mrs. Fibroid," from "Fibroid Street," in "Fibroid, Alabama." Her answers were given in a loud voice, and she struggled to push the doctor away from her as she spoke. Fifteen minutes after the patient's arrival at the hospital, she was transferred to the psychiatric unit via wheelchair. The patient stopped talking as soon as she was seated in the wheelchair. When she arrived on the ward, she was undressed and put to bed. After the ward nurse had completed this routine, the patient smiled at the nurse and thanked her. She asked the nurse where she was. The nurse told her.

The patient was interviewed ten minutes after her arrival on the ward. There was one gap in the patient's account of the episode. She had more difficulty than any of the other patients interviewed in remembering details of what had occurred. With assistance, she was able to reconstruct events of the morning and afternoon of the panic episode. She remembered being at the hairdresser's, and having her hair done. She could not remember what she spoke about, stating several times that the beautician talked to her. She appeared to have no memory of her own participation. The next memory she had was of the arrival of police. She stated that the police brought her to the hospital, but she didn't know why. She gave sketchy details of events that had transpired after her arrival at the hospital. She appeared unable to enlarge on the details. Several times during the interview, the patient stated that she was tired. At no time did she use the word "fibroid" or "operation" during the interview.

When asked what she had thought about during the panic eposide, the patient stated that she could not remember. When asked what she saw, the patient replied, "All I could see was the door." When asked how she had felt, she responded, "All of a sudden I was afraid."

After forty minutes of interviewing, the patient requested that the interview be terminated so that she could sleep. She fell asleep within five minutes.

The patient was diagnosed as "hysteria." She remained in the hospital for two days, after which she was released in her husband's custody.

Three weeks after the panic episode, the husband of this patient was interviewed by telephone to secure biographical data. The husband reported the patient had entered a general hospital for removal of fibroids. According to the husband, she had had an uneventful postoperative course and had been ambulatory. About six days postoperatively, she had developed "complications." She was operated on a second time and had died following the surgical intervention.

## Case 7

The patient was a 19-year-old, Negro female. She was married and the mother of one child. The patient had been employed as a factory worker for three years. She had no previous history of mental illness.

Respondents for this case were the husband and a nephew of the patient. Biographical data were secured from the patient's husband.

According to the patient's husband, there were no changes in the patient's behavior recently. He reported that the patient had been concerned about her health for about one year. She complained of many pains—headaches, back pains, and pains in her side and stomach. When she had gone to doctors, nothing could be found to account for her complaints. Seven or eight months ago she had begun drinking; however, she had not been drinking on the day of the panic episode. The husband stated that the patient did not drink heavily, but that she "liked to get high."

The patient was brought to the hospital by her husband and her nephew. The stated reason for coming to the hospital was for treatment of pain in the patient's side. The patient had a small abrasion on her forehead. She complained of a pain in her leg as well.

The emergency room staff was busy when the patient arrived. She was placed on a stretcher to await treatment. The patient's husband remained with the patient.

The first realization that there was anything unusual in the patient's behavior occurred when the staff and the researcher heard the patient begin to scream, "No! No! Help! Stop! Let me out of here! Stop! Stop! My leg! Help! No! No! Mother! Help!"

Three hospital personnel, the researcher, and research assistant stood in the hall, immobilized momentarily, staring at the patient. The patient's husband was standing a few feet away from the stretcher, looking at the patient. The patient then attempted to get off the stretcher.

The hospital personnel ran to the patient and restrained her with the stretcher blanket. The patient screamed and struggled. The patient was moved to a treatment room, and 50 mg. of Sparine were administered intramuscularly to the patient. The patient screamed and struggled continuously for four minutes. She did not appear to hear the verbalizations of the staff who attempted to speak with her.

One of the nurses who was with the patient asked the patient her age repeatedly during the time that the patient was screaming. After four minutes, the patient said, "Nineteen." She then began screaming again, shouting, "I'm scared! I'm scared! Let me go! Help!" At the end of three minutes, the patient became quieter and looked around the room. A nurse spoke softly to the patient. She told the patient that personnel would remove the patient's clothes and replace them with a hospital gown. The patient cooperated. As the patient's clothes were being changed, she repeated over and over, "I'm scared." She then began to cry.

The nurse asked the patient for her name and address. The patient answered the questions. The nurse asked what had happened. The patient replied that she did not know, then stated, "I'm at a hospital."

The nurse again asked what had happened. The patient stated that she was afraid of her husband, and that he had beaten her before she came to the hospital. The patient repeated this statement over and over for three minutes. At the end of that time, the patient fell asleep, and the researcher left the treatment room.

During this time, the research assistant interviewed the patient's family. Both family members gave the following account of what had occurred earlier.

The patient and her husband went to a local store. The husband went inside; the patient waited outside. A few minutes later, when the husband left the store, he saw his wife lying on the sidewalk, screaming. He attempted to pick her up. She fell down, striking her head. The patient's nephew was walking down the street. He saw his aunt and his uncle. He and two friends assisted the patient's husband in carrying the patient to her house. She screamed and struggled. Her verbalizations were "No! No! Stop! Help!" She screamed about pains in her head, knee, and side. She begged her family not to leave her.

The patient's mother was at home. Husband and mother suggested that the patient go to the hospital. The patient became quieter. She agreed to go. A taxi was called. When it arrived, the patient refused to leave the house. The taxi was dismissed.

The patient was quiet for approximately fifteen minutes. She then became hyperactive. She ran around the house screaming. Another taxi was called, and the patient was forcibly put into the taxi by her husband and nephew.

The patient struggled during the entire trip, striking at the husband and the nephew and attempting to push past them to get out of the cab. She screamed about the pain in her side.

The struggle continued on the sidewalk outside of the hospital. The patient was pulled inside the door. She suddenly became quiet. Her hyperactivity ceased.

The patient's husband told a nurse that the patient had a pain in her side. The nurse assisted the patient onto a stretcher. The patient sat on the stretcher quietly for about five minutes, whereupon she began screaming again.

The patient did not remain at the hospital. After she had fallen asleep, personnel left the room. Approximately one and one-half hours after she had arrived, the patient dressed herself and left the hospital without being seen by hospital personnel.

During the time the patient was observed, her expressed ideation was of pain. She stated also that she had been beaten. She expressed feelings of fear frequently. No specific questions were asked about perceptions. It is interesting to note, however, that her interpretations of perceptions of the panic episode were at variance with data obtained from her family. She perceived their interventions in the panic episode as physical assault by her husband. She did not mention the presence of any other persons during the panic episode.

## PATIENT PROFILES, CASES 1 TO 7

Individual patient profiles were constructed from the analyzed data. Each profile indicated changes of behavior in the patient prior to the panic episode and the length of time during which these changes were noted by significant persons. The experiences of the patients during the panic episode were described operationally. Profiles of each panic patient follow.

PATIENT PROFILE                                                    CASE 1

| Time | Changes in Behavior | Duration |
|------|---------------------|----------|
| Prior to | Increased verbal aggression | 3 months |
| panic | Somatic complaints | 3 months |
| episode | Neglect of personal appearance | 3 months |

### Panic Episode

Operationally, the patient experienced:
1. An abstract thought that excluded all other thought . . High level of anxiety
2. Projection of the abstract idea onto the environment . . Increased anxiety
3. Conversion of anxiety . . . . . . . . . . . . . . . . . . . . . . . . . . . Decreased anxiety
   a. Anger
   b. Aggression
   (Counteraggression from environment) . . . . . . . . . . . . Increased anxiety
4. A sensory-perception detail related to thought was blown up, blotting out all other sensory perceptions . . Increased anxiety
5. Personality disorganization . . . . . . . . . . . . . . . . . . . . . . . Increased anxiety
   a. Increased motor activity
      Reduced sensory perception
      Reduced ability to communicate
   b. Violent motor activity . . . . . . . . . . . . . . . . . . . . . . . . Panic
      Withdrawing
      Loss of sensory perception
      Loss of higher psychic functions

*Panic Episode*

  c. Reduced motor activity ......................Decreased anxiety
     Scattered sensory perception
     Increased, but limited ability to communicate
6. Personality reorganization ........................Decreased anxiety
  a. Reduced motor activity                    Fatigue
  b. Increased sensory perception
  c. Increased ability to communicate
  d. Rationalization of panic episode

## PATIENT PROFILE                                                  CASE 2

| Time | Changes in Behavior | Duration |
|---|---|---|
| Prior to panic episode | Data unavailable | |

*Panic Episode*

Operationally, the patient experienced:
1. Perception of multiple scattered details of environment. High level of anxiety
2. Sensory-perception details blown up, blotting out all
    other sensory perceptions ......................Increased anxiety
3. Personality disorganization ......................Panic
  a. Violent motor activity
  b. Loss of sensory perception
  c. Loss of higher psychic functions
4. Personality reorganization ........................Decreased anxiety
  a. Reduced motor activity
  b. Increased sensory perceptions
  c. Increased ability to communicate
  d. Disorientation about events of panic episode
5. Recurrence of Steps 1 through 4
6. Recurrence of Steps 1 through 4

## PATIENT PROFILE                                                  CASE 3

| Time | Changes in Behavior | Duration |
|---|---|---|
| Prior to panic episode | Increased anxiety | 3 weeks |
| | Decreased communication | 3 weeks |
| | Withdrawal from others | 3 weeks |
| | Decreased ability to function in daily activities | 2 weeks |
| | Insomnia | 4 to 5 days |

*Panic Episode*

Operationally, the patient experienced:
1. Perception of multiple scattered details of environ-
    ment ........................................High level of anxiety
2. Sensory-perception details blown up, blotting out all
    other sensory perceptions ......................Increased anxiety
3. Personality disorganization ......................Panic
  a. Violent motor activity

*Panic Episode*
  b. Loss of sensory perception
  c. Loss of higher psychic functions
4. Personality reorganization ........................ Decreased anxiety
  a. Reduced motor activity                            Fatigue
  b. Increased sensory perceptions
  c. Increased ability to communicate
  d. Disorientation about events of panic episode
5. Recurrence of Steps 1 through 4
6. Recurrence of Steps 1 through 4

PATIENT PROFILE                                          CASE 4

| Time | Changes in Behavior | Duration |
|---|---|---|
| Prior to | Increased anxiety | 1 week |
| panic | Anorexia | 1 week |
| episode | Insomnia | 1 week |
|  | Thanatophobia | 1 week |
|  | Inability to function in daily activities | 2 days |

*Panic Episode*

Data were not complete for this patient. From available data, the patient apparently experienced:
1. A concrete thought blown up, blotting out all other
   thought .................................... Increased anxiety
2. Personality disorganization ...................... Panic
  a. Violent motor activity
  b. Withdrawing
  c. Loss of sensory perception
  d. Loss of higher psychic functions
  (Intervention from environment)
3. Personality reorganization
   (3 hours) .................................... Decreased anxiety
  a. Reduced motor activity
  b. Increased but limited ability to communicate
4. Two alternating concrete thoughts
   (one focused on by others in environment) ........ Alternating
                                                      decreased and
                                                      increased anxiety
5. Recurrence of Steps 1 and 2
6. Frozen-to-the-spot behavior (terror?)
  a. Loss of ability to communicate
  b. Paralysis of action

PATIENT PROFILE                                          CASE 5

| Time | Changes in Behavior | Duration |
|---|---|---|
| Prior to | Increased verbalizations | 6 days |
| panic | Anorexia | 4 days |
| episode | Unpredictable behavior, verbal aggression, gift-giving | 4 days |
|  | Rationalizations of behavior | 4 days |
|  | Absent from work | 2 days |

### Panic Episode

Operationally, the patient experienced:
1. An abstract thought that excluded all other thought . . High level of anxiety
2. Projection of the abstract idea onto the environment . . Increased anxiety
3. Conversion of anxiety . . . . . . . . . . . . . . . . . . . . . . . . . . . Decreased anxiety
   a. Anger
   b. Aggression
   (Counteraggression from environment) . . . . . . . . . . . . Increased anxiety
4. A sensory-perception detail related to thought was
   blown up, blotting out all other sensory perceptions . . Increased anxiety
5. Personality disorganization . . . . . . . . . . . . . . . . . . . . . Increased anxiety
   a. Increased motor activity
   Reduced sensory perception
   Reduced ability to communicate
   b. Violent motor activity . . . . . . . . . . . . . . . . . . . . . . Panic
   Withdrawing
   Loss of sensory perception
   Loss of higher psychic functions
   c. Reduced motor activity . . . . . . . . . . . . . . . . . . . . . . Decreased anxiety
   Scattered sensory perception
   Increased, but limited, ability to communicate
6. Personality reorganization . . . . . . . . . . . . . . . . . . . . . . Decreased anxiety
   a. Reduced motor activity                    Fatigue
   b. Increased sensory perception
   c. Increased ability to communicate
   d. Rationalization of panic episode

## PATIENT PROFILE                                          CASE 6

| Time | Changes in Behavior | Duration |
|---|---|---|
| Prior to | Increased anxiety | 2 months |
| panic | Intermittent periods of amnesia | 1 month |
| episode | Anorexia | 2 weeks |
| | Insomnia | 2 weeks |

### Panic Episode

Operationally, the patient experienced:
1. A concrete thought that excluded all other thought . . . High level of anxiety
2. The concrete thought was blown up . . . . . . . . . . . . . . . Increased anxiety
3. An unrelated (?) sensory-perception detail in the en-
   vironment was blown up, blotting out all other
   sensory perceptions . . . . . . . . . . . . . . . . . . . . . . . . . . Increased anxiety
4. Personality disorganization . . . . . . . . . . . . . . . . . . . . . Increased anxiety
   a. Increased motor activity
   Reduced sensory perception
   Reduced ability to communicate
   b. Violent motor activity . . . . . . . . . . . . . . . . . . . . . . Panic
   Withdrawing
   Loss of sensory perception
   Loss of higher psychic functions
   c. Reduced motor activity . . . . . . . . . . . . . . . . . . . . . . Decreased anxiety
   Scattered, but limited, ability to communicate

*Panic Episode*

5. Personality reorganization
   a. Reduced motor activity
   b. Increased, but limited sensory perceptions
   c. Disorientation
6. Recurrence of Steps 1 through 4
7. Personality reorganization ......................Decreased anxiety
   a. Reduced motor activity
   b. Increased sensory perceptions
   c. Ability to communicate
   d. Total loss of memory of thought that precipitated
      panic episode

PATIENT PROFILE                                              CASE 7

| Time | Changes in Behavior | Duration |
|------|---------------------|----------|
| Prior to panic episode | Somatizing<br>Increased use of alcohol | 1 year<br>7 to 8 months |

*Panic Episode*

Operationally, the patient experienced:
1. A concrete thought blown up, excluding all other
   thought  ......................................Increased anxiety
2. Personality disorganization ......................Increased anxiety
   a. Increased motor activity
      Reduced sensory perception
      Reduced ability to communicate
   b. Violent motor activity .......................Panic
      Withdrawing
      Loss of sensory perception
      Loss of higher psychic functions
   c. Reduced motor activity ......................Decreased anxiety
      Scattered sensory perception
      Increased, but limited, ability to communicate
      Somatizing
3. Personality reorganization ......................Decreased anxiety
   a. Reduced motor activity                        Fatigue
   b. Increased sensory perception
   c. Increased ability to communicate
   d. Rationalization of panic episode
   e. Somatizing

COMPOSITE PROFILE

Patterns of individual panic began to emerge. In all of the cases, patients experienced a high degree of anxiety, which increased to the point at which it was labeled as fear. All the patients became hyperactive, with a common goal of withdrawal. Actions became violent, and there was at least one period of time during which the patients experienced a total lack of recall of thoughts and perceptions. All the patients were able to see and hear what went on in the environment at some time when their behavior was violent. However, most panic participants were unaware of the possibility of communication. All the patients interviewed experienced difficulty in recall of the events following the panic episode. When initially interviewed, each patient said repeatedly, "I can't remember." With difficulty, all except one patient was able to recall a large part of the panic experience. None of the patients was able to recall the panic episode in the order of emergence. Each remembered some fragments of the experience. With assistance they were able to enlarge upon the fragments, then to reconstruct the situation as it occurred. The patients who experienced only one memory gap in events were able to reconstruct the panic episode in sequence more rapidly than the patients who experienced multiple gaps of memory.

Most of the patients experienced more than one period of violent motor activity with concurrent gaps in recall of thoughts and perceptions. This implies increases and decreases in their levels of anxiety, with more than one point in the panic episode in which their personalities disorganized, then reorganized to some extent. In most of the cases, details in the patients' perceptual fields became distorted. These details enlarged until they blotted out all other possible perceptions. It was after this experience that patients described a total loss of contact with their environment.

During the panic portion of the panic episode, the experiences of five of the patients (Cases 1, 2, 3, 5, and 6) were identical. Data were unavailable for Patient 4. Patient 7 reported no distortions of sensory perceptions during the panic episode. The distortion described by this patient was a misinterpretation of what occurred. Because of the difficulty in recall following the episode, it cannot be certain whether this difference in experience occurred, or whether the patient was unable to recall sensory-perception distortion.

All except one patient reported a decrease in the level of anxiety following the panic episode. Almost all the patients described feelings of fatigue, and most fell asleep immediately after the panic episode, whether or not they had received medications.

The individual patient profiles were compared and analyzed. From the analysis, a composite profile of individual panic was constructed. The composite profile, presented operationally, follows.

## COMPOSITE PROFILE                              CASES 1 THROUGH 7

| *Time* | *Changes in Behavior* | *Duration* |
|---|---|---|
| Prior to panic episode | Somatizing | 1 year, 3 months |
| | Changes in daily routine | 3 months, 2 days |
| | Increased level of anxiety | 2 months, 1 week |
| | Changes in communication pattern | 3 weeks, 6 days |
| | Anorexia | 2 weeks, 4 days |
| | Insomnia | 2 weeks, 2 days |

### Panic Episode

Operationally, the individual in panic experiences:
1. A high level of anxiety
2. Distortions of
   a. Thought and/or
   b. Perceptions .................................Increased anxiety
3. Distortions of thought and/or perceptions that are blown up and blot out all other thought and/or perceptions ...............................Increased anxiety
4. Personality disorganization ......................Increased anxiety
   a. Increased motor activity
      Reduced sensory perception
      Reduced ability to communicate
   b. Violent motor activity .......................Panic
      Withdrawing
      Loss of sensory perception
      Loss of higher psychic functions
   c. Reduced motor activity ......................Decreased anxiety
      Scattered sensory perception
      Increased, but limited, ability to communicate
5. a. Reorganization of personality
      (See Step 6)
         or
   b. Recurrence of Steps 1 through 4
6. a. Personality reorganization ....................Decreased anxiety
      (1) Reduced motor activity
      (2) Increased sensory perceptions
      (3) Increased ability to communicate and one or more of the following:
      (4) Rationalization of events of panic episode
      (5) Bewilderment about events of the panic episode
      (6) Somatizing
      (7) Fatigue
         or
   b. A terrorlike state
      (1) Paralysis of motor activity
      (2) Inability to communicate

# PROPOSED OPERATIONAL DEFINITION
# OF PANIC

Panic is a process during which an individual experiences an elevation of his level of anxiety. The individual's usual patterns of anxiety-reduction fail or are blocked by the environment. Anxiety continues to rise until it reaches an intolerable level, experienced by the individual as a feeling of overwhelming fear. Ability to communicate decreases. A detail of thought and/or sensory perception blows up until all other thought and/or sensory perceptions are lost. The personality disorganizes temporarily. There is failure of the higher psychic functions, resulting in disrupted intrapersonal and interpersonal functioning. There is a violent motor reaction, with all energies of the individual directed toward withdrawal.

Following this experience, the personality begins to reorganize. If the personality reorganization is successful, anxiety decreases, sensory perceptions increase, higher psychic functions operate again, and interpersonal and intrapersonal functions resume. If the process of personality reorganization fails, the panic process is repeated until personality reorganization is successfully accomplished.

Operationally outlined, the panic process is:

1. The person experiences a high level of anxiety, but maintains personality organization
2. Anxiety stimulus occurs
   a. Internal
   b. External
      or
   c. Both
3. Person experiences increasing anxiety
4. Person attempts to reduce anxiety
   a. Hyperactive behavior
   b. Somatizing
   c. Aggression
5. Attempts to reduce anxiety fail, or are blocked by the environment
6. Anxiety increases
   a. Increased motor activity
   b. Reduced ability to communicate
   c. Reduced sensory perceptions
   d. A thought and/or concrete perceptual detail is blown up, blots out all other details
7. Personality disorganizes temporarily
   a. Failure of higher psychic functions
   b. Disrupted intrapersonal and interpersonal functioning
   c. Violent motor reaction with goal of withdrawal
8. Personality begins reorganization
   a. Reduced motor activity

     b. Scattered sensory perceptions
     c. Increasing, but limited, ability to communicate
9. Personality reorganizes
     a. Anxiety decreases
     b. Increased sensory perceptions
     c. Ability to communicate
     d. No memory of events of panic episode
or

Recurrence of Steps 2 through 8, one or more times, until personality reorganizes.

# BIBLIOGRAPHY

ARIETI, SILVANO, *Interpretation of Schizophrenia*, Robert Brunner, New York: 1955.

——— "Introductory Notes on the Psychoanalytic Therapy of Schizophrenics," in *Psychotherapy of the Psychoses*, Arthur Burton (ed.), Basic Books, New York: 1961.

BROUSSEAU, A., *Essai Sur La Peur Aux Armées 1914–1918*, Alcan, Paris: 1920.

CALDWELL, J. M., RANSON, S. W., and SACHS, J. G., "Group Panic and Other Mass Disruptive Reactions," *U.S. Armed Forces M. J.*, 1951.

FOREMAN, PAUL B., "Panic Theory," *J. Sociol. and Soc. Res.*, 37:295–304, 1953.

KELLAND, C., "How Men and Women Act Facing Terror," *American Magazine*, Vol. 109, March, 1930.

LA PIERE, R., *Collective Behavior*, McGraw-Hill Book Co., New York: 1938.

MEERLOO, JOOST A. M., *Patterns of Panic*, International Universities Press, New York: 1950.

MULLAHY, PATRICK, *Oedipus: Myth and Complex*. Hermitage House, New York: 1948.

MUNSON, E., *The Management of Men*, Henry Holt and Co., New York: 1921.

PEPLAU, HILDEGARD E., *Interpersonal Relations in Nursing*, G. P. Putnam's Sons, New York: 1952.

QUARANTELLI, ENRICO, "The Behavior of Panic Participants, Sociology and Social Research," *J. Appl. Sociol.*, Vol. 41, 1957.

——— "The Nature and Conditions of Panic," *Am. J. Sociol.* Vol. 60, 1954.

SCHMIDELBERG, W., "The Treatment of Panic in Casualty Area and Clearing Station," *Life and Letters Today*, Vol. 23, 1939.

SCHWARTZ, M. W., and SHOCKLEY, E. L., *The Nurse and the Mental Patient*, Russell Sage Foundation, New York: 1956.

SPIEGEL, ROSE, "Specific Problems of Communication in Psychiatric Conditions," in *American Handbook of Psychiatry*, Silvano Arieti (ed.), Basic Books, New York: 1959.

STRAUSS, ANSELM, "The Literature on Panic," *J. Abnormal and Soc. Psychol.* Vol. 39, 1944.

SULLIVAN, HARRY S., *Conceptions of Modern Psychiatry*, W. W. Norton & Co., New York: 1953.

WOLBERG, LEWIS R., *The Technique of Psychotherapy*, Grune and Stratton, New York: 1954.

# 35 SUMMARY: AN EXPLORATORY INVESTIGATION OF TEACHING A PROBLEM–SOLVING PROCESS IN GROUP THERAPY, TO PATIENTS DIAGNOSED "CHRONIC ALCOHOLISM"[1]

*Anita M. Werner*

*Statement of the Problem.* This study investigated some of the outcomes of experiential teaching of a problem-solving process to a group of patients diagnosed "chronic alcoholism." The following null hypothesis was investigated:

*There is no observable difference in the problem-solving ability, as indicated by the verbal responses, between the patients in the group in which problem-solving is experientially taught and the patients in the group in which a nondirective approach is used.*

*Background of the Study.* Evidence from the study-maker's clinical experience and from reports in the literature supported an assumption that chronic alcoholism results from an inadequate attempt at problem-solving. Teaching problem-solving in a group setting might equip the patients to deal with their difficulties more adequately. The advantages of group therapy with patients diagnosed as chronic alcoholics were supported from the literature.

*Need for the Study.* Alcoholism is becoming an increasingly prominent problem. The need for developing techniques effective in intervening into this condition is urgent.

*Purpose of the Study.* The purpose of this study was to explore and to describe the differential effects of using two approaches to group therapy: experiential teaching of problem-solving and nondirective ap-

[1] Thesis submitted to the Graduate School of Rutgers, The State University of New Jersey, in partial fulfillment of the requirements for the degree of Master of Science, May, 1962.

proach. The findings from this study can be used by clinicians in psychiatric nursing to aid in formulating techniques of nursing intervention that promote learning in patients diagnosed as chronic alcoholics.

*Definition of Terms.* The terms defined for this study were chronic alcoholism, experiential teaching, nondirective approach, learning, and problem-solving. Problem-solving was defined as a nine-step process.

*Assumption.* Three assumptions were presented.

1. Patients diagnosed as chronic alcoholics have experienced inadequate use of problem-solving.

2. When the patients do learn to use adequate problem-solving, they will have more control over their behavior.

3. The presence of a problem-solving ability can be inferred from the products of the process, i.e., the patient's verbalizations.

*Limitations.* The study had the following limitations:

1. Unavailability of facilities having adequate patient population from which to choose a sample of patients who were diagnosed "chronic alcoholism" without other complicating conditions.

2. Lack of psychological testing to ascertain the ability of the patients to learn before and after the study.

3. The small number of patients who met the criteria, necessitating the use of the total universe as a sample.

4. Insufficient time to allow the groups to progress at their own rate in therapy.

5. Inconsistent attendance at meetings.

6. Data-collection methods which were problematic.

7. The small size of the sample, which limits the applicability of the findings.

8. Lack of follow-up interviews.

## REVIEW OF THE LITERATURE

The literature was reviewed in the areas of psychology, psychiatry, sociology, and psychiatric nursing, in relation to etiology, dynamics, and group therapy in chronic alcoholism. The psychological theories of alcoholism include the psychoanalytical theories of unresolved homosexual conflicts, self-destruction, oral fixation, pleasure principle, guilt, and anxiety; the interpersonal theories of insecurity stemming from an unhappy family constellation, dissociative tendencies of the self-system, and the substitutive function of alcohol in place of interpersonal relationships. Some theorists viewed alcoholism as a symptom of an underlying emotional condition; others viewed it largely as a psychological disease. The views of sociologists and physiologists were briefly stated. Support for the study-maker's view that alcoholism is an attempt at problem-solving was provided.

The review also reported on studies and articles on group therapy with persons diagnosed as alcoholic. A variety of methods and techniques was employed in a variety of kinds and sizes of groups. Most often, in spite of the particular technique employed, useful results were reported. No studies were found that employed the teaching of problem-solving as a focus in group therapy.

## METHODOLOGY

This study was carried out in a large county mental hospital where there was no active program for the emotional rehabilitation of patients diagnosed "chronic alcoholism." Patients were selected on the basis of criteria which involved diagnosis, age, sex, length of hospitalization, education, absence of observable brain damage, and the ability to generalize. The final selection of patients as group participants necessitated the use of the total universe. The inconsistent attendance of the control-group members was discussed. The group participants were described in terms of the variables used to select them. The pregroup interview provided information regarding the patient's insight into his illness and his ability to problem-solve. The procedure for the group therapy sessions was described. The introduction of the experimental variable, i.e., teaching problem-solving in the problem-solving group, differentiated this group from the control group. The postgroup interview was described as being similar to the pregroup interview and was used for the purpose of ascertaining change in insight into illness and/or problem-solving ability. An elaboration of the procedure for analysis of the verbatim group data and the pregroup and postgroup interviews was presented. Validity of the study was then described. It was possible to obtain only minimal validation of the study. A jury of experts was asked to analyze portions of the data independently, in an effort to ascertain reliability. The procedure for determining reliability was described. The reliability (89 per cent agreement with the study-maker) was considered to be high for a study of this nature.

## PATTERNS OF PROBLEM–SOLVING IN TWO THERAPEUTIC GROUPS

The data were analyzed to present a description of the problem-solving ability of the patients in each group. The summaries of the group sessions described the important background information necessary in understanding the problem-solving outcomes of the group experience. The sessions were summarized in terms of group content, namely: (1) topics discussed, (2) major themes and concepts, (3) group interaction, and (4) nursing intervention. A comparison of the two groups revealed likenesses in the area of personality dynamics. The groups were also fairly evenly matched on the variables of age, sex, socioeconomic status, race, diagnosis, and previous experience in group therapy. The dissimilarities, however, in the areas of group interaction, topics discussed, and degree of illness, were important differences and contributed to the over-all impression that these two groups were more variant than alike.

Individual profiles of each patient in the groups were summarized from the data collected during the group sessions and the pregroup and postgroup interviews. These profiles presented the problem-solving ability of each patient and the observable changes in this ability over the course of therapy.

# FINDINGS

There was evidence to indicate that the null hypothesis was not supported. There were observable differences between the problem-solving ability of the patients in the problem-solving group and the problem-solving ability of the patients in the control group. The patients in the control group evidenced a slightly greater ability to problem-solve than the patients in the problem-solving group. The control-group patients also evidenced slightly more development in this ability over the course of therapy.

# IMPLICATIONS

Implications were presented in light of theory and clinical nursing practice. There was evidence from the group sessions to support existing theory regarding the etiology and personality dynamics of patients diagnosed "chronic alcoholism." The inferences drawn from the findings were applicable to clinical practice in the areas of the selection of patients for group therapy on the bases of major behavioral patterns and motivation toward learning, readiness to learn in the process of group therapy and its application to teaching processes such as a problem-solving process. The results of this study indicate that the usefulness of a combination of didactic and experiential teaching of problem-solving to patients diagnosed "chronic alcoholism" in fifteen group sessions is strongly questionable. The use of problem-solving as a reliable referential framework for the nurse to use in developing principles of intervention in group therapy was stressed. Six nursing principles were formulated and presented as a basis on which to guide intervention in groups with patients diagnosed "chronic alcoholism."

## RECOMMENDATIONS

It is recommended that further research be conducted in the area of group therapy with patients diagnosed as chronic alcoholics. The following suggestions may provide bases for future clinical research studies in this area.

1. Replicate this study with changes in methodology to overcome the major limitations.

2. Explore the usefulness of seeing patients individually for five to ten sessions before group therapy in order to decrease the time required for the orientation phase.

3. Investigate the differences in the outcomes between seeing patients diagnosed "chronic alcoholism" individually and seeing patients with the same diagnosis in group therapy.

4. Develop a method to measure and control the leader's unwitting or covert influence on a group.

## BIBLIOGRAPHY

AGRIN, ALFRED, "The Georgian Clinic," *Quart. J. Stud. Alcohol*, 21:113–24, 1960.

ALEXANDER, FRANZ, *Fundamentals of Psychoanalysis*, W. W. Norton & Co., New York: 1948.

———— "Views on the Etiology of Alcoholism, The Psychodynamic View," *Alcoholism as a Medical Problem*, H. D. Kruse (ed.), Paul B. Hoeber, New York: 1956, pp. 40–46.

———— and ROSS, HELEN, *Dynamic Psychiatry*, University of Chicago Press, Chicago: 1952.

ALLISON, S. G., "Nondirective Group Therapy of Alcoholics in a State Hospital," *Quart. J. Stud. Alcohol*, 13:596–601, 1952.

ARMSTRONG, JOHN J., and GIBBINS, ROBERT J., "A Psychotherapeutic Technique with Large Groups in the Treatment of Alcoholics," *Quart. J. Stud. Alcohol*, 17:461–78, 1956.

BALES, ROBERT R., "Cultural Differences in Rates of Alcoholism," *Quart. J. Stud. Alcohol*, 6:480–99, 1946.

BATTEGAY, R., "Group Psychotherapy with Alcoholics and Analgesic Addicts," *Internat. J. Group Psychotherapy*, 8:428–34, 1958.

BELL, GORDON R., "Alcohol and Loneliness," *J. Soc. Therapy*, 2:171–81, 1956.

BENEDICT, PAUL, "Psychotherapy of Alcoholism," *Progress in Psychotherapy*,

Vol. 5, pp. 148–55, Jules Masserman and J. L. Moreno (eds.), Grune and Stratton, New York: 1960.

BENNIS, WARREN, "A Critique of Group Therapy Research," *Internat. J. Group Psychotherapy*, 10:63–77, 1960.

BOWMAN, KARL, "The Treatment of Alcoholics," *Quart. J. Stud. Alcohol*, 17:318–24, 1956.

BRUNNER-ORNE, MARTHA, "The Utilization of Group Psychotherapy in Enforced Treatment Programs for Alcoholics and Addicts," *Internat. J. Group Psychotherapy*, 6:272–79, 1956.

——— "Ward Group Sessions with Hospitalized Alcoholics and Motivation for Psychotherapy," *Internat. J. Group Psychotherapy*, 9:219–24.

——— and ORNE, MARTIN T., "Alcoholics," Chapter V in *The Fields of Group Psychotherapy*, S. R. Slavson (ed.), International University Press, New York: 1956, pp. 76–95.

——— and ORNE, MARTIN T., "Directive Group Therapy in the Treatment of Alcoholics: Technique and Rationale," *Internat. J. Group Psychotherapy*, 4:293–302, 1954.

BUTLER, J. DONALD, *Four Philosophies*, Harper and Bros., New York: 1957.

BUTTON, ALAN D., "The Psychodynamics of Alcoholism: A Survey of Eighty-Seven Cases," *Quart. J. Stud. Alcohol*, 17:443–60, 1956.

CHAFETY, MORRIS E., "Practical and Theoretical Considerations in the Psychotherapy of Alcoholism," *Quart. J. Stud. Alcohol*, 20:281–91, 1959.

CLANCY, JOHN, "Procrastination: A Defense Against Sobriety," *Quart. J. Stud. Alcohol*, 22:269–76, 1961.

CLAPP, CHARLES, *Drinking's Not the Problem*, Thomas Crowell Co., New York: 1949.

CLIFTON, STANLEY C., "A Technique for the Initial Interview with Male Alcoholics," *Quart. J. Stud. Alcohol*, 17:89–95, 1956.

CONFER, CHARLES M., "Reasoning as an Associative Process: III. The Role of Verbal Responses in Problem Solving," *J. Gen. Psychol.*, 57:55–68, 1957.

DELEHANTY, E., "State Hospital Care of Alcoholics in Colorado," *J. Dis. Nerv. Sys.*, 8:40–42, 1947.

DENT, JOHN Y., *Anxiety and Its Treatment with Special Reference to Alcoholism*, John Murray, London: 1941, p. 124.

DEWEY, JOHN, *How We Think*, D. C. Heath and Co., New York: 1910, p. 224.

DOLLARD, JOHN, and MILLER, NEAL E., *Personality and Psychotherapy*, McGraw-Hill, New York: 1950, p. 488.

DUGDALE, KATHLEEN, *A Manual of Form for Theses and Term Reports*, Indiana University, Bloomington, Indiana: 1955, p. 58.

DUNCKER, KARL, "On Problem Solving," *Psychological Monographs*, 58:113, 1945.

ENDS, EARL J., and PAGE, CURTIS W., "A Study of Three Types of Group Psychotherapy with Hospitalized Male Inebriates," *Quart. J. Stud. Alcohol*, 18:263–77, 1957.

FORIZS, LORANT, "Brief Intensive Group Psychotherapy for the Treatment of Alcoholics," *Psychiatric Quart. Suppl.*, 29:43–70, 1955.

——— "Motivation of the Alcoholic for Recovery," *Quart. J. Stud. Alcohol*, 19:133–52, 1958.

GLIEDMAN, LESTER H., ROSENTHAL, DAVID, FRANK, JEROME D., et al., "Group Therapy of Alcoholics with Concurrent Group Meetings of Their Wives," *Quart. J. Stud. Alcohol*, 17:633–70, 1956.

HEATH, R. G., "Group Psychotherapy of Alcohol Addiction," *Quart. J. Stud. Alcohol*, 5:555–63, 1945.

HIGGINS, JOHN W., "Psychodynamics in Excessive Drinking of Alcohol," *A.M.A. Arch. Neurol. and Psychiatry*, 69:713, 1953.

HIMWICH, HAROLD E., "Views on the Etiology of Alcoholism, The Organic View," *Alcoholism as a Medical Problem*, H. D. Kruse (ed.), Paul B. Hoeber, New York: 1956.

HODNETT, EDWARD, *The Art of Problem Solving*, Harper Bros., New York: 1955.

HOLLINGSHEAD, AUGUST B., "Views on the Etiology of Alcoholism, The Sociologic View," *Alcoholism as a Medical Problem*, H. D. Kruse (ed.), Paul B. Hoeber, New York: 1956, pp. 56–67.

HORTON, DONALD, "The Functions of Alcohol in Primitive Societies: A Cross Cultural Study," *Quart. J. Stud. Alcohol*, 4:199–320, 1943.

INGRAM, MADELENE E., *Principles and Techniques of Psychiatric Nursing*, W. B. Saunders, Philadelphia: 1955.

JACKSON, JOAN K., "The Definition and Measurement of Alcoholism, H-Technique Scales of Preoccupation with Alcohol and Psychological Involvement," *Quart. J. Stud. Alcohol*, 18:240–62, 1957.

JELLINEK, E. M., *The Disease Concept of Alcoholism*, Hillhouse Press, New Haven, Conn.: 1960, p. 246.

———— "The Problems of Alcohol," *Alcohol, Science, and Society* (Lectures with Discussions as given at Yale Summer School of Alcoholic Studies), pp. 13–29, *Quart. J. Stud. Alcohol*, 15:13–29, 1954.

KANT, FRITZ, *The Treatment of the Alcoholic*, Charles C Thomas, Springfield, Illinois: 1954, p. 531.

KARPMAN, BENJAMIN, *The Hangover*, Charles C Thomas, Springfield Illinois: 1957.

KELLER, MARK, "Definition of Alcoholism," *Quart. J. Stud. Alcohol*, 21:125–33, 1960.

KINGHAM, RICHARD J., "Alcoholism and the Reinforcement Theory of Learning," *Quart. J. Stud. Alcohol*, 19:320–30, 1958.

LERNER, ARTHUR, "An Exploratory Approach in Group Counseling with Male Alcoholic Inmates in a City Jail," *Quart. J. Stud. Alcohol*, 14:427–67, 1953.

LEVY, ROBERT, "The Psychodynamic Functions of Alcohol," *Quart. J. Stud. Alcohol*, 19:649–59, 1958.

MANN, MARTY, *Primer on Alcoholism*, Rinehart and Co., New York: 1950, p. 216.

MARCONI, JUAN T., "The Concept of Alcoholism," *Quart. J. Stud. Alcohol*, 20:216–35, 1959.

MAXWELL, MILTON, "Interpersonal Factors in the Genesis and Treatment of Alcohol Addiction," *Social Forces*, 29:443–48, 1951.

MCCARTHY, R. G., "Group Therapy in an Outpatient Clinic for the Treatment of Alcoholism," *Quart. J. Stud. Alcohol*, 7:98–110, 1946.

MCCORD, WILLIAM, MCCORD, JOAN, and GUDEMAN, JON, "Some Current Theories of Alcoholism: A Longitudinal Evaluation," *Quart. J. Stud. Alcohol*, 20:727–49, 1959.

MENNINGER, KARL A., *Man Against Himself*, Harcourt, Brace and Co., New York: 1938.

MERENESS, DOROTHY, and KARNOSH, LOUIS, *Psychiatry for Nurses*, C. V. Mosby Co., St. Louis: 1958.

MOORE, R. A., and ROMSEUR, FRIEDA, "A Study of the Background of 100

Hospitalized Veterans with Alcoholism," *Quart. J. Stud. Alcohol*, 21:51–67, 1960.

NAVRATI, L., "On the Etiology of Alcoholism," *Quart. J. Stud. Alcohol*, 20:236–44, 1959.

PEPLAU, HILDEGARD E., *Interpersonal Relations in Nursing*, G. P. Putnam's Sons, New York: 1952, p. 330.

PFEFFER, ARNOLD Z., "The Natural History of Alcoholism, Its Onset and Course," *Alcoholism as a Medical Problem*, H. D. Kruse (ed.), Paul B. Hoeber, New York: 1956, pp. 68–77.

PFEFFER, A. Z., FRIEDLAND, P., and WORTIS, H., "Group Therapy with Alcoholics, Preliminary Report," *Quart. J. Stud. Alcohol*, 1:217–51, 1949.

POPE, BENJAMIN, "Attitudes Toward Group Therapy in a Psychiatric Clinic for Alcoholics," *Quart. J. Stud. Alcohol*, 17:233–54, 1956.

POWDERMAKER, FLORENCE B., and FRANK, JEROME D., *Group Psychotherapy*, Harvard University Press, Cambridge, Mass.: 1953, p. 615.

RICHTER, DOROTHEA, "Teaching a Concept of Anxiety to Patients," master's thesis, Rutgers, The State University of New Jersey, 1957.

RILEY, JOHN W., "The Social Implications of Problem Drinking," *Social Forces*, 27:301–5, 1949.

ROGERS, M., "Reference Group Influences on Student Drinking Behavior," *Quart. J. Stud. Alcohol*, 19:244–54, 1958.

SCOTT, EDWARD M., "A Special Type of Group Therapy and Its Application to Alcoholics," *Quart. J. Stud. Alcohol*, 17:288–90, 1956.

——— "The Technique of Psychotherapy with Alcoholics," *Quart. J. Stud. Alcohol*, 22:69–80, 1961.

SHERFEY, M. J., "Psychopathology and Character Structure in Chronic Alcoholism," *Etiology of Chronic Alcoholism*, O. Diethelm (ed.), Charles C Thomas, Springfield, Ill.: 1955, pp. 16–42.

SHOBEN, EDWARD J., "Views on the Etiology of Alcoholism, The Behavioristic View," *Alcoholism as a Medical Problem*, H. D. Kruse (ed.), Paul B. Hoeber, New York: 1956, pp. 47–55.

SMALL, S. MOUCHLY, "The Natural History of Alcoholism, Its Psychopathological Manifestations," *Alcoholism as a Medical Problem*, pp. 78–87, H. D. Kruse (ed.), Paul B. Hoeber, New York: 1956.

STEWART, DAVID A., "Empathy in the Group Therapy of Alcoholics," *Quart. J. Stud. Alcohol*, 15:74–100, 1954.

STRAYER, ROBERT, "Social Integration of Alcoholics Through Prolonged Group Therapy," *Quart. J. Stud. Alcohol*, 22:471–80, 1961.

STRECKER, EDWARD A., "Psychotherapy in Pathological Drinking," *J. A. M. A.*, 147:813–15, 1951.

——— and CHAMBERS, FRANCIS T., *Alcohol, One Man's Meat*, The Macmillan Co., New York: 1938, p. 230.

THOMPSON, CHARLES E., and KOLB, WILLIAM P., "Group Psychotherapy in Association with Alcoholic Anonymous," *Am. J. Psychiat.*, 110:29–33, 1953.

TRAEGER, HARVEY, "How You Can Help the Alcoholic Offender," *Fed. Probation*, 22:25–30, 1958.

VOGEL, SIDNEY, "Some Aspects of Group Psychotherapy with Alcoholics," *Internat. J. Group Psychotherapy*, 7:302–9, 1957.

WALLERSTEIN, ROBERT S., *Hospital Treatment of Alcoholism*, Basic Books, New York: 1957, p. 212.

WASHBURNE, CHANDLER, "Alcohol, Self, and the Group," *Quart. J. Stud. Alcohol*, 17:108–23, 1956.

WEINSTEIN, EDWIN A., "Discussion of Etiological Views," *Alcoholism as a Medical Problem*, H. D. Kruse (ed.), Paul B. Hoeber, New York: 1956, pp. 60–62.

WHITE, R., *The Abnormal Personality*, The Ronald Press, New York: 1950.

WILLIAMS, LINCOLN, *Tomorrow Will Be Sober*, Harper and Bros., New York: 1960, p. 207.

ZWERLING, ISRAEL, and ROSENBAUM, MILTON, "Alcoholic Addiction and Personality," *American Handbook of Psychiatry*, Silvano Arieti (ed.), Basic Books, New York: 1959, Vol. 1, pp. 623–44.

# 36 ABSTRACT: MARRIAGE AND MENTAL ILLNESS [1]

*Shirley A. Smoyak*

An understanding of the nature of interpersonal dynamics between marriage partners, in which one of the pair is psychotic, is vital to understanding mental illness. Both husbands and wives, in order to clarify their interpersonal processes, need to cooperate with professional persons in the field of psychiatry. One way to obtain a description of the marital interaction patterns and integrations is through psychotherapy. Another method is through a more direct, shorter, investigative approach using two specific instruments. The latter method was applied in this research, in which the focus was comparing and analyzing discrepant views about self, other persons, and marriage in a sample of marriage partners in which the husbands were psychotic.

The purpose of this study was twofold: (1) to contribute to the general body of knowledge about marriage and mental illness, particularly in the area of reciprocal views of married couples, and (2) to stimulate the cooperative efforts of public health nurses and hospital nurses toward improving total family health care by demonstrating a method of eliciting discrepant views, using two specific tools. Hospital nurses and public health nurses jointly might use this method to quickly assess the areas in which there is need for predischarge counseling of both hospitalized and nonhospitalized marital pairs. This method could also be used before beginning long-range therapy with a patient or married couple, or as a means of measuring progress during the course of psychotherapy.

In developing the research problem, three major theoretical frames

[1] Thesis submitted to the Graduate School of Rutgers, The State University of New Jersey, in partial fulfillment of the requirements for the degree of Master of Science, May 1959.

248—

of reference were most helpful. These theoretical frameworks were complementariness of patterns, role theory, and interpersonal theory. In studying the marriages, a dyadic, rather than the usual monadic method was designed. Responses of *pairs* to the research instruments were analyzed. One instrument was the Interpersonal Check List, which was developed and tested by a group of social psychologists. It contains 128 adjectives and phrases describing personality. The other instrument was the Marriage Interview Guide, developed by the researcher. It consists of a series of inquiries about role expectations and performances, and marriage problems.

A large county psychiatric hospital was the setting for the study. The sample consisted of ten male patients, diagnosed as psychotic and presently hospitalized, and their nonhospitalized spouses. These husbands and wives, in separate, private interviews with the researcher, were asked to complete the Interpersonal Check List and respond to the Marriage Interview Guide. After the interviews with each couple had been completed, the researcher made a clinical assessment of the mental health and integration of the pair.

Discrepant views of marriage partners emerged when their perceptions of self, other persons, and marriage were compared. There were significantly more disagreements about descriptions of personalities of husbands. Both instruments resulted in a fairly equal distribution of discrepant responses among items or questions. Marital pairs were ranked according to percentage of disagreement on both instruments. The correlation between the check list and the interview guide was high.

Analysis of the data showed an inverse relationship between the quality of marital integration and the amount of disagreements between husbands and wives about views of self, other persons, and marriage. Highly integrated couples had lower amounts of disagreement, while poorly integrated couples had high discrepancies.

Some recommendations for future research include (1) applying this design to larger samples, in order to increase the range of variability of marriage patterns, (2) conducting longitudinal studies to examine changes and shifts in unstable roles, especially in marriages in which one or both partners are diagnosed as manic-depressive, and (3) testing the hypothesis that mental illness occurs in either mate when there is an abrupt shift in, or interruption of, the established marriage integration pattern.

## BIBLIOGRAPHY

ACKERMAN, N., *The Psychodynamics of Family Life*. Basic Books, New York: 1958.

250—CLINICAL RESEARCH

BRIM, O., JR., "Attitude and Content-Intensity and Probability Expectations," *Am. Sociol. Rev.*, 20:68–76, 1955.

BUERKLE, J., and BADGLEY, R., "Couple Role-Taking: The Yale Marital Interaction Battery," *Marriage and Family Living*, 21:53–58.

CHASSAN, J., "On the Unreliability of Reliability and Some Other Consequences of the Assumption of Probabilistic Patient States," *Psychiatry*, 20:163–73, 1957.

CLAUSEN, J., and YARROW, M., "Paths to the Mental Hospital," *J. Soc. Issues*, 11:25–32, 1955.

CLAUSEN, J., et al., "The Impact of Mental Illness: Research Formulation," *J. Soc. Issues*, 11:6–11, 1955.

COLE, N., BRANCH, C., and SHAW, O., "Mental Illness," *A.M.A. Arch. Neurol. and Psychiat.*, 77:393–99, 1957.

COUCH, C., "The Use of the Concept 'Role' and Its Derivatives in a Study of Marriage," *Marriage and Family Living*, 20:353–58, 1958.

CRIST, J., "Marriage Counseling Involving a Passive Husband and an Aggressive Wife," *Marriage and Family Living*, 20:121–28, 1958.

DEASY, L., and QUINN, O., "The Wife of the Mental Patient and the Hospital Psychiatrist," *J. Soc. Issues*, 11:49–60, 1955.

DEUTSCH, M., and SOLOMON, L., "Some Methodological Suggestions for Research in a Family Counseling Setting," *Marriage and Family Living*, 20:21–27, 1958.

DINITZ, S., MANGUS, A., and PASAMANICK, B., "Integration and Conflict in Self-Other Conceptions as Factors in Mental Illness," *Sociometry*, 20:44–45, 1959.

DORNBUSCH, S., and SCHMID, C., *A Primer of Social Statistics*, McGraw-Hill Book Company, New York: 1955.

EDWARDS, A., *Statistical Methods for the Behavioral Sciences*. Rinehart & Company, New York: 1955.

EISENSTEIN, V. (ed.), *Neurotic Interaction in Marriage*. Basic Books, New York: 1956.

FEDERIGHI, E., "The Use of Chi-Square in Small Samples," *Am. Sociol. Rev.*, 15:770–80, 1950.

FREEMAN, H., and SIMMONS, O., "Wives, Mothers, and the Post-Hospital Performance of Mental Patients," *Social Forces*, 37:153–59, 1958.

GOVACCHINI, P., "Mutual Adaptation in Various Object Relationships," *Internat. J. Psychoanalysis*, 39:547–54, 1958.

HEWITT, L., "Student Perceptions of Traits Desired in Themselves as Dating and Marriage Partners," *Marriage and Family Living*, XX (November, 1958).

HOBART, C., "Disillusionment in Marriage, and Romanticism," *Marriage and Family Living*, 20:156–63, 1958.

HUNTINGTON, R., "II. The Personality-Interaction Approach to Study of the Marital Relationship," *Marriage and Family Living*, 20:43–47, 1958.

JAHODA, M., DEUTSCH, M., and COOK, S., *Research Methods in Social Relationships, Part One: Basic Processes*, The Dryden Press, New York: 1951.

KAPLAN, A., and WOLF, L., "The Role of the Family in Relation to the Institutionalized Mental Patient," *Mental Hygiene*, 38:634–39, 1954.

LA FORGE, R., and SUCZEK, R., "The Interpersonal Dimensions of Personality: III. An Interpersonal Check List," *J. Personality*, 24:94–112, 1955.

LEARY, T., *Interpersonal Diagnosis of Personality*. The Ronald Press, New York: 1957.

—— *Multilevel Measurement of Interpersonal Behavior, A Manual*, Psychological Consultation Service, Berkeley, California: 1956.

—— "The Theory of Measurement Methodology of Interpersonal Communications," *Psychiatry*, 18:147–61, 1955.

LEVINE, N., "The Mental Patient in the Community from the Viewpoint of the Family Agency," *Mental Hygiene*, 31:278–85, 1947.

LEVINSON, S., and WITHEY, M., "Sessions with Relatives of Mental Hospital Patients," *Mental Hygiene*, 39:118–25, 1955.

LIDZ, T., *et al.*, "Patient-Family Hospital Interrelationships" in Greenblatt, M., Levinson, D., and Williams, R., *The Patient and the Mental Hospital*. The Free Press, Glencoe, Ill.: 1957, pp. 535–45.

MANGUS, A., "Family Impacts on Mental Health," *Marriage and Family Living*, 19:256–62, 1957.

MITTLEMANN, B., "Analysis of Reciprocal Neurotic Patterns in Family Relationships," in *Neurotic Interaction in Marriage*, V. Eisenstein (ed.), Basic Books, New York: 1956, pp. 81–101.

PETTIT, L., "Attitudes of Relatives of Long Hospitalized Mental Patients Regarding Convalescent Leave," *Mental Hygiene*, Vol. 40, April, 1956.

RILEY, M., and RILEY, J. W., JR., "The Dyad, or Subject-Object Pair," in Riley, M., Riley, J. W., Jr., and Toby, J., *Scale Analysis*. Rutgers University Press, New Brunswick, N.J.: 1954, pp. 150–80.

SARBIN, T., "Role Theory," in *Handbook of Social Psychology*. G. Lindzey (ed.), Addison-Wesley Publishing Co., Cambridge, Mass.: 1954: Vol. I, pp. 223–58.

SCHWARTZ, C., "Perspectives on Deviance—Wives' Definitions of their Husbands' Mental Illness," *Psychiatry*, 20:257–93, 1957.

SCOTT, B., "My Psychotherapy Helped My Entire Family," *Marriage and Family Living*, 20:128–32, 1958.

SPIEGEL, J., "The Resolution of Role Conflict Within the Family," in Greenblatt, M., Levinson, D., and Williams, R., *The Patient and the Mental Hospital*, The Free Press, Glencoe, Ill.: 1957, pp. 545–65.

STANTON, A., and SCHWARTZ, M., *The Mental Hospital*, Basic Books, New York: 1954.

STEINMANN, A., "Lack of Communication Between Men and Women," *Marriage and Family Living*, 20:350–53, 1958.

SULLIVAN, H. S., *Clinical Studies in Psychiatry*, W. W. Norton & Co., New York: 1956.

—— *The Interpersonal Theory of Psychiatry*, W. W. Norton & Co., New York: 1953.

—— *The Psychiatric Interview*, W. W. Norton & Co., New York: 1954.

WARD, A., and JONES, G., "Helping the Families of Our Mentally Sick," *Mental Hygiene*, 38:576–84, 1954.

YARROW, M., *et al.*, "The Psychological Meaning of Mental Illness in the Family," *J. Soc. Issues*, 11(4):12–24, 1955.

YARROW, M., CLAUSEN, J., and ROBBINS, P., "The Social Meaning of Mental Illness," *J. Soc. Issues*, 11(4):33–48, 1955.

ZELDITCH, JR., M., "Role Differentiation in the Nuclear Family," in Parsons, T., and Bales, R., *Family—Socialization and Interaction Process*, The Free Press, Glencoe, Ill.: 1955, pp. 307–53.

# 37 THE "PROBLEM" PATIENT

*Betty H. Newsom, Gloria Oden, and Ura A. L. Lazaroff*

## Problem Statement

This was a study of responses of nurses about those characteristics of hospitalized patients that result in their being labeled "problem" patients.

## Subproblems

1. What category of characteristics of "problem patients" was cited most frequently by nurse-respondents?
2. What category of characteristics of "problem patients" was cited least frequently by nurse-respondents?
3. What percentage of nurse-respondents caring for patients on given wards designated the same patients as "problems"?
4. What percentage of nurse-respondents caring for patients on given wards designated different patients as "problems"?
5. What percentage of responses by nurse-respondents selecting the same patient as a "problem" were similar?
6. What percentage of responses by nurse-respondents selecting the same patient as a "problem" were different?

## Purpose

The purpose of this study was to determine the characteristics of a "problem patient" and to analyze those characteristics described by nurses.

252—

The results of this study could be used as a focus to determine the reasons for the specific problem areas in the nurse-patient situation.

## LITERATURE REVIEW

Virtually every nursing textbook that has been published discusses problems related to patient care. Earlier texts deal almost exclusively with problems related to physical care of patients.[1] Within the last fifteen years, however, various publications[2] have placed increasing emphasis upon the nurse's role in the prevention and reduction of patient anxiety, recognizing it as another source of problems in nursing care.

Any professional nurse working in the hospital setting has heard the familiar refrain, "He's a problem patient," or "He's an ideal patient." What do nurses mean when they use these labels? Generalizations are made in the literature regarding problems arising in the nurse-patient relationship, but the study-makers found no evidence that systematic studies have been undertaken to determine what constitutes a problem patient. Haberstein and Christ[3] state that patients who refuse to accept orders, who are "neurotic," or who are demanding are listed as "problem" patients. Conversely, the "ideal" patient is one who takes care of his own person, cooperates with the staff in the operation of the hospital, is productive in his efforts, and is able to get along with other people.[4] This description of the ideal patient appears to be so optimistic as to practically eliminate his chances of becoming a hospitalized individual, and so unlikely to exist in reality that nurses would rarely expect to find such a patient on the ward.

Burton[5] refers to the problem patient as the "bad" patient and cites demands, avoidance of obeying, disobedience, questioning treatments, complaints, interference with nursing routine, lack of cooperation, and rejection of treatments and medications as the major areas of nurse-patient problems. Schwartz and Shockley[6] write that the problem patient fre-

---

[1] Nightingale, F., *Notes on Nursing*.

[2] For examples, see Shafer, K. N., Sawyer, J. K. McCluskey, A. M., and Lifgren, E. A., *Medical Surgical Nursing*, 2nd ed., pp. 3–9; Harmer, B., and Henderson, V., *Textbook of the Principles and Practice of Nursing*, p. vi, and "Every Aspect of Nursing" contained herein.

[3] Haberstein, R. W., and Christ, E. A., *Professionalizer, Traditionalizer and Utilizer*, p. 162.

[4] Reissman, L., and Roher, J. H., *Change and Dilemma in the Nursing Profession*, p. 145.

[5] Burton, G., *Personal, Impersonal and Interpersonal Relationships*, pp. 21–25.

[6] Schwartz, M. S., and Shockley, E. L., *The Nurse and the Mental Patient*, pp. 72–79.

quently becomes labeled as such because of insistent and persistent demands made upon the nurse.

Ingles,[7] in a series of case studies, describes such qualities as untidiness, uncooperativeness, and ungratefulness, as major characteristics of "bad" patients. Schwartz,[8] through conferences with student nurses and hospital staff, compiled a list of characteristics of uncooperative "problem" patients, patients who do not recognize that help is being given, patients who refuse to accept their illnesses, unappreciative patients, and patients who do not understand. Lack of understanding included language barriers, mental retardation, and hostility of unknown origin.

Highley and Norris[9] published a study of students who dislike certain patients. The nurses' dislikes of certain characteristics in patients are similar to the descriptions of characteristics of problem patients cited by other authors. Complaints, demands, overdependence, untidiness, disobedience, and uncooperativeness were mentioned as major areas of dislike by nurses.

The review of the literature resulted in discovering a collection of descriptive terms, the majority of which were categorizations. Specific characteristics frequently overlapped within categories. A clear and concise answer to "What are the characteristics of a problem patient?" did not emerge. Where, then, can the answer be found? The study-makers went directly to nurses and asked them to describe a problem patient. From their responses, and from a review of the literature, a check list (see p. 265) was developed which systematically categorized those characteristics that constitute the problem patient. From the responses obtained on the check list, the answer to "What is a problem patient?" emerged.

The value of this study lies in its utilization by future investigators. They will attempt, hopefully, to determine the causes of specific problem areas in the nurse-patient relationship and to achieve, through therapeutic intervention, improved professional nursing care.

## ASSUMPTIONS

1. Nurses have the ability to specify and to generalize.

2. Certain patients present problems to nurses and are labeled as problems patients.

[7] Ingles, T., "The Worst Patient on the Floor," p. 99; "Margaret—An Uncooperative Patient," p. 289; "Mr. Parker—A Bad Patient," p. 209.

[8] Schwartz, D., "Uncooperative Patients?" pp. 75–77.

[9] Highley, B. L., and Norris, C., "When a Student Dislikes A Patient," pp. 1163–66.

3. Nurses use labels and can specify to some degree their reasons for doing so.

## LIMITATIONS

1. The study-maker may unwittingly alter the response of the nurses.

2. The responses of the nurses may be modified if they know that the study-maker is a psychiatric nurse.

3. The nurse-respondent may not be motivated to answer questions judiciously.

## DEFINITIONS

1. *Nurse*—an individual who is a graduate of a professional nursing school, is registered by or has applied for registration to a state board of nurse examiners, and is engaged in nursing practice in a hospital.

2. *Patient*—an adult person who is confined in a hospital as a recipient of professional services.

3. *Problem*—the human behavior that is viewed by the nurse as difficult, perplexing, uncertain, or maladjusted.

4. *Problem patient*—a patient whose presence in the hospital is viewed by the nurse as a problem.

5. *Label*—a term or phrase attached by the nurse by way of classification of patient behavior.

6. *Response*—in the instrument sample, a phrase or word said in reply to a statement; in the study sample, a "check," an encircled item, an additional written comment on a questionnaire.

7. *Characteristic*—a trait, quality, or property distinguishing an individual type of patient.

## METHODOLOGY

### 1. DESCRIPTION OF STUDY SETTINGS

Arrangements were made with a metropolitan public hospital in conducting this research. The study-makers collected data from registered nurses on fifteen wards in this hospital from 8:30 A.M., to 12:00 noon on the following dates: instrument sample, 2/22, 2/23, 2/24, 1961; study sample, 3/1, 3/2, 3/3, 1961.

## 2. CRITERIA FOR SELECTION OF RESPONDENTS

Every registered nurse who was on duty on the medical, surgical, or maternity wards during the designated time was selected if the nurse spoke English; was available, i.e., accessible to the study-maker and on the ward at the time of data collection; and was willing to participate. One return visit was made to each ward to interview any registered nurse who had been off duty or unavailable at the time the data were collected on that ward. The same procedure was used for both samples.

## 3. STUDY-MAKERS

This study was conducted by three graduate fellows. These nurses were enrolled in the initial year of education in the Graduate Program in Advanced Psychiatric Nursing at Rutger's University.

## 4. COLLECTION OF DATA: INSTRUMENT SAMPLE

a. Orientation to charge nurse by the study-maker:

I am Miss ———. I am a graduate student at Rutgers University doing a small study as part of my course requirements. I would like to spend about five minutes with you and each of your registered nurses. When would this be convenient for you?

b. Orientation to registered nurse by the study-maker:

I am Miss ———. I am a graduate student at Rutgers University conducting a preliminary study about patients. All information will be kept confidential. You will not be identified.

    c. Instrument question: Following orientation each registered nurse was asked to "describe a problem patient." If the nurse-respondent asked for further elaboration, the study-maker replied, "Think of a problem patient you have had. Describe him to me." A technique for further elaboration was used when the nurse's response appeared vague. The study-maker asked, "Anything else?" or "In what way?" After receiving the nurse's response, the study-maker thanked her for her cooperation.

    d. Recording the data: Data collected for the instrument sample were recorded on index cards (see p. 264). The nurse respondent's verbatim descriptions were recorded on these cards during the interview.

## 5. PROCESSING THE DATA: INSTRUMENT SAMPLE

The following procedure was used in processing the data of the instrument sample.

a. The study-makers transferred individual descriptions to separate pieces of paper.

b. The study-makers grouped similar descriptions together.

c. Step b was repeated to evaluate and regroup descriptions as necessary.

d. Each study-maker independently examined the groups of responses, named tentative categories in writing, and specified questionable descriptions in each group of responses.

e. The study-makers compared independent categorizations, discussed reasons for change within categories, and reached 100 per cent agreement on descriptions in each category. (Each category was defined.)

f. These categories were then formulated into an instrument (check list). This instrument was used to collect data in the study sample. The category titles with definitions were omitted from the instrument (check list) in order to elicit responses of specific characteristics of the "problem patient." At the end of the check list, the nurse was given the opportunity to state the characteristic(s) that may have been omitted. This was categorized "Other."

## 6. COLLECTION OF DATA: STUDY SAMPLE

a. Orientation to charge nurse:

I am Miss ————. I am a graduate student at Rutgers University collecting the final data for the study begun here last week. I am studying problem patients. The information you give me may help solve some of the problems of nurses. I would like to spend a few minutes with you and each of your graduate nurses. When would it be convenient?

b. Orientation to registered nurse:

I am Miss ————. I am a graduate student at Rutgers University collecting the final data for my study. I am studying problem patients. The information you give me may help solve some of the problems of nurses. All information will be kept confidential. You will not be identified by name.

c. Designation of problem patients: The study-maker asked that the nurse-respondent look at the ward Kardex. The study-maker asked, "In your opinion, which three patients on the ward at the present time are problem patients?" If the nurse said there were no problem patients on the ward, the study-maker asked, "No problem patients?" (in order to infer doubt). Then, if the nurse could not designate three patients as "problem patients," one or two patients were accepted.

d. Study question: The nurse-respondent was given the study instrument (see p. 266) and asked to check all the characteristics about "problem patient" X which make him or her a problem patient; then, to circle the outstanding characteristic of the patient which makes him a problem. The nurse-respondent was then asked to add any problem characteristic that was not included in the questionnaire in the space indicated "Other." This procedure was used for acquiring responses from each nurse. After completion of the checking, the nurse-respondent was thanked for her cooperation.

e. Recording the data: study sample: The study-maker recorded the identity of data in the following manner on the instrument.

| Patient | Code Number | |
|---------|-------------|-------------|
| Date | Ward # | |
| Medical | Surgical | Obstetrical |

Study-maker A coded the nurses on the instrument as A-1 to A-100 after each nurse-respondent had completed the checking. Study-maker B coded the nurse as B-1 to B-100 and study-maker C coded the nurse as C-1 to C-100. The head nurse was indicated with an asterisk (*) after the code number. All patients were identified by name.

## 7. PROCESSING THE DATA: STUDY SAMPLE

Each item (i.e., check, circle, or written-in response) was entered from each check list to a master work sheet (see p. 269).

## 8. ANALYSIS OF THE DATA

A total of 34 nurse-respondents completed check lists out of a possible 42 nurses employed full-time on the wards selected for the study. Eight nurses did not meet the criteria established by the study-makers.

On every ward selected for the study, at least one patient was designated as a "problem" by each of the nurse-respondents. Seventeen nurse-respondents named three "problem patients," 14 nurse-respondents named two "problem patients," and 3 nurse-respondents named one patient as a "problem."

A total of 82 check lists were completed with a total of 62 patients designated as "problems." The distribution is indicated in Table 1.

TABLE 1. DISTRIBUTION OF NURSE–RESPONDENTS AND OF PATIENTS DESIGNATED AS "PROBLEMS" ACCORDING TO SERVICE AND WARD

| Service | Wards | Number of Nurse-Respondents | Number of Patients Designated |
|---------|-------|------------------------------|-------------------------------|
| Obstetrics | 1 | 3 | 3 |
| | 2 | 1 | 3 |
| | 3 | 1 | 2 |
| | 4 | 3 | 3 |
| Surgical | 5 | 2 | 3 |
| | 6 | 1 | 3 |
| | 7 | 2 | 5 |
| | 8 | 2 | 3 |
| Medical | 9 | 2 | 4 |
| | 10 | 2 | 4 |
| | 11 | 4 | 4 |
| | 12 | 2 | 4 |
| | 13 | 3 | 7 |
| | 14 | 4 | 9 |
| | 15 | 2 | 5 |

FINDINGS AND INTERPRETATIONS

Table 2 indicates the frequency with which problem characteristics were cited within categories. In over-all ranking, "complaints" were the problem category most frequently designated by nurse-respondents.[10] It is interesting to note that while "lack of cooperation" ranked first in actual number of times that it was designated as a problem by nurse-respondents, it ranked seventh out of the eight categories in ratio to possible responses (see p. 260). Its over-all ranking was fifth. Numerically, "complaints" were cited as the fourth most frequent source of problems with patients, while being rated as the most frequent source of problems in the ratio. "Interference from the outside" was the category cited least often by nurse-respondents.

[10] Over-all ranking was computed by adding the ranks of each of the categories according to the "number of characteristics actually cited" plus the "ratio of actual responses : possible responses." Totals were interpreted by ranking the lowest score as first, the second lowest score as second, etc. (See Table 2.)

TABLE 2. FREQUENCY OF RESPONSES OF CHARACTERISTICS OF "PROBLEM PATIENTS" BY CATEGORY

| Category | No. of Characteristics Cited | No. of Responses Possible | Ratio of Actual Responses to Possible Responses | Over-all Rank |
|---|---|---|---|---|
| Communication | 69 | 328 | 21.0 | 6 |
| Complaint | 119 | 410 | 29.0 | 1 |
| Demand | 94 | 410 | 22.9 | 3 |
| Interference from outside | 57 | 492 | 11.6 | 8 |
| Overt emotional behavior | 82 | 574 | 14.3 | 7 |
| Physical care | 147 | 738 | 19.9 | 4 |
| Interaction | 147 | 656 | 22.4 | 2 |
| Lack of cooperation | 156 | 1148 | 13.6 | 5 |

Table 3 shows the percentage of total responses in each category according to the service on which patients were treated. It was noted that communication problems ranked third on obstetrical wards. This might be due to the influx of young non–English-speaking immigrants to the city. On the medical service, the chronic illnesses of patients were seen by nurse-respondents as one of the primary characteristics that made patients a "problem."

TABLE 3. PER CENT OF RESPONSES OF CHARACTERISTICS OF "PROBLEM PATIENTS" BY CATEGORY ACCORDING TO SERVICE ON WHICH PATIENTS WERE BEING TREATED

| Category of Problem Patient Characteristics | Per Cent of Responses According to Service | | |
|---|---|---|---|
| | Obstetrics | Medical | Surgical |
| Communication | 15 | 10 | 5 |
| Demand | 21 | 8 | 12 |
| Complaint | 12 | 12 | 15 |
| Interference | 11 | 6 | 7 |
| Overt emotional behavior | 14 | 10 | 9 |
| Physical care | 6 | 22 | 14 |
| Interaction | 4 | 14 | 21 |
| Lack of cooperation | 17 | 18 | 17 |
| Total per cent of checks | 100 | 100 | 100 |
| Total number of checks | 66 | 397 | 408 |

Each nurse-respondent indicated the outstanding characteristic of the individual patient that made him a "problem." Table 4 shows the number of times that characteristics of "problem" patients within categories were cited as outstanding. Lack of cooperation was designated most frequently as the outstanding characteristic.

TABLE 4. OUTSTANDING CHARACTERISTIC OF "PROBLEM PATIENT" AS DESIGNATED BY NURSE RESPONDENTS

| Category | Number | Per Cent |
|---|---|---|
| Communication | 16 | 18.6 |
| Complaint | 12 | 14.0 |
| Demand | 6 | 7.0 |
| Interference from outside | 4 | 4.7 |
| Overt emotional problems | 8 | 9.3 |
| Physical care | 13 | 15.0 |
| Interaction | 6 | 7.0 |
| Lack of cooperation | 21 | 24.4 |
| | 86* | 100.0 |

* Four nurse-respondents designated two problems per patient as outstanding.

In Table 5, the percentage of nurse-respondents caring for patients on the same ward who designated the same patients or who designated different patients as "problems" is indicated. Generally, nurses working on

TABLE 5. PERCENTAGE OF NURSE–RESPONDENTS DESIGNATING THE SAME PATIENTS AND DESIGNATING DIFFERENT PATIENTS AS "PROBLEMS" ACCORDING TO THE NUMBER OF NURSES ON GIVEN WARDS

| | Wards with | | | |
|---|---|---|---|---|
| | 4 Nurses | 3 Nurses | 2 Nurses | 1 Nurse |
| Nurses designating the same patients as "problems" | | | | |
| All nurses | 0 | 31 | 20 | |
| ¾ of nurses | 15 | | | |
| ⅔ of nurses | | 15 | | |
| ½ of nurses | 23 | | | |
| Nurses designating different patients as "problems" | 62 | 54 | 80 | 100 |
| Number of patients designated as "problems" | 13 | 13 | 26 | 8 |

the same ward did not agree about the patients they viewed as "problems," indicating that nurses' perceptions of "problem patients" are varied.

Table 6 indicates the percentage of responses by nurse-respondents who selected the same patient as a "problem" for similar or for different reasons. If two or more nurses attributed the same characteristic to a patient, the responses were considered to be similar. In general, even when nurses select the same patient as a problem, they tended to select him for different reasons. Fourteen of the sixteen patients selected by two or more nurses were selected for different reasons more than 50 per cent of the time. This gives further indication that nurses' perceptions of problem patients are varied. In two instances when agreement exceeded 50 per cent, agreement was 79 per cent in one case and 60 per cent in the other.

## Conclusions

The characteristics of "problem patients" according to the frequency of responses fell primarily into the categories of "lack of cooperation," "interaction," "physical care," and "complaints." However, in over-all ranking after equally weighting each category and considering the frequency of responses, the results indicate "complaints," "interaction," "demands," and "physical care," are the serial order of occurrences. It was also found that there was wide variance of views among nurses as to what constitutes a "problem patient." The type service on which the nurse works influences her designation of problem characteristics. Generally, nurses working on the same ward did not agree about the patients they viewed as problems. Even when nurses selected the same patient as a problem, they tended to select him for different reasons.

## Summary

This study was done to determine the characteristics of "problem patients" as viewed by nurses. The basic assumption that certain patients present problems to nurses and are labeled problem patients was validated by the nurses' responses to the check list. Statistical and descriptive findings are presented to show that nurses have individual views of specific "problem patients" which are not shared by other nurses.

## Implication for Further Research

The research shows that there is a difference between the problem of "complaints," which ranked highest, and the problem of "lack of co-

TABLE 6. PERCENTAGE OF SIMILAR RESPONSES AND DIFFERENT RESPONSES BY NURSE-RESPONDENTS WHO SELECTED THE SAME PATIENT AS A "PROBLEM"

|  | | | | | | | | | Patients | | | | | | | |
|---|---|---|---|---|---|---|---|---|---|---|---|---|---|---|---|---|
|  | A | B | C | D | E | F | G | H | I | J | K | L | M | N | O | P |
| Number of nurses selecting same patient | 3 | 3 | 3 | 3 | 2 | 2 | 2 | 2 | 3 | 3 | 2 | 2 | 2 | 2 | 2 | 2 |
| Per cent of similar responses | 20 | 44 | 9 | 79 | 42 | 35 | 12.5 | 43 | 60 | 33 | 42 | 48 | 33 | 44 | 29 | 29 |
| Per cent of different responses | 80 | 56 | 91 | 21 | 58 | 65 | 87.5 | 57 | 40 | 67 | 58 | 52 | 67 | 56 | 71 | 71 |
| Total types of characteristics designated | 15 | 9 | 11 | 43 | 19 | 17 | 8 | 28 | 20 | 18 | 12 | 23 | 12 | 16 | 17 | 7 |

—263

operation," which is cited most frequently. Which of these characteristics is the greater problem to nurses? What changes in the hospital setting could eliminate some of the problems?

The research indicates that problems of interpersonal relationships occur frequently. What are the underlying reasons for the existing problem areas in the nurse-patient relationship? What intervention can reduce these problems? What changes in nursing education would increase awareness of existing problems and deal with reducing or solving these problems?

Nurses view patients in a highly individualistic way. Is this due primarily to differences in the personalities of nurses? Would increased self-awareness on the part of the nurse eliminate some of the problems of the nurse-patient relationship?

This endeavor indicates that emotional problems are rarely cited as problem characteristics. Do nurses fail to recognize these problems? Is more emphasis upon the psychiatric aspects of nursing necessary in the general hospital?

The research indicates that problems of language barriers are significant. Should increased emphasis on learning foreign languages be considered in nursing education?

What additional analysis of the existing data could be done to further explore the problem areas of the nurse-patient relationship?

## Data Collection Card
### Instrument Sample

1. Describe a problem patient.        Ward_____

*Elaboration:*
   Think of a problem patient you have had.     Date_____
   Describe him to me.

## CHECK LIST OF POSSIBLE "PROBLEM PATIENT" CHARACTERISTICS

*Communication*—presents some difficulty in the interchange of thoughts or opinions.

Has a language barrier
Has an intelligence level that restricts understanding
Misinterprets instructions
Cannot read or write

*Complaint*—verbalizes discontent, makes formal accusations or withholds approval.

Reports nurses to the doctor
States he is not getting the proper treatment
States he is not getting the proper service
Is resentful
Does not show appreciation of nurses' efforts

*Demand*—makes insistent requests which the nurse cannot or will not meet.

Asks questions frequently
Wants nurse to come immediately
Wants things that are not ordered
Wants things that are not necessary
Orders nurses around

*Interference from the outside*—environment from outside the hospital which creates problem areas in nursing-care intervention.

Does not have visitors
Has visitors who criticize patient's care
Has visitors who monopolize nurse's time
Has personal problems which interfere with nursing care
Is ready for discharge, but family doesn't want to take patient
Is ready for discharge, but patient has no place to go

*Overt emotional behavior*—behavior that the nurse recognizes as requiring psychiatric-nursing intervention.

Is depressed
Cries frequently
Is disoriented
Is apprehensive
Is too mentally disturbed for regular ward
Won't talk
Is extremely frightened

*Physical care*—characteristic(s) of the patient's physical state (illness and/or state of cleanliness) that present a problem to the nurse.

Is untidy
Is incontinent
Has poor personal hygiene
Has an odor
Requires extensive nursing care
Is acutely ill
Is chronically ill
Is terminally ill
Is senile

*Interaction*—unable to get along with others—verbalizes direct disrespect and contempt for nurses and/or patients in the group setting. These verbalizations are not related to the patient's illness.

Argues with nurses

Argues with other patients
Agitates other patients
Is grouchy
Antagonizes nurses
Lies
Uses profane languages
Is noisy

*Lack of cooperation*—refuses to work with the nurse and other personnel regarding health.

Doesn't follow doctor's orders regarding treatment
Doesn't follow doctor's orders regarding diet
Doesn't follow doctor's orders regarding medicine
Refuses examinations
Refuses medicine
Refuses treatment
Won't follow instructions
Is able to help self, but refuses to do so
Does as he pleases
Does not follow hospital rules
Won't accept illness
Is too helpful
Refuses to keep covers on self while in bed
Disregards principles of safety
Other

## CHECK LIST OF "PROBLEM PATIENT" CHARACTERISTICS

Patient_____          Code Number_____

Date_____          Ward_____

Medical_____     Surgical_____     Obstetrical_____

Step I.  Check those characteristics of the patient that make him a problem.
Step II.  Circle the outstanding characteristic of the patient that makes him a problem.
Step III.  Space is provided to add any problem characteristic that is not included in the questionnaire.

| | |
|---|---|
| Has a language barrier | |
| Has an intelligence level that restricts understanding | |
| Misinterprets instructions | |
| Cannot read or write | |
| Reports nurses to the doctor | |
| States he is not getting the proper treatment | |
| States he is not getting the proper service | |
| Is resentful | |

## CHECK LIST OF "PROBLEM PATIENT" CHARACTERISTICS

| | |
|---|---|
| Does not show appreciation of nurses' efforts | |
| Asks questions frequently | |
| Wants nurse to come immediately | |
| Wants things that are not ordered | |
| Wants things that are not necessary | |
| Orders nurses around | |
| Does not have visitors | |
| Has visitors who criticize patient's care | |
| Has visitors who monopolize nurse's time | |
| Has personal problems which interfere with nursing care | |
| Is ready for discharge, but family doesn't want to take patient | |
| Is ready for discharge, but patient has no place to go | |
| Is depressed | |
| Cries frequently | |
| Is disoriented | |
| Is apprehensive | |
| Is too mentally disturbed for regular ward | |
| Won't talk | |
| Is extremely frightened | |
| Is untidy | |
| Is incontinent | |
| Has poor personal hygiene | |
| Has an odor | |
| Requires extensive nursing care | |
| Is acutely ill | |
| Is chronically ill | |
| Is terminally ill | |

## CHECK LIST OF "PROBLEM PATIENT" CHARACTERISTICS

| | |
|---|---|
| Is senile | |
| Argues with nurses | |
| Argues with other patients | |
| Agitates other patients | |
| Is grouchy | |
| Antagonizes nurses | |
| Lies | |
| Uses profane language | |
| Is noisy | |
| Doesn't follow doctor's orders regarding treatment | |
| Doesn't follow doctor's orders regarding diet | |
| Doesn't follow doctor's orders regarding medicine | |
| Refuses examinations | |
| Refuses medicine | |
| Refuses treatment | |
| Won't follow instructions | |
| Is able to help self, but refuses to do so | |
| Does as he pleases | |
| Does not follow hospital rules | |
| Won't accept illness | |
| Is too helpful | |
| Refuses to keep covers on self while in bed | |
| Disregards principles of safety | |
| Other | |

MASTER WORK SHEET EXAMPLE

| | WARD | | | | | | | | | | | | | | | | | | |
|---|---|---|---|---|---|---|---|---|---|---|---|---|---|---|---|---|---|---|---|
| | 1 (O.B.) | | | | | | | | | 2 (O.B.) | | | 3 Surg. | | 4 (Surg.) | | | | |
| Responses of Nurses | Jones | | | Smith | | | Patient Brown | | | Green | Black | White | Day | Night | Blue | | | Gray | Gold |
| (x—Head Nurse) | A2 | A3 | A8 | A2 | A3 | A8 | A2 | A3 | A8 | A7 | A7 | A7 | A9 | A9 | A1 | A4 | A10 | A10 | A10 |
| x (Head Nurse) | x | | | x | | | x | | | | | | x | x | | | x | x | x |
| **I. COMMUNICATION** | | | | | | | | | | | | | | | | | | | |
| 1. Language barrier | ✓ | | | | | | | | | | ✓ | | ✓ | | | | | | |
| 2. Intelligence level | | | | ✓ | ✓ | | | | | ✓ | ✓ | ✓ | | | ✓ | ✓ | | ✓ | |
| 3. Misinterprets instruction | | | ✓ | | | | | | | | ✓ | | | | ✓ | | ✓ | ✓ | |
| 4. Cannot read or write | | | | | | | | | | | ✓ | | | | | | | | |
| *Subtotal* | 1 | | 1 | 1 | 1 | | | | | 1 | 4 | 1 | 1 | | 2 | 1 | 1 | 2 | |
| **II. COMPLAINT** | | | | | | | | | | | | | | | | | | | |
| 1. Reports nurses | | | | | | | | | | | | | | ✓ | ✓ | ✓ | ✓ | | |
| 2. States not getting proper treatment | | | | | | | | | | | | | | | ✓ | ✓ | ✓ | | |
| 3. States not getting proper service | | | | | | | | | | | | | | | ✓ | ✓ | ✓ | | |
| 4. Is resentful | | | ✓ | | | | ✓ | | | ✓ | | | | ✓ | ✓ | ✓ | ✓ | | |
| 5. Shows no appreciation | | | ✓ | | ✓ | | | | | ✓ | | | | | ✓ | ✓ | ✓ | | |
| *Subtotal* | | | 2 | | 1 | | 1 | | | 2 | | | | 2 | 5 | 5 | 5 | | |

# BIBLIOGRAPHY

BURTON, G., *Personal, Impersonal and Interpersonal Relationships*, Springer Publishing Company, New York: 1958.

HABERSTIEN, R. W., and CHRIST, E. A., *Professionalizer, Traditionalizer and Utilizer*, University of Missouri, Columbia, Missouri: 1955.

HARMER, BERTHA, and HENDERSON, VIRGINIA, *Textbook of the Principles and Practice of Nursing*, The Macmillan Co., New York: 1955.

HIGHLEY, B. L., and NORRIS, C., "When A Student Dislikes A Patient," *Am. J. Nursing*, September, 1957.

HUGHES, E. C., HUGHES, H. M., and DEUTSCHER, I., *Twenty Thousand Nurses Tell Their Story*, J. B. Lippincott Co., Philadelphia: 1958.

INGLES, T., "The Worst Patient on the Floor," *Nursing Outlook*, 6(2):99, 1958.

——— "Mr. Parker—A 'Bad' Patient," *Nursing Outlook*, 6(4):209, 1958.

——— "Margaret—An Uncooperative Patient," *Nursing Outlook*, 6(5):289, 1958.

JOURARD, SIDNEY, "How Well Do You Know Your Patients?" *Am. J. Nursing*, November 1959.

NIGHTINGALE, FLORENCE, *Notes on Nursing*, Harrison, London: 1860.

REISSMAN, L., and ROHER, J. H., *Change and Dilemma in the Nursing Profession*, G. P. Putnam's Sons, New York: 1957.

SCHWARTZ, D., "Uncooperative Patients?" *Am. J. Nursing*, January 1958.

SCHWARTZ, M. S., and SHOCKLEY, E. L., *The Nurse and the Mental Patient*, Russell Sage Foundation, New York: 1956.

SELLTIZ, C. M., JAHODA, M., DEUTSCH, M., and COOK, S., *Research Methods in Social Relations*, Henry Holt and Co., New York: 1959.

SHAFER, K. N., SAWYER, J. R., MC CLUSKEY, A. M., and LIFGREN, E. A., *Medical-Surgical Nursing*, 2nd ed. The C. V. Mosby Co., St. Louis: 1961.

# 38 WARD STUDY: THE MEANING OF TOUCH IN INTERPERSONAL COMMUNICATION

*Jane De Augustinis, Rebecca S. Isani, and Fern R. Kumler*

A ward study in the area of nonverbal communication done by the researchers at an earlier date aroused their interest in the use of touch as a means of communication. More specifically, the researchers became interested in the meaning of touch gestures that occur in patient-personnel relations in the psychiatric setting.

> We have unfortunately made too little use of all the avenues of communication with our schizophrenic patients. Body language is particularly effective at certain stages, but we are uncertain in its uses. Furthermore, there is a severe tradition in psychology that psychotherapy is a verbal process and the patient must not be touched. These latter fears, it must be pointed out, are our own and not the patient's.[1]

To use touch therapeutically, the nurse must have knowledge of the various meanings of the touch gestures used. This study is designed to explore these meanings.

## PROBLEM STATEMENT

What are the various meanings of the touch gestures that occur in patient-ward personnel dyadic relationships in the psychiatric setting, and are these meanings to the initiators and recipients similar or dissimilar?

### SUBPROBLEMS

1. What touch gestures are used in patient–ward personnel dyadic relationships?

[1] Burton, A. (ed.), *Psychotherapy of the Psychoses*, p. 180.

2. When touch gestures are used in patient–ward personnel dyadic relationships, what are the meanings of these touch gestures to their initiators?

3. When touch gestures are used in patient–ward personnel dyadic relationships, what are the meanings of these touch gestures to their recipients?

4. When touch gestures are used in patient–ward personnel dyadic relationships, are the meanings of these gestures to the initiators and recipients similar?

5. When touch gestures are used in patient–ward personnel dyadic relationships, are the meanings of these gestures to the initiators and recipients dissimilar?

## REVIEW OF LITERATURE

Literature concerning the use of touch, its developmental aspects, and its interpretation is widely scattered throughout psychiatry, psychiatric nursing, psychology, sociology, and communication journals and texts. Periodicals in the areas of psychiatry, psychology, and nursing were studied through 1955 for theories and studies on the use of touch. The only studies found relevant to the subject were those that dealt with early parent-child interaction and did not deal with dyadic interpretations of touch gestures.

Hofling and Leininger [2] see communication as "a two-way process concerned with conveying a message or an idea between two or more individuals." If touch is to be considered a form of communication, it must convey a message or an idea between two or more persons. Peplau [3] supports this view of touch by stating that the body or parts of it act as "expressional instruments that communicate to others the feelings, wishes, and aspirations of an individual." She goes on to say that these communicative acts are individual and cultural. This view is further supported by Ruesch and Kees,[4] who state, "We have today come to realize that any form of action, whether verbal or nonverbal, has communicative function. As soon as another person interprets a signal with some degree of accuracy, it must be codified in terms that qualify as language."

Touch, then, as a form of nonverbal communication is used in message sending and receiving. The importance of understanding touch as communication is emphasized by Peplau,[5] particularly in regard to nurses. "The

[2] Hofling, C., and Leininger, M. M., *Basic Psychiatric Concepts in Nursing*, p. 40.
[3] Peplau, H. E., *Interpersonal Relations in Nursing*, p. 305.
[4] Ruesch, J., and Kees, W., *Nonverbal Communication*, p. 48.
[5] Peplau, H. E., *op. cit.*, p. 289.

development of consciousness of tools used in nursing includes awareness of means of communcation; spoken language, rational and nonrational expressions of wishes, needs, and desires; and the body gestures." In regard to working with psychiatric patients, Ruesch [6] believes that verbal communication is difficult, if not impossible, if nonverbal perception and expression do not function. He also notes that there is a lack of a vocabulary to describe nonverbal communication and points to the global terms used, such as interaction, support, etc.

## VIEWS ON TOUCH IN EARLY DEVELOPMENTAL PERIODS

Sullivan [7] says that the young infant has a need for contact which constitutes the "very genuine beginnings of purely human or interpersonal needs." This view is supported by Fromm-Reichmann [8] who states that the need for physical contact is innate and consistent from birth. She goes on to say that physical and emotional disturbances are caused by consistent lack of physical contact. In Greenwald's study [9] of the call girl, he observes that, at an early age, they discovered that they could satisfy feelings of loneliness and unworthiness and needs for affection and interest by giving sexual gratification. This physical contact was one way of obtaining the closeness and tenderness they did not receive from the parents. Spiegel [10] describes a patient who had very limited communication with her mother because of a lack of physical closeness. "What's the use of talking? It's futile. All I got from my mother was praise, words, for giving up to my sister. Never a touch, never a hug!"

Touching can be associated with pleasure, satisfaction, and rewards or with anxiety and punishment in infancy and childhood. Sullivan [11] speaks of fondling as a pleasure-giving manipulation of the child which can become associated with rewards, and the refusal of contact and the inflicting of pain and inducement of anxiety as forms of punishment. In a study done on patterns of mothering, Brody [12] notes that the infant's first pleasurable responses involve physical contact and refers to Anna Freud's observation of the "close interrelationship between the infant's need for body contact and the pleasure of functions like sleeping and eating." Ruesch [13] also

[6] Ruesch, J., "General Theory of Communication," *American Handbook of Psychiatry*, p. 901.
[7] Sullivan, H. S., *Interpersonal Theory of Psychiatry*, p. 40.
[8] Fromm-Reichmann, F., *Psychoanalysis and Psychotherapy*, p. 335.
[9] Greenwald, Harold, *The Call Girl*, Ballantine Books, New York, 1958.
[10] Spiegel, R., "Specific Problems of Communication," p. 923.
[11] Sullivan, H. S., *op. cit.*, p. 155.
[12] Brody, S., *Patterns of Mothering*, p. 338.
[13] Ruesch, J., *Disturbed Communication*, p. 90.

states that the infant gains satisfaction and pleasurable sensations when hunger is gratified, and that this process necessitates close contact and handling by the adult, thus forming an association between pleasure and touch. In a comparative study of the tactile experiences of two girls during infancy and their effects on personality development, Ritro and Solnit [14] found that when the feeding-touch experiences were associated with increased discomfort, they became a model for later disturbed object relationships as demonstrated by nursery school behavior. As one of the children studied progressed in therapy, she displayed the desire to touch and be touched.

Touch is also viewed by some as the earliest means of reality contact. Brody [15] says that the infant's perception of reality is first through the skin of the entire body surface. Chambers [16] states that the reality experience of the neonate consists of the inner environment (physiological experience) and the outer environment. She further observes that the environmental stimuli most sharply perceived by the infant are those that respond to his physiological reality—care of the body and satisfaction of needs, which involve tactile manipulation. The mother is usually the one involved in caring for the infant and using touch, and affords him "a stimulation which enlarges and enriches his reality experience."

Nonverbal communication, including touch, is seen as a form of language by Ruesch.[17] He says that with the development of hand-mouth coordination and locomotion, the striped muscles become the principal effector organs, and "action language" is used. This form of language is first used to call attention, to please, or to retaliate. However, says Ruesch, if the parents do not acknowledge action language, the child will not be able to learn it. Critchley [18] views gesture as a primitive component of speech. He states that "a study of the comprehension and development of speech in infants and very young children shows that the baby learns to react to a number of simple gestures and movements made by the mother."

As the individual moves into childhood and the significant phase of acculturation, the use of touch and other nonverbal cues is begun. Murphy [19] points out, "A society has a traditional set of signals or cues to which the child becomes conditioned. He learns what leads to what in

[14] Ritro, S., and Solnit, A., "Influences of Early Mother-Child Interaction on Identification Processes," pp. 64–85.

[15] Brody, S., op. cit., p. 340.

[16] Chambers, J., "Maternal Deprivation and the Concept of Time in Children," pp. 406–19.

[17] Ruesch, J., Disturbed Communication, p. 80.

[18] Critchley, M., The Language of Gestures, pp. 120–21.

[19] In Hall, C. S., and Lindzey, G., Theories of Personality, p. 519.

his particular society." A study of child-rearing in different cultures by Elonen [20] indicates that there is a striking difference between the American and Finnish cultures in the use of touch by parents to demonstrate affection toward their children. She notes that the Finnish infant receives far less fondling and kissing, but that affection is demonstrated through tone of voice, glance of eye, and instructive play. However, Fromm-Reichmann [21] states:

> Among the people of the middle and upper social strata in our Western culture, physical loneliness has become a specific problem, since this culture is governed by so many obsessional taboos with regard to people's touching one another or having their physical privacy threatened in other ways.

## Major Interpretations of Touch

Feldman's theory [22] of touch has an instinctual basis. He states, "Human beings and other members of the animal kingdom come into physical contact with each other for purposes of self-preservation, mating and play." He accepts the proposition that the main drive carried out by the arms and hands is that of "clinging." He says that the arms, hands, and fingers serve a multitude of other purposes, but that all of these other functions are substitutes or derivatives of the instinct to "cling." Feldman believes that gestures originally communicated needs in the struggle for life, and that "most of the gestures and other bodily movements express the same drive at the present time as they did at the time of their origin, though some of them went through certain modifications, became 'culturized.' "

Touch is seen by some authors as a means of reality contact and testing. Wolfe [23] states, "The hand is both a tool of learning about the outside world and as an organ of spatial sensibility can be considered the fundamental vehicle of the structure of thought. Spatial differentiation goes with physical as well as mental balance." According to Schachtel,[24] "Kant described touch as the only sense of immediate outer perception, hence also the most important and the one that informs with the greatest certitude." Descartes also considered touch to be the most reliable sense. Schachtel further points out that "children want to touch everything in order to get really acquainted with it, and when the adult does not feel

[20] Elonen, A. S., "The Effect of Child Rearing on Behavior in Different Cultures," pp. 505–12.
[21] Fromm-Reichmann, F., op. cit., p. 336.
[22] Feldman, S., Mannerisms of Speech and Gestures, pp. 197–225.
[23] In Ruesch, J., and Kees, W., op. cit., p. 40.
[24] Schachtel, E. G., Metamorphosis, pp. 141–42.

quite sure whether his senses may not be playing a trick on him, he touches an object to make sure of its really being there." Schwartz and Shockley [25] specifically refer to the use of touch in the nurse-patient relationship. They point out that the patient may need to touch and be touched by the nurse to reassure him that the nurse is a "real" person.

Some authors say simply that there is a human need for physical contact which must be filled. Already mentioned in this respect is the need for physical contact of the call girls studied by Greenwald. Sullivan [26] points out the desire to touch one another and to be physically close. Schwartz and Shockley [27] say that behavior having a sexual aspect may be an indicant that a psychiatric patient wants a simple physical contact and to form a relationship to reduce his isolation and loneliness. Spiegel [28] supports this, stating that "the schizophrenic patient may express some of his longings for closeness by means of direct body-language."

The primary focus of the present study was upon the use of touch in communication. Critchley [29] mentions a group of gestures that have a universal interpretation, which he says constitute a "silent lingua franca" that is comprehensible to all, regardless of age, race, religion, social status, or mental and cultural level. He believes that these can be used to deal with simple propositions and emotional themes, which can be expressed verbally only with great difficulty. Ruesch is one of the foremost exponents of the communicative ability of nonverbal gestures. As he and Kees [30] point out,

> In interpersonal meeting, gestures and actions tend to have a more mandatory function; they direct or shape the other person's behavior, whereas words serve a more explanatory function. . . . By means of duality of verbal and nonverbal communication, the human being is able to create impressions based upon differences between the things he says in words and the things he communicates through action.

They go on to say that the individual may respond selectively to the verbal component, to the nonverbal component, or to an integration of the two in a fuller interpretation of the message. More specifically, they [31] say that

> . . . when someone wishes to appraise others in the terms of friendliness or hospitality, one of his major cues is the physical distance maintained. This

[25] Schwartz, M. S., and Shockley, E. L., *The Nurse and the Mental Patient*, p. 253.
[26] Cited in Mullahy, P., *Oedipus: Myth and Complex*, p. 281.
[27] Schwartz, S., and Shockley, E. L., *op. cit.*, pp. 157–66.
[28] Spiegel, R., *op. cit.*, pp. 936–37.
[29] Critchley, M., *op. cit.*, p. 116.
[30] Reusch, J., and Kees, W., *op. cit.*, p. 86.
[31] *Ibid.*, p. 82.

may range from actual touch to various spans of distance, indicating familiarity or strangeness, or intimacy.

Ruesch and Kees also indicate that there may be nonverbal invitations to decrease or increase distance. "Some, through a skillful exposure of the skin, invite touch; others, because of an overly immaculate countenance, exert a forbidding influence." [32]

Present abilities and past experiences of the individual may influence his interpretation of the touch gesture. Meredith [33] says,

> . . . even if all our processes of communication were technically perfect there must still be a failure of those cases in which the mind of the recipient is such that it cannot take in the message in the form in which it is given. The communicator needs, in relation to the recipient, not only a knowledge of the latter's objective needs—what information he has to supply—but also an ability to project himself into the mind of the recipient and influence his readiness and aptitude for the message.

Peplau [34] indicates aspects involving the individual's past:

> When the nurse is viewed as a figure, symbolic of past experience, values and feelings held in relation to the older experience are reactivated and enter into the patient's expectations of the nurse. The behavior of the nurse—her appearance, mode of action, body gesture, manner of speaking—will be evaluated in terms of the patient's past experience.

There are three general schools of thought on the use of touch in therapy. The first strongly advocates the use of touch, the second is strongly against any use of touch, while the third school indicates that the use of touch may be valuable when the therapist is aware of the patient's dynamics and of the possible interpretations of the touch gesture.

The techniques of Rosen and Sechehaye involve the use of close contact with their patients. The schizophrenic girl analyzed by Sechehaye [35] indicated a sense of security when she was with her therapist, especially when they sat together on the couch and the therapist put her arm around the patient's shoulder. "Oh, what joy, what relief to feel the life, the warmth, the reality!" Sechehaye used many touch gestures with this girl in various "mothering" activities. Greenhill [36] says that physical contact seems to act as a powerful catalyst in communication. He maintains that nursing procedures involving physical contact can strengthen the verbal interaction between the nurse and her patient. Robinson [37] argues for the

[32] Loc. cit.
[33] Cited in Soddy, K., Mental Health and Infant Development, p. 286.
[34] Peplau, H. E., op. cit., p. 36.
[35] Sechehaye, M., Autobiography of a Schizophrenic Girl, p. 256.
[36] Greenhill, M., "Interviewing With a Purpose," pp. 1259–62.
[37] Robinson, A., "Communication with Schizophrenic Patients," pp. 1120–23.

use of love as a tool in communicating with schizophrenic patients. She gives an example of an instance when she used touch in tying a patient's shoelaces, and there was subsequent strengthening of the relationship.

Other authors advise strongly against the use of touch in therapy. Wolberg[38] states, "It goes without saying that physical contact with the patient is absolutely taboo. Touching, stroking or kissing the patient may mobilize sexual feelings in the patient and therapist, or bring forth violent outbursts of anger." He goes on to say that the therapist must not respond to the physical approach of a patient, but must encourage the patient to verbalize the feelings. Matheney and Topalis[39] show a picture of a nurse half-embracing a patient and state, "Intimate relationships with patients are not conducive to a therapeutic atmosphere." Render and Weiss[40] further caution that "women nurses, especially young students, should not touch a male patient; merely walk beside him with a male aide or nurse."

The third group of authors indicate that touch should be used with care. Fromm-Reichmann[41] says,

> As to the fourth goal of human satisfaction, the avoidance of physical loneliness, it goes without saying that the patient should not be used for its achievement. This does not advocate that the psychiatrist be an obsessional denizen of our culture, wherein touching another person or being touched by him is considered taboo unless there is an intimate relationship. The contrary is true. At times it may be indicated and wise to shake hands with a patient or, in the case of a very disturbed person, to touch him reassuringly or not to refuse his gesture of seeking affection and closeness. However, it is always recommended that one be thrifty with the expression of any physical contact.

Varley[42] believes that the therapist must know the patient's dynamics to understand the meaning the gesture may have. "A physical gesture may convey better than words to some patients the therapist's knowledge and acceptance of their emotional turmoil. To other patients even a minimum of physical contact may be very frightening and must be avoided." She further points out that the therapist is schooled in verbal communication, but that it is difficult to learn and use nonverbal communication with competence. Schwartz and Shockley[43] also state, "The nurse must determine when closeness is acceptable and when it is not; she must determine

[38] Wolberg, L. R., *The Technique of Psychotherapy*, p. 352.

[39] Matheney, R., and Topalis, M., *Psychiatric Nursing*, p. 95.

[40] Render, H. W., and Weiss, O. M., *Nurse Patient Relationships in Psychiatry*, p. 161.

[41] Fromm-Reichmann, F., *Principles of Intensive Psychotherapy*, p. 12.

[42] Varley, B. K., "Reaching Out, Therapy with Schizophrenic Patients," pp. 407–16.

[43] Schwartz, S., and Shockley, E. L., *op. cit.*, p. 253.

how the patient might interpret and respond to it." They also indicate that when personnel can accept the patient's behavior that has a sexual aspect as an expression of the need for physical contact, then personnel can accept the patient more and try to meet some of the needs, while setting the limits.[44]

Steele and Manfreda [45] believe that the nurse may sometimes give reassurance through the use of touch. However, they point out, some touch gestures may be very threatening to certain patients, particularly those who have homosexual tendencies and those patients who fear that they have homosexual tendencies and avoid a close relationship of any kind with a member of the same sex. Hofling and Leininger [46] emphasize,

> . . . the actions, the gestures, and the spoken words of the patient and the nurse are important because each takes clues from the other. The nurse takes such clues to determine her interaction with the patient. On the other hand, the patient determines his actions and decisions by what the nurse is communicating to him. There exists a sensitive interplay of feeling between them.

Therefore, the nurse must be aware of the clues given in touch gestures and their possible meanings for the patient.

The researchers involved in this study agreed with the school of thought that advocates the use of touch, but with foresight and knowledge about the patient and the possible interpretations of touch. There is a time when touching may be a valuable avenue of communication, but the value of its use must not be based on intuitive guesswork. The researchers believed that the value of touch as an avenue of communication would be revealed to some extent by this study.

## PURPOSE

This study may provide psychiatric workers with information on the possible interpretation of touch used in communication. This knowledge may then encourage insightful evaluation of the use of touch gestures in the psychiatric setting.

## DEFINITIONS

*Meanings*—the verbalized interpretations of the message indicated by the touch gesture.

---

[44] *Ibid.*, pp. 157–66.
[45] Steele, K. M., and Manfreda, M. L., *Psychiatric Nursing*, p. 110.
[46] Hofling, C., and Leininger, M. M., *op. cit.*, p. 43.

*Touch gestures*—movements of the head, body, or limbs involving physical contact that express an idea or feeling and which are used alone or in conjunction with verbalizations.

*Patients*—individuals receiving care in a psychiatric hospital.

*Ward-personnel*—the individuals employed by a hospital to render direct care to patients on a ward.

*Patient–ward personnel dyadic relationships*—two-person interactions between a patient and one of the ward personnel.

*Initiators*—individuals who originate the act of movement of head, body, or limbs that involves physical contact with another individual.

*Recipients*—individuals who receive the act of movement of head, body, or limbs that involves physical contact with another individual.

*Similar response*—the responses of the initiator and recipient that had a correspondence of meaning as determined by the judgment of three researchers.

*Dissimilar response*—the responses of the initiator and recipient that had a lack of correspondence of meaning as determined by the judgment of three researchers.

## ASSUMPTIONS

1. Nonverbal communication, including touch gestures, has purpose, is meaningful, and can be understood.

2. Touch gestures and the setting in which they occur can be accurately observed and recorded by the researchers.

3. The inherent meanings of the touch gestures can be derived using the methodology outlined in this study.

## LIMITATIONS

1. The sample consisted only of female patients and personnel and, thus, the findings could not be generalized to the total hospital population.

2. The presence of the researchers on the ward affected the patterns of interaction.

3. A limited number of personnel was on each ward and a limited number of wards were available to the researchers; hence, the sample was small.

4. The researchers had a limited amount of time for data collection, consequently, no pretesting of the technique was done.

5. Knowledge of the researchers' professional status may have influenced the respondents' answers to the interview questions.

## METHODOLOGY

The following presents the methodology designed to collect the data necessary to answer the research questions.

### SETTING FOR THE STUDY

Arrangements were made with a psychiatric hospital for three fifth-year graduate fellows in the Master of Science Program in Advanced Psychiatric Nursing at Rutgers, The State University of New Jersey, to do research in the hospital. Four wards, staffed with nonprofessional female personnel and populated with chronically ill female patients were made available to the researchers for this study. The study, which began on March 14, 1962, and ended on April 13, 1962, involved a total of six hours of observation and interviewing periods, and a total of three one-hour periods in which the three researchers administered a questionnaire to patients and personnel.

### INTRODUCTION OF RESEARCHERS TO THE WARD

Ward personnel were informed that registered nurses from Rutgers, The State University, would be observing interaction on the ward and would be conducting brief interviews. No other information was offered initially. If questioned by ward personnel or patients, the reply was, "I am studying interaction on the ward." When introducing herself to the respondents for the interview, the researcher said, "I am a registered nurse studying interaction on the ward, and I would like to ask you a few questions."

A member of the faculty of the college of nursing served as a fourth researcher for observation and interviewing.

### METHOD OF RECORDING AND INTERVIEWING

1. Observations of patient–ward personnel dyadic relationships involving touch gestures were recorded on 5- by 8-inch cards (see p. 299).

2. Double observers were used, and each recorded observations of each dyadic relationship.

3. One observer interviewed the initiator and one observer interviewed the recipient of the gesture. (For interview questions, see p. 299).

4. Observers alternated interviewing patient and personnel,[47] i.e., the observer who interviewed the patient in one recorded dyadic relationship interviewed personnel in the next recorded dyadic relationship.

5. Verbatim responses and nonverbal cues during the interview were recorded on 5- by 8-inch cards.

6. The respondents were interviewed immediately after the completion of the interaction, i.e., when one or both respondents turned to a new task or dyadic relationship.

7. Unless the new task was judged by the observer as an emergency task to be completed without interruption, the observer interrupted the respondent for the interview.

8. In the event that the prospective respondent became involved in a task that could not be interrupted, the data were retained to be processed with the data of those relationships in which only one respondent was willing to be interviewed.

9. In the event that the answer to question 1 in the interview was "no," the alternative question was asked of the respondent.

10. The data from the observation and interview periods were used to compose the questionnaire.

## DEVELOPMENT AND ADMINISTRATION OF QUESTIONNAIRE

1. After four periods of observation and interviewing, the researchers reviewed the data collected to gain information that would aid in selecting questions for a questionnaire.

2. The researchers then designed a questionnaire (see p. 300) consisting of direct, open questions.

3. The questions were designed to answer the research questions and to obtain as nearly as possible the same type of data obtained by observation and interviewing.

4. The researchers recorded verbatim responses to the questionnaire.

5. If the respondents were vague in their responses or did not understand the question, the researcher asked for description of concrete examples (see p. 300).

[47] This technique was used to reduce the possibility of interviewers developing stereotyped perceptions and attitudes toward respondents. For further explanation of interviewer bias, see Selltiz, Claire, et al., Research Methods in Social Relations, pp. 583–87.

## SELECTION OF RESPONDENTS FOR OBSERVATION AND INTERVIEWING

1. The initiator and recipient of a touch gesture in a patient–ward dyadic relationship observed during the time specified by the researchers were chosen for interviews.

2. The respondents had the ability to respond verbally, in the English language, to questions.

3. In the event that the same gesture occurred repeatedly in the same dyadic relationship during the observation hour, the researchers recorded only two such observations and interviews.

4. In the event that only one member of the dyadic relationship was willing to respond, the data were retained to be processed separately from the data recorded of complete dyadic relationships.

5. The respondents were observed between the hours of 7:30 A.M. and 4:00 P.M., according to an observation schedule (see p. 301).

6. The researchers obtained a time schedule of the working hours of the ward personnel and varied the observation periods so that (a) the personnel on both day and evening shifts would be observed and (b) a number of different ward personnel would be observed.

7. The respondents selected for observation and interviewing were selected from all four wards.

## SELECTION OF RESPONDENTS FOR THE QUESTIONNAIRE

1. Any female patient from the available wards who was willing and able to respond in the English language was chosen.

2. The number of patients and personnel who completed the questionnaire was limited by the time available to the researchers.

3. Any of the female personnel from the available wards who were willing to be interviewed by the researchers were chosen as respondents to the questionnaire.

## DATA PROCESSING (see p. 281)

### OBSERVATION AND INTERVIEW DATA

Responses were transferred from the data-collection cards onto a large basic worksheet. These data were classified into two main sections—one relating to the initiator of the touch gesture and one relating to the recipient of the gesture. The dyadic relationship was maintained in the recording except for the cases in which a response was not given. All three study-makers agreed on the categories (see p. 303) into which the types and interpretations of gestures were classified. In addition, the study-makers validated the meaning as similar or dissimilar and indicated this on the worksheet.

### QUESTIONNAIRE DATA

The responses from the questionnaire were recorded on another basic worksheet (see p. 302). The worksheet was divided into two main sections. One section included personnel responses as initiators and recipients, and one section included patient responses as initiators and recipients. Once again, the study-makers agreed on the categories used to classify the types of gestures and the interpretations of gestures.

## Summary of Methodology

Initially, the researchers planned to record data on two of the available wards by using the observation and brief-interview technique. However, during the fourth period of observation and interviewing on the two wards chosen, the personnel stayed in the office and avoided all communication with the patients. The reasons for the actions of the personnel were not implicitly clear to the researchers. Therefore, assuming that the action might be related to the presence of the researchers and the misinterpretation by personnel of the purpose of the researchers, the observation and interview technique was extended to include the other available wards for the final two hours of observation and interviewing.

Respondents for the observations and brief-interview technique were chosen on the following criteria: (1) They had been the initiator or the recipient of a touch gesture in a patient–ward personnel dyadic relationship. (2) They were willing and able to respond in the English language.

Using the data obtained during the initial four hours of research, a questionnaire was developed. Originally, it was planned that the questionnaire would be administered on the third and fourth available wards. However, since the observation and interviewing had been extended to include all the wards, the questionnaire was also administered on all the wards available to the researchers. The selection of respondents for the questionnaire was based on the willingness and ability of the respondents to reply in the English language to all of the questions.

The collected data were processed and tallied on worksheets. Separate worksheets were used for the data obtained from the two techniques used for data collection. An analysis of the data from the worksheets and the incidental findings follow.

## ANALYSIS

In order to answer the research questions, as much data as possible was analyzed to include the responses of both the initiators and recipients of touch gestures or to include both the nurse [48] or recipient. The analysis of the observation and interview data is shown first and followed by the analysis of the questionnaire data. The analysis of incidental findings from observation, interviewing, and the questionnaire concludes the analysis.

TABLE 7. INITIATORS' AND RECIPIENTS' AWARENESS OF TOUCH AT TIME OF OCCURRENCE

| | Initiator | | Recipient | |
|---|---|---|---|---|
| Touch | Nurse | Patient | Nurse | Patient |
| Noticed | 20 | 4 | 5 | 11 |
| Not noticed | 0 | 2 | 0 | 8 |
| No answer | 2 | 0 | 1 | 3 |
| Total | 22 | 6 | 6 | 22 |
| Total observations = 28 | | | | |

*Findings and Interpretations:* This table shows that nurses initiated touch in the majority (79 per cent) of the observations and that most cases in which the nurse responded she noticed the touch regardless of whether she was the initiator or recipient of the gesture. The patients reported not noticing touch both as initiators and recipients of the gestures. At least slighly over one-third (36 per cent) of the gestures initiated by the nurses were reported as not noticed by the patient-recipients. The data on patient-initiated touching are small in quantity for generalization, but seem further to indicate a possibility that patients were less aware of touch as initiators than were nurses.

It seems that nurses initiated touch gestures much more frequently than did patients and that nurses were more aware of touch than were patients. This is an indication that if the nurse used touch to convey a message to the patient, only about one-half of the patients consciously noted any form of message.

[48] The terms "nurse" and "personnel" are used interchangeably and include references to attendants, practical nurses, and registered nurses.

## TABLE 8. INITIATORS' AUTOMATIC OR THOUGHTFUL *
## USE OF TOUCH

|  | Initiator | |
| --- | --- | --- |
|  | Nurse | Patient |
| Automatic use | 12 | 2 |
| Thoughtful use | 7 | 2 |
| No answer | 3 | 2 |
| Total | 22 | 6 |

Total number of gestures initiated = 28

* Thoughtful use indicated by answering, "Yes, I thought about it before I touched," Question 2.

*Findings and Interpretations.* About one-half (55 per cent) of the nurses' use of touch was automatic while less than one-third (32 per cent) of the nurses' use of touch was thoughtful. It seems that nurses most frequently initiated touch automatically as an avenue of communication. Data on patient-initiated touch are insufficient for generalization, but they also offer indications that patients as initiators thought about touch before touching about as frequently (one-third of the time) as nurses as initiators.

It seems that much less than one-half of the initiated gestures were used as an avenue of communication to convey premeditated, purposeful messages.

## TABLE 9. RECIPIENTS WHO THOUGHT ABOUT TOUCH *

| Thought about | Nurse | Patient |
| --- | --- | --- |
| Yes | 5 | 4 |
| No | 0 | 4 |
| No answer | 1 | 3 |
| Total recipients | 6 | 11 |

* Includes only those recipients (17) who noticed the gestures.

*Findings and Interpretations.* Of the patient recipients who noticed being touched, approximately 36 per cent, or more than one-third but less than one-half, of them thought about having been touched. Table 7 shows that only about one-half of the patient recipients noticed having been touched. Nurses, however, responded that they noticed having been touched (refer to Table 7) in nearly all the cases and that they also thought about having been touched in nearly all the cases. As a matter of fact, all the nurses who responded to whether they noticed and thought about it said that they did notice and think about having been touched. This would seem to indicate that nurses were not only more aware of touch as recipients than were patients, but also that nurses, as recipients, gave more conscious thought to the meaning of touch gestures than did patients.

TABLE 10. PATIENT-PERSONNEL INTERPRETATIONS OF TOUCH COMPARED ACCORDING TO TYPES OF TOUCH GESTURES USED

| Interpretations | Hand Touches | | Embraces | | Holding Hands | | Holding Arms to Sides | | Adjust Clothes | | Arm in Arm | | Total | |
|---|---|---|---|---|---|---|---|---|---|---|---|---|---|---|
| | No. | % | No. | % | No. | % | No. | % | No. | % | No. | % | No. | % |
| **Showing tender feelings** | | | | | | | | | | | | | | |
| Pt. | 5 | 70 | 1 | 33 | 0 | 0 | 0 | 0 | 0 | 0 | 0 | 0 | 6 | 46 |
| Pers. | 5 | 50 | 2 | 40 | 2 | 66 | 0 | 0 | 0 | 0 | 1 | 100 | 10 | 43 |
| **Gaining attention** | | | | | | | | | | | | | | |
| Pt. | 1 | 14 | 2 | 66 | 0 | 0 | 0 | 0 | 0 | 0 | 0 | 0 | 3 | 23 |
| Pers. | 2 | 20 | 0 | 0 | 0 | 0 | 0 | 0 | 0 | 0 | 0 | 0 | 2 | 8 |
| **Instigating an action** | | | | | | | | | | | | | | |
| Pt. | 1 | 14 | 0 | 0 | 1 | 100 | 1 | 100 | 1 | 100 | 0 | 0 | 4 | 30 |
| Pers. | 1 | 10 | 1 | 20 | 1 | 33 | 2 | 100 | 2 | 100 | 0 | 0 | 7 | 30 |
| **Other** | | | | | | | | | | | | | | |
| Pt. | 0 | 0 | 0 | 0 | 0 | 0 | 0 | 0 | 0 | 0 | 0 | 0 | 0 | 0 |
| Pers. | 2 | 20 | 2 | 40 | 0 | 0 | 0 | 0 | 0 | 0 | 0 | 0 | 4 | 17 |
| **Total** | | | | | | | | | | | | | | |
| Pt. | 7 | 100 | 3 | 100 | 1 | 100 | 1 | 100 | 1 | 100 | 0 | 0 | 13 | |
| Pers. | 10 | 100 | 5 | 100 | 3 | 100 | 2 | 100 | 2 | 100 | 1 | 100 | 23 | |

*Findings and Interpretations.* The largest group of gestures was interpreted by personnel and patients as "tender feelings," while "instigating an action" was the second largest category. The greatest differences between patient and personnel interpretations of touch gestures were in the "gaining attention" and "other" categories. All the interpretations classified as "other" (comfort, support, interest) were given by nursing personnel and constituted one of the largest differences in interpretation. Hand touches appear most often to indicate tender feelings to both patients and personnel.

## TABLE 11. SIMILAR AND DISSIMILAR—INTERPRETATION BY INITIATOR AND RECIPIENT *

| Question 3 † Interpretation By Recipients | Patient Initiator | Personnel Initiator | Total |
|---|---|---|---|
| Similar | 2 | 4 | 6 |
| Dissimilar | 2 | 3 | 5 |
| Neither | 0 | 1 | 1 |
| Total | 4 | 8 | 12 |

* Includes only patient-personnel dyadic relationships in which the touch gesture used was noticed and interpreted by each.

† Initiators were asked what they wanted to indicate, and recipients were asked what the initiators indicated to them.

## TABLE 12

| Question 4 * Interpretation | Nurse Initiator |
|---|---|
| Similar | 2 |
| Dissimilar | 2 |
| Neither | 1 |
| Total | 5 |

* "When someone (description of gesture) another person, what do you think it indicates?" Patient-personnel dyadic relationships in which the touch gesture used was not noticed by patient and answer was given to Question 4. (No instances of patient initiators.)

*Findings and Interpretations.* When the initiator and recipient gave an interpretation to the same touch gesture, the interpretation was similar in approximately one-half of the cases. There was no apparent difference whether a member of the personnel or patient group was the initiator as to the similarity or dissimilarity of interpretations. This would indicate that in any single instance there is an equal chance for a touch gesture to be interpreted correctly or interpreted incorrectly.

### QUESTIONNAIRE DATA

Limited by time, the researchers were unable to test and revise the questionnaire so that sufficient data could be recorded for a detailed statistical analysis. However, the following tables reveal that a greater variety of gestures were described in the questionnaire data than were observed during the initial observation and interview periods. There was also a greater variety of interpretations of the use of touch in the questionnaire data. These tables also indicate that patients did not offer as much descriptive information on the types of touch gestures or on the interpretations of touch as did personnel.

Since the respondents offered more than one interpretation and described more than one type of gesture, but did not match specific gestures with specific interpretations, the numbers in Tables 13 and 14 indicate the number of times that a category was mentioned by the total number of

TABLE 13. LISTING OF DESCRIPTIONS OF TOUCH GESTURES BY PERSONNEL AND PATIENTS AS INITIATORS AND RECIPIENTS

| | Personnel | | Patients | |
|---|---|---|---|---|
| Gestures Described | Initiator | Recipient | Initiator | Recipient |
| Hand touches | 5 | 9 | 2 | 1 |
| Embraces | 0 | 5 | 1 | 0 |
| Holding hands | 3 | 2 | 0 | 0 |
| Shaking hands | 1 | 1 | 0 | 0 |
| Utilitarian | 5 | 0 | 0 | 0 |
| Restraining or, instigating actions | 3 | 0 | 0 | 3 |
| Kissing | 0 | 2 | 1 | 0 |
| Crying on shoulder | 0 | 1 | 0 | 0 |
| Grabbing hair | 0 | 0 | 1 | 0 |
| Hitting with fist | 0 | 0 | 1 | 0 |
| Accidental | 0 | 0 | 1 | 0 |
| Total number of descriptions of gestures | 17 | 20 | 7 | 4 |

TABLE 14. LISTING OF INTERPRETATIONS OF TOUCH GESTURES BY PERSONNEL AND PATIENTS AS INITIATORS AND RECIPIENTS

| | Personnel | | Patients | |
|---|---|---|---|---|
| Interpretations | Initiator | Recipient | Initiator | Recipient |
| Express tender feeling | 3 | 4 | 2 | 1 |
| Gain attention | 3 | 7 | 3 | 1 |
| Instigate an action | 4 | 0 | 1 | 1 |
| Punitive or restraining | 2 | 0 | 0 | 0 |
| Aggressive feelings | 0 | 1 | 1 | 0 |
| Reality testing | 0 | 1 | 0 | 0 |
| Reality orienting | 3 | 0 | 0 | 0 |
| Others | 2 | 1 | 0 | 0 |
| Total number of interpretations | 17 | 14 | 7 | 3 |

respondents. The total number of respondents for the questionnaire was 18. The total number of patient respondents was 9, and the total number of personnel respondents was also 9.

TABLE 15. NUMBER OF PATIENTS * WHO GAVE INTERPRE-TATIONS OF TOUCH GESTURES AS INITIATORS AND RECIPIENTS

|  | Initiator | Recipient |
|---|---|---|
| Gave interpretations | 6 | 2 |
| Did not give interpretation | 3 | 7 |
| Total patients | 9 | 9 |

* All the personnel gave interpretations of touch gestures initiated and received.

TABLE 16. NUMBER OF PATIENTS * WHO INITIATED OR RECEIVED TOUCH GESTURES

|  | Initiator | Recipient |
|---|---|---|
| Yes | 7 | 5 |
| No | 2 | 3 |
| Not noticed | 0 | 1 |
| Total | 9 | 9 |

* All the personnel responded that they were initiators and recipients of touch gestures.

Findings and Interpretations: Table 13 indicates the variety of gestures that were described by patients and personnel. The personnel reported being the initiators particularly of hand touches, holding hands, and utilitarian gestures. They also reported as being the recipients of hand touches and holding hands. They mentioned their use of restraining actions, and the patients agreed that they were the recipients of these. The more openly expressive gestures, such as kissing and embracing, were only initiated by the patients. The variety of gestures reported in the questionnaire was greater than that noted by observation and in interviews. (Utilitarian gestures, kissing, crying on shoulder, and accidental touch appeared for the first time in the questionnaire.) Some types of gestures were mentioned by both personnel and patients, while others were noted by personnel *only* or patients *only*.

Table 14, the classification of gestures by categories of interpretation, indicates a greater range of interpretations by personnel. Gestures expressing tender feeling or seeking attention were reported by both patients and personnel —in the position of both initiators and recipients. This indicates some similarity of interpretation. In the questionnaire, new interpretations of gestures appeared which had not been mentioned in the interview. (These were punitive, aggressive feelings, reality testing, and reality orienting.)

An important finding from Table 15 is that two-thirds of the patients gave interpretations of their gestures when they themselves were the initiators. On the other hand, when these gestures were initiated by others, less than one-third of the patients gave interpretations of the gestures. The patients seemingly have difficulty interpreting the gestures of others.

From Table 16, it can be seen that not all the patients answering the questionnaire reported that they do touch personnel and are in turn touched by them. More mentioned themselves as initiators than as recipients. Nearly one-fourth of the respondents, however, denied receiving or initiating touch. This table indicates that the patients are more aware of their own gestures than those directed toward them.

## INCIDENTAL FINDINGS

During the observation and interview periods, the researchers noted a great deal of data which seemed pertinent to understanding the meaning and use of touch in the psychiatric setting. The incidental findings seemed to fall into three general categories: (1) Observations regarding the use of touch which seemed to be directly related to the presence of the researchers and the methodology used by the researchers. (2) Observations of the researchers regarding the frequency of the use of touch by certain patients and personnel. (3) The implied, but not directly verbalized, data by the respondents which seemed to support the incidental observations.

It was noted that personnel who were interviewed during the initial observation and interview periods seemed to alter their attitude toward the use of touch gestures. Many of the personnel who were hesitant and guarded during an initial interview appeared to be trying to note the researcher's attitude about touching patients. The alteration in the use of touch by certain of the personnel seemed to be related to what they thought was the positive or negative attitude of the researchers. After the initial interview, some of the personnel began touching almost every patient with whom they communicated verbally. Other personnel, after the initial interview, were observed to begin the initiation of a touch gesture and suddenly stop just before physical contact with the patient. Frequently, patients who appeared guarded and hesitant during the initial part of the interview changed their answers in the latter part of the interview. The change in answers was from such replies as, "No, I don't know," "I didn't notice," and "No meaning" to "Oh yes, she always does that. We're friends" or "She likes me."

The researchers wondered how much of the alteration in the use of touch by personnel and how much of the hesitancy and change in replies was due to the authority represented by, or attributed to, the researchers. It was known to each of the respondents that the researchers were registered nurses and that, as such, they represented authority over the respondents. The researchers speculated that many of the terms used by the personnel to interpret the gestures were textbook clichés used to impress the researchers. Terms such as "support," "comfort," and "interest" are non-specific terms which represent, according to textbooks, what personnel are "supposed to do." The speculation that the respondents were influenced by the status of the researchers was strengthened by the fact that although personnel frequently said the gesture was automatic, they offered an interpretation of the gesture that implied the gesture was used with deliberate and thoughtful intent. According to the textbook, personnel are "supposed to have a reason" for their actions toward patients.

In addition to those responses that may have been researcher-influenced, other observations seemed to have pertinent implications regarding the meaning and use of touch in the psychiatric setting. These observations seemed to be independent of researcher influence. It was noted that a few of the personnel and patients gave the appearance of deliberately avoiding touching or being touched by any other person. This observation applied to patient-patient and personnel-personnel dyadic relationships as well as to patient-personnel dyadic relationships. It was also noted that among the patients and personnel who did use touch gestures, there were patterns in the frequency of the use of the gestures initiated toward and received by both patients and personnel. Some of the personnel used touch frequently with certain patients and only rarely touched other patients. On the other hand, some of the personnel were touched frequently, and some were only rarely touched by patients.

Many of the replies to the initial interviews increased the researchers interest in the casual observations regarding the frequency of the use of touch in certain dyadic relationships. In one such relationship, a patient touched one of the personnel on the arm with her hand before initiating verbal interchange. The recipient was observed to recoil from the patient. Her (the recipient's) response to the question, "Did you notice a patient touching you a few minutes ago?" was, "Yes, I did, because of this particular patient." When asked for an interpretation of the gesture, the recipient replied, "She was saying she was ready to go to supper." The patient who initiated the gesture denied using the gesture. Her response was, "No! No! No! I never use touch." Neither the initiator nor the recipient clarified their responses any further. The researchers could only speculate that there must have been a particular meaning to the initiator and recipient that neither was willing, or perhaps neither was able, to verbalize at that time.

Another response indicated possible reasons for the patterns in the use of touch. One initiator said, "Why, I like her. She's the type of person you take to. She's been here so long." In that relationship the initiator (member of the personnel) had put her arm around the patient's shoulder, and the patient responded by putting her arm around the initiator's waist.

Replies such as these seemed to support the researchers' speculation that there were patterns in the frequency of the use or avoidance of touch in dyadic relationships. The specific reasons for these patterns were only implied and needed clarification. The method of observation and brief interviewing did not clarify the specific reasons, since the data were limited to those dyadic relationships in which touch was used and in which the researchers could clearly discern one initiator and one recipient. There were no data on interpretations of touch in relationships in which both people seemed to initiate touch spontaneously in the same instant. Also, there were no data on the interpretation of touch by people who avoided being either initiator or recipient of touch gestures.

The researchers had many questions which they hoped would be answered by respondents in their responses to the questionnaire developed from the observation and interview data. It was planned that the questionnaire would reveal some interpretations of touch by respondents who never touched or were never touched as well as the interpretations of touch by respondents who touched or were touched. The researchers further hoped that replies to the questionnaire would provide data which would yield clues to the many possible variables which influenced the initiation and interpretation of touch gestures.

In the questionnaire data, the researchers did include variables they thought might influence the use and interpretations of touch. However, the number of respondents was so small and the variables included such a wide range of information that it was not useful in the data analysis. For instance, the age range for the nine patient respondents was from 21 to 71 years, and the age range for the nine personnel respondents was from 18 to 55 years. The patients' length of stay in the hospital ranged from 1 to 23 years, and the length of employment for personnel was from 2 months to 10 years. However, the questionnaire data did reveal many other clues which seemed to indicate the reasons for the use or avoidance of touch. Much of these data revealed what seemed to the researchers to be incongruities between the gestures used and the interpretations of such gestures.

Frequently, gestures the personnel and patients described seemed to indicate to the researchers punitive action by personnel, but they were not interpreted as such by the respondents. Personnel described touching overactive and assaultive patients in order to put them into seclusion, but personnel then said they used touch to indicate interest in the patients. One patient, who said she never touches nurses, described nurses as hitting her with a hairbrush. This same patient offered no interpretation of the meanings of touch. Two other patients who offered no interpretations of touch said that they only touched nurses to fight with them. One of these patients indicated that she touched the nurses only when they slapped her first. The other patient said that nurses never touched her, and she never touched the "nice nurses" and described her touch as "hitting" the nurses. One other patient said she only touched nurses accidentally when "brushing against them" or to get their attention, but said that she didn't know what the nurses indicated by touch because they only touched her when "grabbing" her collar or "tearing" her sleeve. Another patient said that she only touched one nurse to show affection when the nurse left the ward, but nurses never touched her because "women just don't touch each other." Only one of the personnel mentioned that patients touched them when they were assaultive or overactive. Neither the patient-respondents nor personnel-respondents ever used the words "anger" or "hostile" in their interpretations of touching, although many of the instances noted would suggest that these interpretations might have been appropriately used by both patient and personnel respondents.

The previous data indicate that in patient-personnel dyadic relationships, some patients touch but are never touched; some never touch but are touched; some never touch and are never touched; and some touch and are touched. While the patients did not offer explicit reasons for avoiding touching nurses, such comments as "I don't bother with them" followed by descriptions of gestures which suggested punitive actions indicate the possibility that the types of previous experiences with nurses who initiated touch or responded to touch influenced the patients' reaction to the use of touch as an initiator. The comment that "women don't touch" suggests a cultural basis for the use or avoidance of touch.

Personnel responses such as, "They hug you when they want mothering" or "They cling to you when they're frightened" provide a clue that the developmental level, as well as the individual developmental experiences, of the patient might be an important variable in interpreting the use of touch gestures. Another clue to the use of touch was provided by such personnel descriptions as, "They touch your hair to see if it's as soft as it looks" or "They touch your uniform to see if it's as starched as it looks." The researchers categorized these responses as indicating reality testing which is important at certain developmental levels of growth.

The personnel respondents were more explicit about reasons for using and avoiding touch than were patient respondents. All the personnel described instances of touching and being touched, and many indicated thoughtful use of touch, although some indicated that they touched patients only out of necessity, which may or may not have indicated thoughtful use. In one such response, the nurse described touching only in the performance of utilitarian functions such as bathing, feeding, dressing, and combing hair. She interpreted the touching as "showing interest" and noted that she never touched patients who "can do for themselves." Other personnel said that they avoided touching patients who verbalized a dislike of being touched; patients who were sexually perverted; patients who were diagnosed as paranoid; and overactive and assaultive patients.

The researchers found that personnel were more verbal and elaborate in the variety of gestures described and in the number of interpretations of gestures. The reasons for the patients' meager responses could possibly indicate that (1) they had lost their descriptive skills as a result of illness or lack of practice in describing and/or (2) they were unwilling or unable to verbalize to strangers and/or (3) the questionnaire did not illicit adequate data because of its form and/or limited scope. The same lack of descriptive data was apparent in the results of the observation and interview technique.

All the incidental findings suggest that the methodology used and the limited amount of time available to the researchers influenced the amount and type of data collected. Even so, the data collected provided many clues to the use and meaning of touch in the psychiatric setting. The incidental findings indicate that (1) there are definite patterns in the use of touch by both patients and personnel; (2) both patients and personnel, wittingly or unwittingly, avoid interpreting gestures associated with punitive actions; (3) the overt behavior and diagnosis of the patient influence the nurses' use of touch; (4) the nurse's stereotype of herself and what she is "supposed to do" influences her interpretations of touch gestures; (5) the patient's developmental level and previous experiences with touch, both in and out of the hospital, influence the patient's use of touch; and (6) cultural attitudes may influence the use and interpretations of touch.

## IMPLICATIONS

1. From the data collected in this study, it appears that when touch is used as a form of communication, there is an uncertainty of interpretation that must be considered. With approximately a fifty-fifty chance of a similar interpretation of the touch on the part of the patient as recipient, the nurse as initiator must realize the possibility of her communication being misinterpreted. When the nurse is recipient, she must be aware that her

interpretation of the touch may or may not be correct. Increased awareness and thoughtfulness concerning the use of touch are certainly indicated.

2. The majority of the dissimilarities occurred when the nurse's interpretation included such terms as "interest," "comfort," or "support." In these cases, the patients interpreted the gestures as "getting attention" or "She wanted me to do. . . ." The researchers were not sure exactly what these nurses' terms indicated, or if they indicated the same meaning to all who used them. The vagueness of these terms to those who use them may be a factor in the misinterpretation of these communications, indicating a need for clarification of terms on the part of the individuals who use them.

3. The limited awareness of touch on the part of the patients, particularly as recipients, seems to indicate a high degree of anxiety associated with touch. Therefore, the nurse needs to be aware of the possibility of raising the patient's anxiety when she uses touch.

4. Interpretations of touch given included those that indicated a reality-orientation or reality-testing, such as, "to bring her back from daydreaming" and "to hold her attention." This would indicate that the nurse may utilize touch as a means for aiding the patient in becoming oriented to the reality situation.

5. Personnel indicated that certain patients are not touched, and certain patients indicated a marked dislike toward being touched. It appears, therefore, that the individuality of patients is a factor to be considered in the use of touch.

# RECOMMENDATIONS

1. Further study on the interpretations of touch, using a larger sample, would give more reliable statistics on the possibilities of correct and incorrect interpretations of touch.

2. Definition of concepts used in psychiatric nursing, particularly by nurse educators, would be valuable to workers in the clinical area.

3. Education of psychiatric workers in the area of touch should be included in present programs to increase the awareness and thoughtful use of touch in the psychiatric setting.

4. Investigation into the genesis of the anxiety apparently associated with touch in psychiatric patients may be profitable. The developmental aspects of touch may be studied in this connection.

5. A study on touch used as a means of reality-orientation could divulge

information useful in clinical practice in aiding the reality-testing of patients.

6. Research on the types of patients who touch and are touched would provide much information for the psychiatric worker in the thoughtful use of touch.

# SUMMARY AND CONCLUSIONS

## PROBLEM AND PURPOSE

The study was intended to reveal the various meanings of touch gestures which occurred in patient–ward personnel dyadic relationships and to discover similarities or dissimilarities of meanings of these gestures to the initiators and recipients. The many authors who have written about the use and meaning of touch in the psychiatric setting and elsewhere have expressed divergent views. The purpose of this study was to discover information which would provide psychiatric workers with knowledge that could be used for a more insightful evaluation of the uses of touch.

## FINDINGS RELATED TO THE LITERATURE

Certainly the data revealed the difficulty in verbalizing nonverbal communication as mentioned by Ruesch. The respondents did have difficulty in describing specific meanings of the gestures used. They very frequently used such terms as "interest" and "support" which are nonspecific in meaning. One could easily wonder about these replies and ask such questions as, "Interest in what or whom?" or "Support of what or whom?" The descriptions, especially by patients, were meager. The number of interpretations of touch as a communication of tender feelings and the descriptions of embracing and hand holding, as opposed to the extremely limited number of interpretations by personnel of assaultive touch and the lack of interpretations by patients of described punitive gestures, seem to support the ideas expressed by Sullivan, Brody, Ruesch, and Ritro and Solnit. Touching can be associated with pleasure, satisfaction, and rewards or with anxiety and punishment. The data indicate that when touching is associated with anxiety and punishment, the use of touch may be denied or avoided.

Touch as a means of reality testing and orienting seemed evident when personnel described touching "depressed or daydreaming patients to bring them back" or being touched by patients to test the softness of their hair or the texture of their uniform.

Many of the findings suggest that if touch is used with a patient, it should be used with care and conscious knowledge and intent. This is advocated by Fromm-Reichmann and Varley. In this study, although the nurses responded that they were aware of touching and thought about it at the time it occurred, the patients frequently responded with nonawareness and indicated even more frequently that they did not think about the gesture. Thus, it seems that many times the touch is not interpreted by the patient unless he is asked to do so. Even so, the dissimilarity of interpretations by the initiators and recipients showed that the initiator's intent was similarly interpreted only about 50 per cent of the time. In addition, the same gesture may mean different things to different people, so that the initiator cannot even assume that the recipients will interpret the message similarly on the basis of a popular meaning of the gesture.

The data indicated that cultural prescriptions, developmental levels, developmental experience, and recent personal experiences, all influence the meaning and use of touch. However, further research needs to be done in the psychiatric setting to determine the importance of each variable.

## CONCLUSIONS

1. Touch as a form of nonverbal communication involves an element of risk. Even with conscious knowledge of its initiation, the initiator's message may be similarly interpreted by the recipient only about one-half of the time.

2. Patients were more aware of initiating than receiving touch gestures. The researchers hypothesize that it is possible that the experience of being touched is more anxiety-producing for some people than the experience of touching.

3. Experiences of pleasure and satisfaction related to touch are more apt to be in awareness and interpreted by people who frequently use touch than an experience of touch associated with anxiety and punishment.

4. There are patterns in the use of touch gestures. Some people touch and are touched, some people never touch and are never touched, some people touch, but are never touched, and some people never touch, but are touched. It is possible that some people use touch to express only anger and aggression, while other people use touch to express only tender feelings.

5. Specific touch gestures do not have universal meanings.

6. Cultural prescriptions, developmental level, developmental experiences, and recent personal experiences, all influence the use and interpretation of touch.

## TOOL FOR RECORDING OBSERVATION AND INTERVIEWING DATA (5- by 8-inch card)

*Side One*

| |
|---|
| Observer_____<br>Date_____ Ward_____ Obs. No._____ Partner_____<br>I. Record description of interaction (verbal and nonverbal) and gesture. |

*Side Two*

| |
|---|
| Verbatim recording of response of initiator _____<br>                     or recipient _____<br>Quest. 1<br>Quest. 2<br>Quest. 3<br>Quest. 4 |

### INTERVIEW QUESTIONS

*Questions for Initiator*

1. Did you notice that you (description of gesture) the nurse (or a patient) a few minutes ago?
2. Did you think about (description of gesture) before you did it, or was it automatic?
3. What did you want to indicate to the other person when you used this gesture?

*Alternative Question*

4. When someone (description of gesture) another person, what do you think it indicates?

*Questions for Recipient*

1. Did you notice that the nurse (or a patient) (description of gesture) you a few minutes ago?
2. Did you think about it when the other person (description of gesture) you?
3. What did the other person indicate to you when she used this gesture.

*Alternative Question*

4. When someone (description of gesture) another person, what do you think it indicates?

## Ward Study Questionnaire

*Personnel*

Background data: Age_____ Sex_____

Race _____ Length of employment_____

1. Do you ever touch patients?
2. Are there certain patients you touch frequently? Rarely? Never? Give some examples.
3. In what situations do you touch patients?
4. Are there certain situations in which you don't touch patients? Give some examples.
5. What touch gestures do you use? Give some examples.
6. What do you want to indicate to the patient when you use these touch gestures?
7. Do patients ever touch you?
8. What touch gestures do the patients use?
9. When do you notice patients touching you?
10. What does the patient indicate to you when she (or he) uses these gestures?

*Patients*

Background data: Age_____ Sex_____

Race _____ Length of hospitalization_____

Number of hospitalizations_____

1. Do you ever touch nurses? (If the response is no) Tell me your thoughts about touching nurses.
2. What nurses do you touch? What nurses don't you touch?
3. In what situations do you touch nurses?
4. Are there certain times you don't touch nurses? For instance.
5. What touch gestures do you use? Give me some samples.
6. What do you want to indicate to the nurse when you touch her? Give me an example.
7. Do nurses ever touch you?
8. What touch gestures do the nurses use? Give me an example.
9. When do you notice nurses touching you?
10. What does the nurse indicate to you when she touches you? Give some examples.

# Observation Schedule

| Time | 3/14/62 Team | | 3/16/62 Team | | 3/21/62 Team | | 3/23/62 Team | | 4/4/62 Team | | 4/6/62 Team | |
|---|---|---|---|---|---|---|---|---|---|---|---|---|
| | A | B | A | B | A | B | A | B | A | B | A | B |
| 7:30– 8:30 | | | | | X | X | | | | | | |
| 9:30–10:00 | | | | | | | | | X | X | | |
| 11:00–11:30 | | | | | | | | | | | | |
| 12:30– 1:00 | | | | | | | | | | | | |
| 1:00– 2:00 | | | | | | | | | | | | |
| 2:00– 3:00 | | | | | | | | | | | X | X |
| 3:00– 4:00 | X | X | X | X | | | X | X | | | | |

SAMPLE OF WORKSHEET USED FOR DATA FROM OBSERVATION AND BRIEF INTERVIEWS

| Initiator | | Observations | Patient Responses | | | Personnel Responses | | | Researcher Notes |
|---|---|---|---|---|---|---|---|---|---|
| Pt. | Pers. | | Ques. 3 | Ques. 1 | Ques. 2 | Alternate Ques. 4 | Ques. 3 | Ques. 1 | Ques. 2 | Alternate Ques. 4 | |

## Categories of Touch Gestures

I. Hand touches

These include touches of the hand on head, neck, shoulder, arm, and hand. Examples: Attendant put hand on patient's shoulder. Patient rubbed hand across attendant's arm.

II. Embraces

These include one or both arms placed around the individual. Examples: Nurse threw arms around patient. Patient put arm around nurse's shoulder.

III. Holding hands

Examples: Nurse held out hands, took patient's hands. Nurse leading patient by hand.

IV. Holding arms to sides

Example: Attendant walking with patient in front, holding patient's arms to sides.

V. Adjusting clothes

Examples: Attendant adjusts patient's slip. Attendant fixing patient's skirt.

VI. Arm in arm

Example: Nurse walking up hall with arm crooked in patient's arm.

## Categories of Interpretations of Touch Gestures

I. Tender feelings

Examples: "She likes me." "I want them to know I care." "Friendliness."

II. Gaining attention

Examples: "I want to get her attention." "To get her attention—emphasize the point." "To get a cigarette."

III. Effecting an action

Examples: "So she would come with me." "Wanted me to sit down." "Wanted her to take her sweater off."

IV. Other

Examples: "Show interest." "Give comfort and support when the patient's shy." "I'm interested in her."

# WORKSHEET FOR RECORDING RESPONSES
## TO QUESTIONNAIRE

| | | | | | | | | |
|---|---|---|---|---|---|---|---|---|
| | | *Personnel* | | | | | *View of Patient* | |
| Age | Race | Length | Notice | Type | Interpretation | Notice | Type | Interpretation |
| | | | | | | | | |

| | | | | | | | | |
|---|---|---|---|---|---|---|---|---|
| | | *Patient* | | | | | *View of Personnel* | |
| | | | | | | | | |

# BIBLIOGRAPHY

BRODY, SYLVIA, *Patterns of Mothering*, International Universities Press, New York: 1956.

BURTON, ARTHUR (ed.), *Psychotherapy of the Psychoses*, Basic Books, New York: 1961.

CHAMBERS, JUANITA, "Maternal Deprivation and the Concept of Time in Children," *Am. J. Orthopsychiat.*, Vol. XXI, No. 2.

CRITCHLEY, MAC DONALD, *The Language of Gestures*, Edward Arnold and Co., London: 1939.

ELONEN, ANNA S., "The Effect of Child Rearing or Behavior in Different Cultures," *Am. J. Orthopsychiat.*, Vol. XXI, No. 3.

FELDMAN, SANDOR, *Mannerisms of Speech and Gestures*, International Universities Press, New York: 1959.

FROMM-REICHMANN, FRIEDA, *Principles of Intensive Psychotherapy*, University of Chicago Press, Phoenix Edition, Chicago: 1960.

——— *Psychoanalysis and Psychotherapy*, The University of Chicago Press, Chicago: 1959.

GREENHILL, MAURICE, "Interviewing With a Purpose," *Am. J. Nursing*, Vol. 56, No. 10.

GREENWALD, HAROLD, *The Call Girl*, Ballantine Books, New York: 1958.

HALL, CALVIN S., and LINDZEY, GARDNER, *Theories of Personality*, John Wiley and Sons, New York: 1957.

HOFLING, CHARLES, and LEININGER, MADELINE M., *Basic Psychiatric Concepts in Nursing*, J. B. Lippincott Company, Philadelphia: 1960.

MATHENEY, RUTH, and TOPALIS, MARY, *Psychiatric Nursing*, The C. V. Mosby Company, St. Louis: 1961.

MULLAHY, PATRICK, *Oedipus: Myth and Complex*, Grove Press, New York: 1948.

PEPLAU, HILDEGARD E., *Interpersonal Relations in Nursing*, G. P. Putnam's Sons, New York: 1952.

RITRO, SAMUEL, and SOLNIT, ALBERT, "Influences of Early Mother-Child Interaction on Identification Processes," *The Psychoanalytic Study of the Child*, Vol. XIII, 1958.

ROBINSON, ALICE M., "Communicating with Schizophrenic Patients," *Am. J. Nursing*, 60:1120–23, 1960.

ROSEN, JOHN N., *Direct Analysis*, Grune and Stratton, New York: 1953.

RUESCH, JURGEN, *Disturbed Communication*, W. W. Norton & Co., New York: 1957.

——— "General Theory of Communication," *American Handbook of Psychiatry*, Silvano Arieti (ed.), Basic Books, New York: 1959.

RUESCH, JURGEN, and KEES, WELDON, *Nonverbal Communication*, University of California Press, Berkeley: 1956.

SCHACHTEL, ERNEST G., *Metamorphosis*, Basic Books, New York: 1959.

SCHWARTZ, MORRIS S., and SHOCKLEY, EMMY LANNING, *The Nurse and the Mental Patient*, Russell Sage Foundation, New York: 1956.

SECHEHAYE, MARGUERITE, *Autobiography of a Schizophrenic Girl*, Grune and Stratton, New York: 1951.

SELTIZ, CLAIRE, et al., *Research Methods in Social Relations*, Holt, Rinehart and Winston, New York: 1961.

SODDY, KENNETH (ed.), *Mental Health and Infant Development*, Basic Books, New York: 1956.

SPIEGEL, ROSE, "Specific Problems of Communication," *American Handbook of Psychiatry*, Silvano Arieti (ed.), Basic Books, New York: 1959.

STEELE, KATHERINE MC LEAN, and MANFREDA, MARGUERITE LUCY, *Psychiatric Nursing*, F. A. Davis Co., Philadelphia: 1959.

SULLIVAN, HARRY STACK, *The Interpersonal Theory of Psychiatry*, W. W. Norton & Co., New York: 1953.

VARLEY, BARBARA K., "Reaching Out, Therapy with Schizophrenic Patients," *Am. J. Orthopsychiatry*, 29:407–16, 1959.

WOLBERG, LEWIS R., *The Technique of Psychotherapy*, Grune and Stratton, New York: 1954.

# 39 EFFECTS OF NURSING INTERVENTION IN ANXIETY OF PATIENTS

*Shirley F. Burd*

Anxiety is a key concept for all nurses working in psychiatric facilities. Nursing includes the observation of behavior of patients. Since nurses are aware of the familiar tenet that behavior is purposeful, meaningful, and can be understood, the nurse must explain, at least to herself, what is being observed. Thereupon, the nurse can utilize such explanations or understandings to assist the patient toward health. She can employ the conceptual framework of anxiety—the theory—to explain many of the clinical observations. Further, this conceptual framework gives rise to the formulation of nursing principles. These nursing principles serve as guidelines for the nursing action or intervention.

Since anxiety permeates the life of all persons, the nurse can employ it as one of her conceptual frames of reference in work with all patients. Much of the behavior of patients is coerced by anxiety. It is possible that nurses in psychiatric facilities may be more aware of the problem of anxiety than are nurses in other, nonpsychiatric facilities. Integration of interpersonal and psychiatric nursing theory in the nursing areas of medicine, surgery, obstetrics, and pediatrics is relatively recent in nursing education. Nevertheless, anxiety occurs and determines the behavior of nonpsychiatric patients as well as psychiatric patients.

At this point, the conceptual framework of anxiety might well be briefly reviewed. May [1] has defined anxiety as "apprehension cued off by a threat to some value which the individual holds essential to his existence as a personality." Consider the order of events inherent in his definition:

[1] May, R., *The Meaning of Anxiety*, p. 191.

First, the initial event is that the individual holds some "value." This value is of extreme importance, since it is essential to the individual's "existence as a personality," or security. According to Sullivan,[2] the self-system is an organization of views of the self and of patterns of behavior which operate to prevent and/or reduce anxiety. The "value" in May's definition is an aspect of the self-system as described by Sullivan. Other aspects of the self-system are desires, wishes, and images of the individual. A more general term for classifying these specific aspects of the self-system is "expectations." Prestige and status needs are other "values" as is the biological integrity, i.e., the maintenance of homeostasis through actions and bodily processes. All of the preceding maintain the security, the comfort, of the individual.

Second, the "value" held by the individual is not met but, instead, is threatened. Illness threatens the biological integrity of a person. Frequently, the expectations of self and/or the needs are also threatened or unmet.

The third step in order of May's definition is "the apprehension," used as a synonym for anxiety. Frequently, the terms "fear" and "anxiety" are used synonymously. However, May differentiates between these two concepts when he specifies that fear is object-oriented and anxiety encompasses the entire personality. If this apprehension, the anxiety, is not fear, what is it? At this point, the comprehensive definition and behavioral observations of anxiety by Hays[3] are of value to the conceptualization of anxiety. She has described the behavioral observations according to the four levels of anxiety—mild, moderate, severe, and panic. Included herein are the operations and the variations of the operations. For example, an operation of severe anxiety is that "only details are perceived." The oustanding variation of this operation is that "connections between details are not seen." This dissociation functions as a deterrent to panic and subsequent reorganization of the personality. The patient's perceptual field is reduced. A patient has described these phenomena as "It's like my vision is narrow. I'm not seeing what I should see." Generally, patients do not know that they are anxious, since dissociation and the perceptual field reduction occur. Behavioral observations of severe anxiety may include the repetition of a word or phrase, repeated fingering of an object, and prototaxic mode of experience. (Other variations and behavioral observations are possible within the severe level of anxiety.)

How can the conceptual framework of anxiety be applied in the clinical practice of a nurse? The question demands an answer that is a method or

[2] Sullivan, H. S., *Conceptions of Modern Psychiatry*, pp. 19–24, 46.
[3] Hays, D. R., "Teaching a Concept of Anxiety to Patients," p. 108, for the entire definition.

process, since the critical word is "how." Further, the method of applying the theory needs to be stated in such a manner as to allow for the individual differences of nurses.

The profession of nursing has several conceptual frames of reference for nursing action or intervention. Problem-solving and learning are two of these frameworks. The initial step of these processes is the same. This step suggests that the patient needs to observe and name his anxiety.

Observation and naming of anxiety are the first of several steps toward learning. The ultimate goal is to assist the patient in learning something about his response to, and about whatever initiates the development of, increased levels of anxiety. Subsequently, he will need assistance in ascertaining and using other methods of dealing with the anxiety. This learning or problem-solving approach enables the patient to respond to similar situations in a manner which tends to exclude the possible problems of panic and subsequent personality reorganization.

The nursing-intervention technique in this chapter is the first of a series of techniques. The purpose of the technique is to assist the patient in the achievement of the initial step in learning—recognition and naming of anxiety. It is a series of nursing principles which permit the individual differences in clinical practice by nurses. Some of these differences are included as illustrations of the various steps. Generally, the steps of the technique occur in order.

A small sample of nurse-patient data was collected from twenty-nine students in order to study further the nature and effects of the general approach described by Peplau.[4] These students were learning counseling techniques and the application of the following principles relevant to observation of effects of anxiety in a series of interviews.

## INTERPERSONAL TECHNIQUE OF NURSING: RECOGNITION AND NAMING OF ANXIETY

1. *In counseling, the nurse takes the direction in communication easiest for the patient to follow.*

The interview content is determined by the patient's selection of subject(s) based upon his or her needs at the time of the interview. The patient's needs are primary. Given the opportunity, patients will discuss their problems. The nurse makes a verbatim record of all communication between herself and the patient. This record includes verbal and nonverbal communication between patient and nurse as well as whatever environ-

[4] Peplau, H. E., "Interpersonal Techniques: The Crux of Psychiatric Nursing," pp. 50–54.

mental stimuli impinge on the interview situation. The nurse's comments and questions are in accord with the conceptual framework of learning. Early in the interview series, the nurse's comments and questions are selected to assist the patient in describing his observations of whatever his selected subject is as it relates to the patient. Open comments such as, "tell me," "describe," or "what" encourage description.

When the nurse is moving from the technical to the counseling role or is combining these roles, she also adheres to this principle. This combination of roles occurs in all settings wherein nursing is practiced. Patients have a wide range of problems. They frequently need some information about themeselves and their illness. If this need for information is unmet, the problem of anxiety soon becomes apparent. The nurse can initiate this anxiety if she violates this initial principle of the technique. One of the common ways this principle is violated is in the social chatting that goes on between nurse and patient. The patient is thereby burdened by the daily information dispensed about other patients or the nurse's family and activities. This social chatting prevents discussion of the patient's problems and the possible learning about and solution of the problems.

Obviously, the nurse cannot make a verbatim record of the communication when she is simultaneously using both the technical or mother-surrogate and counseling roles. She can make an occasional note of her observations and significant verbalizations in the same way she jots down the vital sign information ascertained in the course of her care of the patient.

2. *In counseling, the nurse repeatedly assesses the patient's level of anxiety to determine the subsequent nursing intervention.*

Assessment of anxiety requires that the nurse (a) analyze her observations of the patient according to known theory and (b) formulate the level of the patient's anxiety, if increased. The Hays specification of behavioral cues is one theoretical framework available for analysis of observations of the manifestations of anxiety. Some critical questions based on this theory must be answered. "What behavioral observations am I making?" "Does the concept of anxiety explain these observations?" "What level of anxiety is the patient experiencing?"

The theory of the various types of dissociation is another basis for analysis of thought content affected by anxiety. Do the patient's verbalized thoughts indicate any evidence of selective inattention or dissociation, i.e., denial, parataxic distortion, prototaxic or parataxic modes of experience, dreams, direct statements, etc.? What are these evidences of dissociation?

Where on the continuum of anxiety does (do) this (these) evidence(s) of selective inattention or dissociation occur according to this theory?

Sullivan's view [5] regarding the empathic linkage of anxiety is another basis for analyzing anxiety on the feeling level. "Am I feeling anxious? If so, is the anxiety originating with me?" If the answer is in the negative, the nurse usually assumes that the anxiety is originating with the patient, when her preceding analysis of the patient's behavior and verbalized thoughts indicates evidence of severe anxiety. This analysis related to empathic linkage of anxiety requires that the nurse know, or at least is beginning to learn, something regarding her own response to anxiety.

After the nurse has answered the preceding critical questions, she is able to determine whether the patient is experiencing the problem of anxiety. She is able to specify the level of anxiety and the behavioral, thought, and/or feeling cues that indicate this level. The cues and the level of anxiety can be substantiated with verbatim data and its relationship to known explanatory theory by peers, faculty, and consultants in seminar and/or conferences.

3. *Whenever the patient is anxious, the nurse assists the patient with the recognition and naming of the anxiety in order to initiate the patient's learning and/or problem-solving.*

Since the patient's perception of his own anxiety may be dissociated, the nurse questions the patient regarding his anxiety in order to bring this aspect of the situation into his perceptual range. The application of this principle may take the form of direct and precise communication— "Are you anxious?" Another nurse may be concerned with the circumvention of the possibility of autistic invention by the patient. Her question would be, "I notice that you (observation of the patient). Are you anxious?" Still another nurse may use, "Are you uncomfortable now?" Note that this question does not use a form of the word "anxiety." This nurse is requesting validation of the patient's anxiety as are the other nurses. She is asking about the present situation. Further, this question utilizes a lay term for anxiety. The nurse is expected to be able to specify the reason for her selection of words in the use of this and the other nursing principles.

Since the preceding nursing intervention requires an affirmative or negative response by the patient, what does the nurse do with this response? Acceptance of whatever the patient's response might be is a vague answer

[5] Sullivan, H. S., *Conceptions of Modern Psychiatry*, pp. 17, 20, 89; *The Interpersonal Theory of Psychiatry*, pp. 41–43.

to the question. What does this acceptance mean? Does the affirmative or negative response affect acceptance as demonstrated by the subsequent nursing intervention? Two contributory nursing principles are required to answer these questions.

(a) *When the patient does not affirm the presence of anxiety, the nurse follows the direction principle* [6] *and refocuses the patient to a previous discussion subject.*

The following example will illustrate one nurse's application of this principle:

> (Previous content: Patient has been rapidly speaking of several persons. The connection between these persons appears to be the word, "upset," as used by patient regarding each person. Patient repeatedly sits in chair for five minutes and walks about room for one to three minutes continuing this rapid speech. Three cigarettes were lit—one from the other and were all in the ashtray at one time.)
> *Nurse:* Mr. M., are you upset now?
> *Patient:* Upset? I never get upset. I'm as strong as the Rock of Gibraltar. (Patient arises and begins walking about room in silence.)
> *Nurse:* You were describing Ann when she became upset.
> *Patient:* Oh, yes, Ann—Well . . . (content regarding Ann being upset).

In the preceding example, the nurse used the patient's term when she asked whether the patient was presently anxious. The patient denied the anxiety. The nurse waited for the patient to continue his pattern of walking and talking to reduce his anxiety. He walked but discontinued the speech. The nurse's next comment encouraged the patient's use of the security operation of talking as it reminded him of the previous subject as related to the theme. Thereupon, the patient refocused and used both his security operations.

(b) *When the patient does affirm the presence of anxiety, the nurse steers the discussion to a description of the patient's observations of his present experience of anxiety as the initial step in learning.*

> (Previous content: Mr. O was speaking of a member of the hospital personnel in a rapid and derogatory manner. He repeatedly readjusted the position of his chair. His face was flushed and he rolled and unrolled his shirtsleeves often.)
> *Nurse:* Mr. O., are you anxious now?
> *Mr. O.:* Of course, I'm anxious. Anybody would be anxious living in this place. (Shirtsleeves were rolled up again. Silence.)
> *Nurse:* Tell me about being anxious.
> *Mr. O.:* I get so annoyed when I have to ask and wait for someone. It happens all day long. I have to ask to have the bathroom door opened or wait until someone resolves it be open. I can't decide if I want to go to OT, Recreation, Canteen. I must go. Someone else decided. Of course,

[6] Previously described as principle 1 of nurse's interpersonal technique of nursing.

I get anxious, glower at people, and get a red face, and I'll have a coronary yet. I haven't made a decision for myself since coming here—for help, I'm told. Anybody would get anxious in this place. (Sigh.) Now some of the other men sit around and wait for the white uniform to tell them it's time to . . . . (Description of other patients followed. During this section of interview, speech rate decreased, facial flushing subsided, shirtsleeves were buttoned, and posture in chair became more relaxed.)

In the preceding example, the nurse's initial comment requested validation of her interpretation of the patient's verbal and nonverbal communication. Mr. O. affirmed this interpretation. Since the experience of anxiety is not exactly the same from person to person, the nurse's open comment served to encourage description of Mr. O.'s observations of self and allow him to select any aspect (actions, including dynamics, thoughts, and feelings) of this experience for discussion. Further, this comment indicated that the nurse was willing to listen even when the response of Mr. O. to his anxiety indicated aggression. Other possible nurse comments requesting description include, "What is the anxiety like to you?" "Describe this anxiety," and "What do you notice when you're anxious?

In order to study the application and effects of a general approach to anxiety, based on the foregoing interpersonal technique of nursing, a form for data collection was set up. This form requested information of each interview with each patient. The areas of information requested included (1) the nurse's assessment of anxiety, (2) the observations indicating anxiety, (3) whether or not the nurse asked, "Are you anxious?" or a similar question, and (4) the patient's reply when the nurse asked the foregoing question. These forms were distributed for completion to nineteen undergraduate students and ten graduate students.

The nineteen undergraduate students were enrolled in their first collegiate nursing course—psychiatric nursing—during the fall semester. Their knowledge of the theory of anxiety and the nursing intervention was, for the most part, nil. This freshman course included a nurse-patient relationship for each student. Three hours of seminar for the study of these relationships followed each clinical hour with the patients. The data submitted by these students came from these initial nurse-patient relationships.

The ten graduate students were enrolled in the clinical specialty program of psychiatric nursing. Four of these ten students were enrolled in the initial course of this master's level program. Three of these four students submitted data from their first nurse-patient relationship. These data represented the students' initial experience with the theory and interpersonal nursing technique as previously described. This initial experience was not viewed as a limitation, since these nurses were assumed to be entering a career of nursing specialty, committed to the task of learning. The fourth graduate student in the initial year of the program was cognizant of and had used the theory and some aspects of the nursing technique during the nurse-patient relationships of her various undergraduate programs and the subsequent work experience prior to master's level study. The other six graduate students were enrolled in the initial semester of the second year of the master's program. The prior year of education had included recurring experiences with the theory and its application in clinical practice.

Data from four undergraduate students were discarded, since the students had not followed directions. Their data forms were incomplete. Evaluation of the student's assessment of anxiety and observations was not possible.

Obviously, a limitation to the study can be noted since the sample of nurses were students rather than specialists in psychiatric nursing. This limitation was that nursing students represented three levels of competency with the theory and the technique. However, it was anticipated that differences in levels of education would reveal a wider scope of the effects of application of the interpersonal technique. It was hypothesized that the proportion of students using the technique fully in a series of interviews would increase as the education and experience in using the technique increased.

Answers to several critical questions were being sought by this study. The questions and results of an analysis of data forms submitted by the twenty-five students are herein presented. Each of the questions was answered through content analysis of the twenty-five data forms.

The initial major question was, Were the students able to observe and assess the anxiety of the patients?

1.1. All twenty-five undergraduate and graduate students are able to make observations that indicated anxiety in their patients. The undergraduates made these observations by the eighth hour of the nurse-patient relationship. All graduate students observed anxiety in their patients during the initial hour of the relationship.

The undergraduate and three of the graduate students made observations in the same sequence as the faculty, generally, introduced explanatory theory in the teaching seminars. Initially, the observations were behavioral and followed the Hays' classification. Second, observations of thought and perceptual problems were added to the behavioral cues. Last, the observations included empathic observation of anxiety. This sequence of observations was not discernible when data forms from seven graduate students were reviewed. These students had prior experience with the theoretical framework and the interpersonal technique. Their data forms evidenced the integration and use of learning products when appropriate to the clinical setting.

1.2. Twenty-two of the twenty-five students (88 per cent) were able to assess anxiety correctly by the completion of the semester's course. Five of the fifteen undergraduate students (33.33 per cent) were able to assess anxiety correctly in all interviews following initial observation of the problem. Seven of these students (46.67 per cent) had occasional errors in the assessment of anxiety. The remaining three undergraduates (20 per cent) made errors in assessment of all interviews. These students made no observations of their patients indicating dissociation, reduced perceptual field, or empathic linkage of anxiety, as did their twelve peers. Nine of the ten graduate students (90 per cent) were able to assess anxiety correctly in all interviews regardless of the number of observations for any one interview. The tenth graduate student made occasional errors in the initial seven interviews.

When errors were made, they represented the student's underassessment of anxiety level. Moderate and severe anxiety were assessed as mild and moderate levels, respectively.

1.3. When did the students make their initial observations of patients' anxiety?

Seventeen of the twenty-two students (82 per cent) observed anxiety in the initial interview. Seven of the twelve undergraduates (58.33 per cent) made such observations in this first interview. The other five undergraduates (41.67 per cent) made their initial observations of anxiety between the second and sixth interviews. Generally, the assessments were moderate and severe levels of anxiety; none of the patients experienced the panic level of anxiety during the interviews.

A difference between the content submitted on data forms of undergraduates and graduate students was discernible. Repeatedly, ten of the twelve undergraduates and one graduate student recorded observations and assessed anxiety as though their respective patients were in mild or severe levels of anxiety *throughout* the hour of the nurse-patient interview. No change of anxiety level was indicated for any one hour. However, nine of the graduate students and two undergraduates made multiple entries of observations which indicated change in anxiety level *within* an interview. These multiple entries for each interview indicate that the anxiety level was reduced as the interview progressed. A severe level of anxiety became moderate or a moderate level became mild. The patients were more comfortable at the end of an interview than at the beginning. All eleven of these students making multiple entries for interviews were included in the sample employing the interpersonal technique consistently.

Some examples of mild, moderate, and severe levels of anxiety as generalized by students follow. Mild anxiety was reported as "[Patient is] describing with more specificity than previously." The earlier interviews had been assessed as being characterized by moderate and severe levels. Moderate anxiety was described as "Patient is aware of and able to make verbal connections [between thoughts] and slight swinging of foot; diaphoresis; selective attention and content focused on two topics in the hour; occasional restlessness in chair; speech rate moderate; no empathic communication of anxiety observed." A student described severe anxiety as "Patient's verbal content consisted of scattered details. Behaviorally, he (1) changed position frequently, (2) cracked knuckles, (3) broke fingernails, (4) puffed cigarettes constantly, (5) rolled empty cigarette package into a ball and played with it, (6) took out a strip of gum and chewed rapidly. The patient also got up and took a walk—returned in five minutes."

The second major question for analysis was, Was the interpersonal technique employed consistently by the students?

Consistent use of the nursing intervention was defined as the application of all three principles whenever the nurse assessed at least a severe level of anxiety. The use of the principle could occur when the assessment was of moderate anxiety.

2.1. All students able to assess anxiety correctly applied all of the interpersonal technique, including, "Are you anxious?" or a similar question. Sixteen of these twenty-five students (72 per cent) comprised the "consistency" sample. The remaining six students did not consistently use the technique when appropriate to the assessment.

Seven of the twelve undergraduates and nine of the ten graduates constituted the "consistency" sample. Twelve of these sixteen students (75 per cent) initiated use of the nursing question by the conclusion of the third interview following initial accurate observation and assessment of anxiety in their respective patients. These twelve students included five undergraduate and seven graduate students. Two of the undergraduates asked the nursing question during the initial interview in an unwitting fashion, since they had no knowledge of the theory at that time in the course. The other four students (25 per cent) asked this question during the fifth interview following initial accurate assessment.

2.2. The hypothesis that the proportion of students using the technique fully in a series of interviews would increase as the education and experience in using the technique increased was confirmed. The undergraduate and graduate student ratios using the technique fully were 7:15 and 9:10, respectively.

The third major question was, What are the effects of consistent nursing intervention—the use of the interpersonal technique?

The patient responses to the sixteen students who consistently asked the nursing question, "Are you anxious?" following accurate observation and assessment of anxiety, were subjected to a content analysis. These responses were classified in three sequential categories or phases. These phases were denial, ambivalence, and awareness of anxiety by the patient.

3.1. The *denial* phase of patient's response to the nursing intervention took several forms. Some examples of verbal denial indicated by students were "No," "No, I'm all right, thank you," "No, I don't know," "No, this chair is wiggling but it's all right," "I feel pretty good," "No, I'm not uncomfortable, I have slippers on," "No, I feel great," and "No, I'm fine, thank you." Denial was also expressed as verbal avoidance of the question. A complete change of topic focus by the patient illustrates this verbal avoidance. "They make you wear underwear in here. They think you need long underwear, wear a heavy pair of pants." Occasionally, a patient would combine nonverbal and verbal avoidance of the question. In such a situation the patient would walk away from the nurse, return within the subsequent five minutes and resume the interview on another topic.

Two undergraduates and a graduate student submitted data indicating that their patient's responses did not move from the denial phase to any subsequent phase. The similarity in the content on these three data forms is that these patients had little skill in describing their observations and the students asked the nursing question only once per interviewer.

3.2. The *ambivalent* category and phase of patient responses begins with the initial affirmative reply to the nursing question, "Are you anxious?" This category of response contains a combination of denial and affirmative responses. A typical series of patient responses to the nursing questions follows:

1. Yes. They put something in my shot shouldn't have been there.
2. I'm uneasy, I dunno.
3. No. Like I said in 1947 . . .
4. I suffer all kinds of rheumatic pains.
5. You just don't get enough sleep around here. . . .
6. Yes, I really am. . . .

7. Sometimes. . . .
8. Not as comfortable as I once was.
9. These floors are nuts. Dull oatmeal white with gold in them. And those windows.

Eight of the thirteen patients affirming anxiety (62 per cent) gave their initial affirmative response in the first interview *after* initiation of the nursing intervention. Two patients (15 per cent) affirmed anxiety in the fourth interview. Another two patients did so during the fifth interview. The final patient (8 per cent) affirmed anxiety in the sixth interview.

Five of the seven undergraduates submitted data forms indicating that their patient responses terminated within this ambivalent phase. Again, these students tended to ask the nursing question only once per interview. One student asked it twice in an interview. Another student used the question twice in each of three interviews.

Three graduate students also submitted data indicating that the patient's awareness of anxiety had terminated in the ambivalent phase. One of the students submitted a wealth of verbatim data which permitted analysis for other problems that would continue the combination of denial and acceptance responses found in the ambivalent phase. The nurse had a communication problem which appeared to prevent the patient from moving on to the awareness phase. The student used the lay term "uncomfortable" when she didn't use a form of the word "anxiety." The patient used "nervous" to indicate the state of being anxious. Throughout the data, the nurse used, "Are you anxious?" "Are you uncomfortable?" or "Are you nervous?" No pattern was discernible regarding the number of times either lay term was used. Neither term was used consistently. Whenever the nurse employed the patient's term for anxiety in her question, the patient's response was in the affirmative. Whenever the nurse employed her own lay term, the patient's response was denial. At no time was there clarification of the similar usage of the two terms or their relationship to anxiety. The nurse's inconsistency in selection of words determined and continued the ambivalence of the patient's responses.

3.3. The third category or phase of patient response is that of *awareness* of the anxiety. The patient's responses indicate that he knows that he is uneasy, uncomfortable, anxious, or whatever the term being used at the time of the anxiety. The patient affirms the presence of anxiety whenever asked, or else he initiates the discussion of anxiety.

Initially, the patient affirms the presence of anxiety when queried. Typical affirmative comments include: "Well, certain things are upsetting me lately" (followed by description of "things"); "I am, I just didn't want to talk anymore. I didn't know what to talk about, and now I'm worried about being transferred" (followed by description of being "worried"); and, "Yes, I feel like something's wrong with my body. I have low blood pressure, anemia, and a type of nervous disorder. Now my respirations appear to change from time to time. . . ."

The affirmation of anxiety is followed by the unsolicited comments by the patient that he was or is anxious. No longer is the problem of anxiety dissociated or selectivity inattentive. The patient notices what the nurse has noticed. He introduces the subject *before* the nurse asks the usual question. The patient is modeling some of his observations of self after the behavior of the nurse. The patient is completing the recognition of the problem. Some typical comments include, "I'm a little nervous today"; "I'd like to mention I feel a little uneasy"; and "I was so upset yesterday" (followed by description of the subject). These comments initiate the patient's description of the problem of anxiety and the clarification of the various terms used synonymously with the term "anxiety."

Five of the nine graduate students submitted data indicating that their patients' responses terminated within the awareness category and phase of anxiety. The initiation of this phase occurred, on an average, during the tenth interview. The range of the initiation of this phase was between the third and seventeenth hours of interview following initial use of the technique in its entirety.

What has been ascertained by this small study of students' use of an interpersonal technique during the psychiatric nursing courses on the 100, 500, and 600 levels of collegiate education? Three major findings have been abstracted.

First, freshmen nursing students enrolled in this initial nursing course, psychiatric nursing, can develop beginning competency in using part or all of an interpersonal technique. Differences indicating the trend toward sophistication of clinical competency in the knowledge of the theory and its clinical application—the technique—are evident in the perusal of undergraduate and graduate students' data.

Second, the earlier students gain theoretical knowledge and clinical competency in each of the principles of the technique, the earlier the patient gains awareness of his own anxiety and can begin some learning and problem-solving. The patients literally do not know that they are anxious. They need help in gaining this awareness of anxiety.

Third, when patients do receive consistent assistance from the nurse as she uses the interpersonal technique, their responses generally move through the sequential phases of denial, ambivalence, and awareness of anxiety. Within the awareness phase, the patients affirm the anxiety when queried and then initiate the discussion of the problem, the second step in learning.

The implication of this study pertains to all areas of nursing education. Since anxiety occurs in all persons, it presents a nursing problem in all specialty areas of nursing. The undergraduate students have developed beginning competency with part or all of the interpersonal technique during the initial nursing course in their professional education. This competency of the undergraduate nursing students could undergo further refinement during the brief and long-term contacts that students have with nonpsychiatric patients. The student would need faculty members who were competent in using the interpersonal technique and/or willing to obtain readily available consultation of faculty within the school who were adept in the technique.

The general approach, the technique for responding to anxiety described by Peplau,[7] needs to be refined in terms of the patient's response phases of denial, ambivalence, and acceptance of anxiety. This study has indicated the presence of these phases.

This chapter has printed a small study of nursing intervention in anxiety of patients. Data from the nurse-patient relationships of students enrolled in 100, 500, and 600 level courses in psychiatric nursing were studied to ascertain the effects of the interpersonal techniques of nursing intervention.

# BIBLIOGRAPHY

HAYS, DOROTHEA R., "Teaching a Concept of Anxiety to Patients," *Nursing Research*, 10(2):108–13, 1957.
MAY, ROLLO, *The Meaning of Anxiety*, The Ronald Press, New York: 1950.
PEPLAU, HILDEGARD E., "Interpersonal Techniques: Crux of Psychiatric Nursing," *Am. J. Nursing*, 62(6):50–54, 1962.
SULLIVAN, HARRY STACK, *Conceptions of Modern Psychiatry*, W. W. Norton & Co., New York: 1953.
——— *The Interpersonal Theory of Psychiatry*, W. W. Norton & Co., New York: 1953.

---

[7] *Op. cit.*, p. 54.

# SECTION

# IV

## CONCEPTUAL FRAMEWORKS

# 40 A WORKING DEFINITION OF ANXIETY

*Hildegard E. Peplau*

The term "anxiety" is a key concept in psychiatric work. It can be defined by specifying the operations associated with it as these have been observed, inferred, and formulated from the experiences of experts. These operations help nurses to use this concept to explain observations of human behavior and from such understanding to determine the actions the nurse can take to help in the use or reduction of anxiety—in the nurse or in the person.

## A. WHAT IS ANXIETY?

The essential characteristic of anxiety has been variously stated.

1. Anxiety is an energy. As such, it cannot be observed directly; therefore, its presence must be inferred from its effect on behavior, since only the energy transformations can be observed.

2. Anxiety is a secondary behavior which follows the startle generically in infants and often experientially in adults.

3. "Anxiety is the subjective experience of the organism in the catastrophic condition." [1]

4. "Anxiety is an emotion without a specific object." [2]

5. "Thus, anxiety is the basic underlying reaction—the generic term; and fear is the expression of the same capacity in its specific, objectivated form." [3]

[1] May, R., *The Meaning of Anxiety*, p. 49, quoting Kurt Goldstein.
[2] *Ibid.*, p. 54.
[3] *Ibid.*, p. 205.

6. Anxiety is an inability to know an emergent threat which will be felt as prevention of ability of the organism to "actualize its own nature" to achieve "self-realization." [4]

7. "Anxiety is the apprehension cued off by a threat to some value which the individual holds essential to his existence as a personality." [5]

8. ". . . anxiety is a signal of danger to self-respect, to one's standing in the eyes of the significant persons present even if they are only ideal figures from childhood. . . ." [6]

## B. HOW IS ANXIETY EXPERIENCED?

1. Anxiety is usually experienced as one of its effects, as listed under Section D in this chapter.

2. People can learn to notice and name as anxiety its early manifestations such as: "vague discomfort," "an exceedingly painful experience," "as disintegration of self . . . a dissolution of the existence of his personality," "diffuse apprehension," uncertainty, a "profoundly irrational experience," "feelings of helplessness or impotence." [7]

3. When fear becomes anxiety, there is "a change from the perception of the threat as coming from a specific object [definable source] to an apprehension which engulfs the whole personality so that the person feels his very existence is endangered." [8]

## C. WHAT CAUSES ANXIETY?

1. *Any threat to the security of an individual produces anxiety.* Such threats fall mainly into two categories:
(a) Threats to biological integrity, i.e., threats to the tendency of the human organism toward maintenance of homeostasis through such processes as temperature control, vasomotor stability, etc., and through actions taken to meet bodily needs.
(b) Threats to the self-system,[9] i.e., threats to the tendency of an individual toward maintaining established views of self and the values and patterns of behavior he uses to resist changes in self-views.

[4] *Ibid.,* pp. 50, 232.
[5] *Ibid.,* p. 191.
[6] Sullivan, H. S., *The Psychiatric Interview,* p. 219.
[7] May, R., *op. cit.,* pp. 18, 43, 53.
[8] *Ibid.,* p. 55.
[9] According to Sullivan, the self arises in interpersonal situations and is organized as a system of views of self and patterns of behavior in order to prevent, reduce, or relieve anxiety; the self-system is seen, therefore, as the antianxiety system.

These threats include: [10]

(1) Expectations (wishes, desires, wants, images, etc.) that are held by an individual and then are not met, nor are in accord with what actually happens in a situation in which those expectations are operative.

(2) Needs for prestige, status, and deference that are operative and then are not met in the situation.

2. *Anxiety is always communicated interpersonally.* One anxious person communicates it to another person or persons in a situation; the latter empathically observe [11] the anxiety.

## D. WHAT EFFECTS OF ANXIETY UPON BEHAVIOR CAN BE OBSERVED?

1. *Effects upon biochemical functioning.*[12] Epinephrine is released into the organism.

2. *Effects upon physiological functioning.* These effects are dependent upon the degree of anxiety; in general, mild and moderate anxiety heighten use of capacities; whereas, severe and panic degrees paralyze or overwork capacities and structures.

Increased heart rate
Increased rate and depth of respiration
Rapid, extreme shifts in
    body temperature
    blood pressure
    menstrual flow[13]
    urinary urgency
    dryness of mouth
    loss of appetite
    "cold sweat"

[10] The threats indicated in this section have been variously stated:
    any threats to existence (Goldstein)
    any inability to cope with the demands of the environment
    any inability to actualize capacities (Goldstein)
    any threat to values identical with the subject's existence (Horney)
    any threat of nonbeing (Tillich)
    any threat of nonbelonging (Koffka)
    when confronted with the possibility of freedom (Kierkegaard)
    individuation and the possibility of becoming able as compared to impotent (Fromm, E.)
[11] Empathic observation—the ability to feel in oneself feelings the same as, or similar to those experienced by another person in the situation.
[12] For example, see Ruikel, M., and Solomon, H. C., "Chemical Theories of Psychosis."
[13] Gregory, B. A. J. C., "The Menstrual Cycle and Its Disorders in Psychiatric Patients."

dilation of pupils
release of sugar by liver

### 3. *Effects upon the ability of anxious person to observe.*[14]

*Degree*

| | |
|---|---|
| + Mild level | Person is alerted, sees, hears, grasps more than previously. |
| ++ Moderate level | Person's perceptual field is narrowed, sees, hears, grasps less, but can attend to more if directed to do so (selective inattention). |
| +++ Severe level | Person's perceptual field is greatly reduced—the focus is on a detail or on many scattered details (prototaxic mode). |
| ++++ Panic level | Panic, awe, dread, terror, uncanniness—the detail previously focused upon is "blown up" (i.e., becomes an exclusive focus plus elaboration) or the speed of the scatter is greatly increased. |

### 4. *Effects upon ability to focus attention on the contents of awareness.*

| | |
|---|---|
| + Mild level | Awareness and alert attention are possible; skill in seeing relations (connections) can be used. |
| ++ to +++ Moderate level to severe level | Selective inattention, i.e., fails to notice what goes on in situations peripheral to the immediate focus but can notice if attention is pointed there by another observer. |
| +++ to ++++ Severe level to panic level | Dissociating tendencies operate to prevent panic, i.e., the person does not notice what goes on in a situation (specifically communication with reference to self). There is inability to do so even when attention is pointed in this direction by another observer. |

### 5. *Effects upon learning and adaptation.*[15]

| | |
|---|---|
| + to ++ | If the person has well-developed skill, he is able to use all of the steps in the process of learning, i.e., is able to<br>observe<br>describe<br>analyze<br>formulate meanings and relations<br>validate with another person<br>test<br>integrate<br>use the learning product |
| +++ to ++++ | With or without skill the behavior of the person |

[14] May, Rollo, *op. cit.*, p. 51, quoting Kurt Goldstein ". . . it seems as if, in proportion to the increase of anxiety, the objects and contents [of awareness] disappear more and more."

[15] As defined by Peplau, H. E., "Experiential Teaching," pp. 884–86.

will be oriented toward getting immediate relief; adaptive patterns (i.e., automatic behavior which does not require thought) are used to relieve, reduce, or prevent greater anxiety.

6. *Effects upon major patterns of behavior.* As a result of anxiety, and of the need to adapt behavior in order to avoid, reduce, or relieve anxiety, *four major patterns* [16] are used to transform the energy of anxiety. These conversion patterns are

(a) *"Acting-out" behavior*
   (1) overt, e.g., using anger, then locating details to justify the anger and to prevent recognition of the anxiety and its causes.
   (2) covert, e.g., using resentment.
(b) *Somatizing*, i.e., various "psychosomatic" disorders.
(c) *"Freezing-to-the-spot"* behavior, e.g., withdrawal, depression.
(d) *Using the anxiety in the service of learning.* This requires enduring the anxiety while searching out causes and struggling with the problem; considerable help is often needed to experience success and to develop this pattern to replace the other patterns of behavior.

## BIBLIOGRAPHY

GREGORY, B. A. J. C., "The Menstrual Cycle and Its Disorders in Psychiatric Patients," *J. Psychosomatic Res.*, 2:61–79, 1957.

MAY, ROLLO, *The Meaning of Anxiety*, The Ronald Press, New York: 1950.

PEPLAU, HILDEGARD E., "Experiential Teaching," *Am. J. Nursing*, Vol. 57, No. 7, July, 1957.

——— *Interpersonal Relations in Nursing*, G. P. Putnam's Sons, New York: 1952.

RINKEL, MAX, and SOLOMON, HARRY C., "Chemical Theories of Psychosis," *J. Clin. Exper. Psychol.*, 18:323–24, 1957.

SULLIVAN, HARRY S., *The Psychiatric Interview*, W. W. Norton & Co., New York: 1954.

[16] These have also been stated as (a) fight, (b) helplessness, (c) flight, and (d) conflict.

# 41 PROCESS OF CHANGE

*Shirley F. Burd*

Change is a process consisting of the phases of need, formulation, and acceptance, utilizing a concept of anxiety and a process and concept of learning.[1]

1. NEED PHASE
    1.1 Need for change
    1.2 Recognition of this need
    1.3 Increase in anxiety level    1.41 Aggression
    1.4 Conversion of the energy                *or*
        of anxiety ─────────→ 1.4.2 Withdrawal
                                            *or*
                                    1.4.3 Somatization
                                            *or*

    The process ends here if any of these conversion patterns is utilized

2. FORMULATION PHASE
    2.1 Use of the learning process
        2.1.1 Observation (of 1.2)
        2.1.2 Description (of 1.2)
        2.1.3 Analysis
        2.1.4 Formulation of a learning product
        2.1.5 Validation of the learning product (solves 1.2 and 2.1.1)
3. ACCEPTANCE PHASE
    3.1 Leadership (role and function) assumed
        3.1.1 Communication with other persons
                re preceding phases (including collaboration)

[1] The underlying assumption is that the change is constructive, in type, rather than destructive.

328—

3.1.2 Increase of anxiety level (of these persons)

3.1.3.1 Aggression ⎤ The process
3.1.3 Conversion of the　　　　　or　　　　　ends here if
　energy of anxiety　3.1.3.2 Withdrawal ⎬ any of these
　(of these persons)　　　　or　　　　　conversion
　　　　　3.1.3.3 Somatization ⎦ patterns is
　　　　　　　or　　　　　　utilized

Use of learning process

3.2 Further validation of the learning product (solves the need for change for the increased number of persons—3.1.1)

3.3 Use of the learning product

3.4 Analysis of use of the learning product

3.5 Revision of the learning product
　acceptance of the needed elements
　rejection of the incompatible elements (may cause an increase in anxiety and use of conversion patterns)

3.6 Use of the revised learning product (solve the need for change—1.1)

3.7 New needs arise

# BIBLIOGRAPHY

CRUZE, WENDALL W., *Psychology in Nursing*, McGraw-Hill Book Co., New York: 1955, p. 354.

———— *Psychology for College Students*, Prentice-Hall, New York: 1951, p. 515.

FRIEDMAN, RONALD, et al., *Principles of Sociology: A Text with Readings*, Henry Holt and Co., New York: 1956, pp. 320–35, 452, 522, 523.

GREEN, ARNOLD, *Sociology*, McGraw-Hill Book Co., New York: 1952, pp. 504–5.

HAMILTON, GORDON, *Theory and Practice of Social Case Work*, 2nd ed., Columbia University Press, New York: 1951, p. 26.

HAYS, DOROTHEA RICHTER, "Criteria for Favorable Change," mimeographed paper, College of Nursing, Rutgers, The State University of New Jersey, 1957.

OGBURN, W. F., *Encyclopedia of the Social Sciences*, The Macmillan Co., New York: 1931, Vol. 3, p. 331.

# 42

# THE DEVELOPMENT OF AN OPERATIONAL DEFINITION USING THE PROCESS OF LEARNING AS A GUIDE

*Shirley F. Burd*

A concept is a term defined operationally so as to explain observations of behavior, in part, and to provide a structure for collecting more data so as to secure a complete and valid explanation. An operational definition provides statements of all observed behaviors (or inferences that classify all possible variations of each behavior) that are associated with the term, in the order in which such behaviors emerge in the observed.

| Steps in the Process of Learning [1] | Steps in the Process of the Development of an Operational Definition | Competencies Demonstrated |
|---|---|---|
| 1. Observation | *Phase I: Collection of data*<br>1.1 Select a concept from data of nurse-patient interviews, nurse-patient seminars, and/or conferences. | Ability to notice a possible term to be defined. |
| | 1.2 Review the literature, using an index approach, for established definitions of the selected concept.<br>  1.2.1 The type of literature reviewed will cover at least three different disciplines (including your own) and a dictionary reference.<br>  1.2.2 Note additional definitions in the literature as you read for other purposes. | Ability to use an index approach to review literature. |
| 2. Description | *Phase II: Description of data*<br>2.1 Record the one- or two-sentence definitions [2] on 5- by 8-inch white paper making a carbon for personal files. | Ability to follow directions. |

[1] See p. 333.

[2] Use one- or two-sentence definitions for the initial eight or ten definitions. Thereafter, one might use longer descriptive comments of authors re the concept. Defer the use of long descriptive comments until the ninth or eleventh definition.

330—

| Steps in the Process of Learning | Steps in the Process of the Development of an Operational Definition | Competencies Demonstrated |
|---|---|---|
| | 2.1.1 Do the preceding in *legible* handwriting. Use the following form: Concept's name, date collected, your name, biographical reference, publishing company, etc., page and quotation.<br>2.1.2 Record eight to twelve definitions from the literature in the foregoing manner. | Ability to select succinct, pertinent, defining statements which suggest operations of the concept. |
| 3. Analysis | *Phase III: Analysis of data*<br>3.1 Analyze the collected data:<br>  3.1.1 Review all definitions collected re one concept.<br>  3.1.2 List all the suggested behaviors connected with each concept.<br>  3.1.3 Sort data from Step 2 to show order of emerging operations [3] (inferred and observed).<br>  3.1.4 Retrospectively consider your own clinical experience in order to fill in gaps in definition of the concept.<br>3.2 Decide whether to discard some or all definitions and return to Step 1. | Ability to abstract the operations.<br>Ability to reorder the operations.<br>Ability to compare and sort the operations.<br>Ability to discriminate differences and similarities.<br>Ability to evaluate the preceding intellectual operations.<br>Ability to make a decision. |
| 4. Formulation | *Phase IV: Formulation of operational definition*<br>4.1 Review results of Step 3.1 and write your formulation of the emerging operations of the concept:<br>  4.1.1 in sequence<br>  4.1.2 in general terms<br><br>4.2 Write a one-sentence definition of the concept using the operations on colored 5- by 8-inch paper. Use the following form: Concept, date submitted, your name. Sentence definition. The sequence of emerging behaviors (performances).<br>4.3 Staple the 5- by 8-inch colored paper on top of the white papers (refer to 2.1 through 2.3). Submit both the original and carbon copies. The carbon copy will be returned. | Ability to give form and structure to preceding intellectual operations.<br>Ability to restate the operations in clear and direct communication.<br>Ability to generalize by summarizing.<br><br>Ability to follow directions.<br><br>Ability to follow directions. |
| 5. Validation | *Phase V: Validation of formulation*<br>5.1 Check the formulation (refer to 4.2) with someone else.[4] | Ability to check with someone else. |

[3] The terms "operation(s)," "behavior(s)," and "step(s)" are used synonymously within this process.

[4] Instructor in conference. Place on your conference agenda after the carbon copy with instructor's comments has been read by student.

| Steps in the Process of Learning | Steps in the Process of the Development of an Operational Definition | Competencies Demonstrated |
|---|---|---|
| | 5.2 Review areas of agreement and disagreement with that person. | Ability to reach agreement on difference re formulation. |
| | 5.3 Reformulate as necessary, according to the previous steps (5.1 and 5.2) and perhaps the steps of observation through validation.[5] | Ability to precisely state disagreeing issue(s). |
| 6. Test | Phase VI: Determination of formulation's application<br>6.1 Determine the method(s) of the concept's application in clinical practice of psychiatric nursing.<br>6.2 Validate 6.1 with at least one other person. | |
| 7. Use | Phase VII: Application of the formulation<br>7.1 Use the validated formulation and method of application as foresight in clinical practice, psychiatric nursing. | |

[5] Increased number of persons used for validation will increase the validity of the formulation.

# 43 PROCESS AND CONCEPT OF LEARNING

*Hildegard E. Peplau*

Learning is an active process which utilizes the thinking and perceiving abilities and knowledge previously acquired for three major purposes: (1) acquiring new knowledge to explain events, (2) facilitating change, and (3) solving problems.

| Steps in learning as a concept and as a process | Operations, performances, behaviors, separate skills, associated with each step in learning. (Major use of the perceptual processes—see, hear, smell, touch, etc.) | Examples of statements by the nurse to facilitate development of each step in a patient, in the total sequence of the process of learning |
|---|---|---|
| 1. To observe: The ability to notice what went on or what goes on now. | To see with one's eyes<br>To hear<br>To feel using empathic observation<br>To feel using tactile senses | What do you see?<br>What is that noise?<br>Are you uncomfortable?<br>Do you have something to say to me?<br>Could I share the thought with you or is it private?<br>Tell me about yourself.<br>What happened?<br>I don't follow.<br>Tell me, what did you notice?<br>You noticed what?<br>Did you see this happen?<br>Who was with you?<br>When did this occur?<br>What is the color?<br>Where were you?<br>Tell me.<br>Then what?<br>Go on.<br>Give me a blow-by-blow description.<br>Tell me every detail from the beginning. |

*Assumption:* The patient can describe the situation as he or she viewed it with encouragement and assistance from a person who can focus exclusively on the situation of the patient.

| Learning | Operations | Nurse Statements<br>Who, What, When, Which, Where |
|---|---|---|
| 2. To describe: The ability to recall and tell the details and circumstances of a particular event or experience. | Increased verbalization<br>Greater recall<br>Enumeration of details<br>Focus on details of one event | Tell me about the feeling.<br>What name would you give to your feeling?<br>Tell me more.<br>Then what?<br>Go on, —<br>Give me an example.<br>Who are they?<br>What about that?<br>For instance?<br>Describe that further.<br>Give me a blow-by-blow account of that.<br>What did you feel at the time?<br>What happened just before?<br>Which was it?<br>Who was the person?<br>What did you say?<br>What did your comment evoke in the other?<br><br>Use nurse statements of observation step, as well. |
| 3. To analyze: The ability to review and to work over the raw data with another person. | | Explain.<br>Help me to understand that!<br>What do you mean?<br>What do you see as the reason?<br>What was the significance of that event?<br>What are the common elements in these two situations?<br>What is the connection?<br>Boil this down to the one important aspect.<br>What caused this?<br>What was your part in it?<br>In what way did you participate?<br>In what way did you reach this decision?<br>What caused this feeling?<br>(I expected you at 8:30; you were late; that caused my anger.)<br>Have you had this feeling before?<br>Is there anything similar in this situation to your previous experience? |
| Step 3 may occur simultaneously with Step 4. | | |

Within the Operations column for Step 2:

Movement of patient's general and ambiguous terms for person(s) and nurse's question words assisting patient to be specific

| Patient's terms | Nurse's Question Words |
|---|---|
| 1. Everybody<br>They<br>Them<br>Technicians | Who? |
| 2. The nurses<br>The doctors | Which? |
| 3. The ones who work from 8–4 (narrowing) | What are their names? |
| 4. Miss Jones (specific name) | |

Within the Operations column for Step 3:

Examples of the kinds of analysis used by the nurse.

Identify needs
Decode key symbols
Distinguish literal and figurative
Sort and classify
  1. Impressions
  2. Speculations
  3. Thematic abstractions
  4. Hypotheses
  5. Generalizing
Compare
Summarize
Sequence
Application of concepts
Application of personality theory as a frame of reference
*Formulating relations* resulting from the foregoing:
  1. Cause and effect
  2. Temporal
  3. Thematic
  4. Spatial

| Learning | Operations | Nurse Statements Who, What, When, Which, Where |
|---|---|---|
| 4. To formulate: The ability to give form and structure, to restate in a clear, direct way, the connections resulting from Step 3 (analysis). | Restatement of data in light of Step 3<br>Verbal or written result of analysis of data | State the essence of this situation in a sentence or so.<br>What did you feel?<br>What did you think?<br>What did you do?<br>Tell it to me in a sentence or so.<br>Tell me again.<br>Was there a discrepancy between what you felt, thought, and did?<br>What would you say was the problem?<br>What name would you give to the patterns of your behavior as you interacted with another person? |
| 5. To validate (by consensus): The ability to check with another person and to reach agreement as to the result of Step 4 (formulation), or to state clearly the issue if there is divergence in the formulations of the two persons. | Checking with, comparing notes of two or more people | Is this what you mean?<br>Let me restate. Is this what you were saying?<br>Do you go along with this?<br>Is this what you believe?<br>It seems that—Is this the way it appears to you?<br>Is it that you feel angry when people tell you what to do?<br>Am I correct in concluding that—?<br>Are you saying—? |
| | *Pt.:* Are you anxious?<br>(Pt. trying to validate.)<br>*N.:* (Is anxious.) No, I'm not. Yes, I could say I am. What called my anxiety to your attention? | |
| 6. To test: The ability to try out the result of Step 4 (formulation) in situations with people, things, etc., for utility, completeness. | | (Set up situations where patient can try out new behavior patterns.)<br><br>Now that you have thought about this and come to this conclusion, why don't you try it out?<br><br>What would you do if a situation like this came up again?<br><br>In what way can you use this conclusion to prevent repeating this mistake?<br><br>In what way will this conclusion help you in the future?<br><br>What difference will it make now that you know this? |

| Learning | Operations | Nurse Statements Who, What, When, Which, Where |
|---|---|---|
| 7. To integrate: The ability to see the new in relation to or as an integral part of the old; to add to previously acquired usable knowledge for active use by the person. | Enmeshing the new with the old | |
| 8. To utilize: The ability to use the result of Step 4, (formulation) as foresight. | | (Set up situations where patient can use new behavior patterns.) |

# 44 THE PROCESS OF THEME ABSTRACTION

*Shirley F. Burd*

A theme is a recurring relation, view, or opinion held with respect to some aspect of living. It is the central idea inherent in many verbal and non-verbal details, rather than the details of verbalized material. The process of theme abstraction is as follows:

### PHASE 1: DURING THE ON-GOING INTERPERSONAL SITUATION

1.1 An interpersonal situation exists which includes:
    1.1.1 a minimum of two individuals;
    1.1.2 verbal communication;
    1.1.3 nonverbal communication;
    1.1.4 verbatim recording of interaction data, the unverbalized thoughts, feelings, and actions of the recorder (Individual A) and the non-verbal communication of Individual B.
1.2 Content of the interaction [1] suggests a theme.
*or*
1.3 Individual A does not recognize the theme of the interaction or its cues.
1.4 Individual A identifies (in thought) the cues in the interaction which suggest the theme and initiates the abreaction of operation 1.3.
1.5 Individual A names (in thought) the theme.
1.6 Individual A asks B for validation of the thoughts of operations 1.4 and 1.5.
1.7 Individual B
    1.7.1 consensually validates with Individual A;
*or*
    1.7.2 cooperates with individual A in mutually observing, describing, analyzing, formulating and validating another theme;
    1.7.3 avoids the above cooperative learning process due to conflict.

---

[1] Segments and/or total interaction content.

### Phase 2: After the Interpersonal Situation

2.1 Individual A reviews the verbatim data, etc.[2] of the interaction for cues and/or theme previously unidentified [3] *immediately* after leaving the interpersonal situation.

2.2 Individual A recognizes cues that suggest a theme of segments and/or total interaction content, through use of his thought process re former experiences with the cue(s) and/or theme.

2.3 Individual A seeks validation of cue(s) and theme with his colleagues and expert counselor in interpersonal relations.

2.4 Individual A seeks validation of the formulations (validated) of operation #3, with Individual B at the succeeding interpersonal situation.

2.5 Individual B

   2.5.1 consensually validates with Individual A;

   *or*

   2.5.2 cooperates with Individual A in mutually observing, describing, analyzing, formulating, and validating another theme;

   *or*

   2.5.3 avoids the above cooperative learning process due to conflict.

## BIBLIOGRAPHY

BERELSON, BERNARD, *Content Analysis in Communication Research*, The Free Press, Glencoe, Ill.: 1952.

BREGG, ELIZABETH A., LEDDY, MARY C., and MACKENZIE, LILLIAN G., "A Study on the Nurse's Concept of Death," master's thesis, Columbia University, New York: 1953.

CHILD, IRVIN L., POTTER, E. H., and LEVINE, E. M., "Children's Textbooks and Personality Development: An Exploration in the Social Psychology of Education," *Psychological Monographs*, 60(3):3, 1946.

COX, JOYCE E., DAVIS, M. E., FERNANDEZ, T. M., JOHANNESON, L., and TOSIELLO, F. C., *Trends and Directions*, master's thesis, Columbia University, New York: 1953.

FARLEY, SHIRLEY, "Family Views on Mental Illness," master's thesis, Graduate School, Rutgers, The State University of New Jersey, 1957.

KELLY, GEORGE A., *The Psychology of Personal Constructs*, W. W. Norton & Co., New York: 1955.

PEPLAU, HILDEGARD E., "Themes in Nursing Situations: Power," *Am. J. Nursing*, 53:1221–23, 1953.

——— "Themes in Nursing Situation: Safety," *Am. J. Nursing*, 53:1343–46, 1953.

---

[2] Refer to 1.4.
[3] Refer to 1.3.

# 45

## RÉSUMÉ[1] OF ARIETI'S THEORY OF PALEOLOGIC[2]

*Bettijean Richter*

Silvano Arieti has deduced a theory of schizophrenia, from an extensive review of the literature on thinking and from his own clinical observations of persons diagnosed schizophrenic. No controlled study of his predictions was found in the review of the literature.

According to Rabin and King,[3] such a study had not been made at the time of their review of the literature. This study was designated as an exploratory investigation of Arieti's theory in regard to some structural differences between hebephrenic schizophrenic thought processes and nonschizophrenic patterns of thought. If the indicators of thought process selected for study suggest categorical differentiation between the two thought patterns, further research with more sophisticated experimental design would be warranted. Such research might aid in a clearer definition of schizophrenia.

For the sake of clarity, a discussion of the theory of Arieti including definition of his terms [4] follows.

Arieti hypothesizes that teleologic regression, or a tendency toward a reverse hierarchy of responses, operates under given conditions. This

---

[1] Included in Richter, B., "Exploratory Empirical Testing of Arieti's Theory of Paleologic," master's thesis, Graduate School, Rutgers, The State University of New Jersey, May, 1960, pp. 3-31.

[2] Silvano Arieti, *Interpretation of Schizophrenia*, pp. 541.

[3] Rabin, A. I., and King, G. F., "Psychological Studies," *Schizophrenia: A Review of the Syndrome*, p. 241.

[4] The study-maker's wording of definitions is used except where quotation marks or other clues indicate Arieti's exact wording. In all cases the view of Arieti has been maintained.

phenomenon is viewed as having a teleologic base in the sense that it grows out of purposeful, although unconscious, withdrawal of a person. Such withdrawal occurs from levels of behavior that have been associated with severe anxiety. "Tendency," as used by Arieti, is defined as a propensity toward an occurrence, but lacks the immutability of a law. Arieti differentiates response and behavioral response. The term "response" is used by Arieti to indicate the formal central process responsible for the observed "behavioral response." The more dynamic "behavioral response" is a unique manifestation dependent on numerous individual experiences, perceptions, and interpretations. These aspects of response comprise the specific differences (i.e., relatively stable differences within a specific individual) to be observed in behavior plus the accidents (or unnecessary temporary aspects of the observed behavior). The central process constitutes the genus (or similarities) of the observed phenomenon.

Arieti states that only as the formal and the dynamic aspects of any process are understood is its meaning clear. He states that the American school of psychology has done little work in the area of formal mechanisms. This implies that the American school has studied the dynamics of behavior rather than the patterns formed by, or forming, behavior.

The principle of teleologic regression was identified within three areas of schizophrenic behavior. These classes are reason, affect, and socialization. The categorical arrangement differs slightly from the more common division: thinking, feeling, and action. The first difference is that action is divided into the will to act (or not to act) and observable action. The willing of action has been separated from behavior and classified with reason. The second difference is the inclusion of the needs of a person as a social being. These needs are conceived as influencing and being influenced by the thoughts and actions of the person.

In the study reported here,[5] the portion of Arieti's theory that is immediately significant is only a segment of the material in the category named "reason." The material includes descriptions of the principles of denotation, connotation, association, and logic. Denotation refers to the absence of conceptual meaning for a term. Connotation is defined as the presence of conceptual meaning of a term. Association refers to any way in which two ideas can be related. Logic is the process that provides direction to thinking. These principles of denotation, connotation, association, and logic which are central to this study are elaborated in the following paragraphs.

Arieti proposes a basic assumption in regard to schizophrenic retreat

[5] See n. 1.

from reason. This assumption can be stated as follows: Assuming a continuum with mathematical thinking at one extreme, as the most typical example of pure logical Aristotelian thought, then schizophrenic thinking is at the other extreme, with all possible gradations between the two. Paleologic is a pattern of thinking that utilizes denotation, literal connotation, verbalization, and predicate identification. Aristotelian logic tends more to utilize literal and symbolic connotation, association by similarity, and subject identification.

Arieti supports his assumption that Aristotelian logic is, per se, less archaic than and also superior to other logic. He presents data from anthropological studies of primitive cultures, dream content analyses, and analyses of thought content of young children and of myths. He also indicates the influence which acceptance of the theory of evolution had in his deductions. An important point to keep in mind is that Arieti regards thinking as a cultural,[6] and not a psychological, problem.

Some of the reasons cited for the inferiority of paleologic are (1) paleologic thought is less reliable (he [Arieti] supports this inference, but the data will be excluded in this chapter) and (2) it induces errors and perpetuation of those errors that could be avoided with Aristotelian thought.

This statement that paleologic is more archaic than Aristotelian logic rests on deductions made from the works of Levy-Bruhl, Cassirer, Piaget, Werner, Storch, and numerous others. These works were examined in light of evolutionary and biological theories as well as within a cultural context.

Arieti postulated that although emotional need and the amount of distortion to be seen in the reasoning process will not vary proportionally, the greater the emotional intensity, the greater may be the need to resort to intellectual distortion.

He regards the need for rationality to be as powerful as the need to gratify irrational emotions. He infers that, in a situation of severe anxiety, if behavior at a certain level of integration cannot (or does not) bring about the desired results, a strong tendency exists toward behavior at lower levels of integration. This movement toward lower levels of integration occurs to effect the desired results. (He points out that the lower organization usually does not produce the result sought, but it does lower the level of anxiety, at least temporarily.)

To restate the above observations, if a person cannot tolerate the

---

[6] Basic biological minimums are assumed as prerequisite to the cultural considerations.

anxiety that results from use of traditional logic, he retreats to more archaic forms of logic. At this time, the person, in his efforts to explain why certain phenomena occur, organizes his thoughts with nonabstract means, which are the only means available to him.

According to Arieti, it is as difficult to escape from some types of intellectual organization as it is to escape from some emotions. One inference is that the paleologic, resorted to as a defense by the patient, begets more paleologic. Arieti suggests, however, that it is possible to translate archaic thought into Aristotelian thought. The translator needs to understand the *form* of paleologic, some of the verbalized gestalt exhibiting paleologic form, and some of the subjective content of the expressed thought, i.e., some of the autisms.

It was inferred from the information presented in the preceding paragraph that a clinician capable of translating paleologic could assist a patient in reversing the paleologic process. This presupposes minimal somatic and physiological capacities and parallel utilization of the concept of anxiety. The statement, "Changing from some types of intellectual organization to another is difficult," indicates the need for objective assistance. The clinician could provide this aid.

Intellectual organization is defined by Arieti. He states that it is a process that provides some kind of organization of mental activity through which the individual derives an understanding of the situation involved. Arieti has hypothesized that the intellectual process of the schizophrenic exists, but the products appear faulty from the common point of view. This hypothesis suggests the role of socialization in the process of thinking. A common point of view requires identification of subjects, i.e., objects as total units are found to be perfectly similar or similar in essence. When subject identification is utilized, the logical progress would appear to be limited to a few complex nervous pathways. Identification in paleologic requires similarity in functions or attributes which might be stated about two or more objects. The identification does not occur from similarity of essential attributes or functions, but often from accidental ones. For example, a red rose and a red house might be regarded as alike by virtue of the common quality of redness. The possible number of attributes and functions is great for any subject. The number of possible combinations arising from accidental attribute identification are many. These facts suggest that the progression of association would be through numerous pathways in paleologic.

The number of association tracts of the brain available in the human being for facilitation are myriad. This factor favors diversity of association (i.e., paleologic) in the human population rather than commonality. Variations in thought products from culture to culture further support the hypothesis that thinking is a learned rather than a physiological process.

Arieti approaches the problem with the question, Why does a patient accept an idea as reality in spite of the most complete contradictory evidence? Again, he arrives at the same inference. He states that what appears to the majority of a cultural population as forms of irrationality are, in fact, forms of rationality when viewed from the premise of the actor. These apparently irrational forms of rationality are the only means available to a regressed person to interpret phenomena. In other words, a person who has actually withdrawn from abstract thinking because it has become too painful for him to endure (whatever exogenous or endogenous factors "cause" the pain) can no longer utilize the processes of scientific thinking. The withdrawal from scientific thinking is manifest in other situations as well as in the area of injury. During the period of withdrawal, a person functions totally through lower integration levels.

The foregoing discussion of general principles, hypotheses, and assumptions has been provided as a framework for the specific principles which this study tested. In the following paragraphs (1) general principles are stated, (2) terms used in the principles are defined, and (3) each principle is discussed for clarity.

### Three Principles that Underlie the Frequencies Tested in this Study

Von Doramus Principle (as modified by Arieti)
Whereas the normal person accepts identity only upon the basis of identical subjects, the paleologician accepts identity based upon identical predicates.[7]

Principle of Denotation-Connotation (verbalization is included)
Whereas the healthy person in a wakened state is mainly concerned with the connotation and the denotation of a symbol, but capable of shifting his attention from one to another of these three [sic] aspects of a symbol, the person who thinks paleologically is mainly concerned with the denotation and the verbalization, and experiences a total or partial impairment of his ability to connote.[8]

Principle of Association
The normal person associates either by contiguity, if the ideas have a common predicate of contiguity, or by the law of similarity if the associational link is a predicate of quality. The law of similarity is the higher form of association. Paleologicians replace association by similarity with identification by similarity. Later, not only ideas that might be associated by similarity but also ideas that associate by contiguity are no longer associated but are paleologically identified.[9]

[7] Arieti, op. cit., p. 194.
[8] Ibid., p. 210.
[9] Ibid., p. 260.

# CLARIFICATION OF THE FOREGOING PRINCIPLES: DEFINITIONS AND DISCUSSION

Definitions significant to Van Doramus' principle are—

*Predicate:* that part of a statement which says something about a subject, i.e., the qualities or functions of the subject (e.g., a rose is *red*).

*Subject:* that part of a statement about which something is said (e.g., a *rose* is red).

*Identity:* to make identical, i.e., the very same, or equal (e.g., *a rose is a rose*).

(*Note:* Identification needs to be clearly differentiated from "association" which relates two or more substances by judging similar at least one conceptual abstraction for each. For example, "a rose is a flower" is association of a part [rose] with attributes of one whole of which it is a part [flower].)

The Von Doramus principle indicates that a person who thinks paleologically (i.e., with other than Aristotelian logic) will recognize two objects as being identical because each possesses a quality perceived (or, at times, conceived) to be in the other. This quality is not regarded as being necessary to the essence of the subject (as is done in highly scientific thought). The attribute is chosen by subjective considerations and never subsequently exposed to objective considerations by the paleologician, as is done by the poet, artist, or other symbolic thinker (including physicists, theologians, mathematicians). The point cannot be stressed too forcefully that a distinct difference exists between the paleologician and the abstract thinker, although unsophisticated abstractionists may not recognize the difference immediately. For example, a paleologician could identify a wolf and a man through a perceived common quality such as greediness. The abstractionist would abstract the concept "greed" from the concept "wolf" and the concept "a man." He would then associate the two subject concepts rather than identify the two ideas (or objects) as equal or identical.

A thinker who uses traditional logic follows the laws of identity, contradiction, excluded middle, and sufficient reason. The first three of these laws are negated by application of the Von Doramus principle. This can be seen by comparing the principle to the following definitions and examples.

1. According to the *law of identity*, A is always A; never not-A. (The paleologician will say that A *is* not-A when both are perceived by him to contain a quality "x."

2. The *law of contradiction* states that at the same time and place A cannot *be* A and not-A simultaneously if A and not-A are both perceived to contain "x." (An object can be both book and chair to a paleologician if both are green, assuming green is a quality he uses for identification.)

3. The *law of excluded middle* states that either A is A or it is not; in other words, it cannot be *part* this and *part* that. (If the paleologician perceives that A contains "x" and that B contains "x," he will often condense A and B into a single fused perception or conception.)

4. The *law of sufficient reason* is applied by the paleologician but the method he uses is different. In other words, the paleologician does seek the reason for an event. Instead of looking for a valid explanation for the event, however, he looks for an "unreal" motivation or intention as the cause of the event. The "unreal" reason is usually related to personal needs or fears of the paleologician.

Since predicate identification is hypothesized by Arieti as the basis for recognizing paleologic, a description of the categories of predicates follows.

First, there are *predicates of quality*. These are attributes or functions, abstract or concrete, that are contained in the subject. For example, a piece of artificial fruit may have the qualities of roundness, blackness, waxiness, and irregularity. Association by predicates of quality is a normal Aristotelian means of association, if these qualities are essential to the nature of the objects. The paleologician will identify two objects through this method rather than associate them on the basis of similarity through a commonly held necessary quality.

Second, there are *predicates of contiguity*. The first type includes ideas or events or objects that were perceived as occurring together in space. A paleologician will see as identical two objects, terms, and/or perceptions that he experienced simultaneously in space or time.

In summary, the Von Doramus principle modified by Arieti differentiates paleologic, as seen in persons diagnosed schizophrenic, from Aristotelian logic, seen in "normal" persons. The basis for differentiation is identification. The paleologician identifies through any of a large group of attributes that characterize the two subjects. The normal individual identifies only if the subjects are identical actually or essentially. In normal thought the opportunity for identification is limited, since all or any essential pattern of the attributes must be identical in both objects (subjects).

Definitions useful to the understanding of the meaning of the denotation-connotation principle are—

*Denotation:* The process by which a term is used as the object that is meant as a particular physical entity.

*Connotation:* The process by which the term signifies the concept represented by the term, rather than the object in its concreteness. There are two classifications of connotation.

*Literal connotation:* the conceptualization is limited to the ordinary meaning.

*Symbolic connotation:* the quality abstracted may be applied through association in another context, i.e., figuratively or metaphorically.

*Verbalization:* The process by which a term represents only the form, letter, or sound rather than possessing any meaning value; e.g., "cat" and "rat" can be associated more easily than "cat" and "kitten" when verbalization is the process used.

It should be recalled at this point that the important differentiation between paleologic and Aristotelian logic rests on the ability of the normal person not only to connote but to shift from one aspect of a symbol to another. The abilities to connote and especially to shift are absent in a paleologician.

The points on the continuum of thought of which denotation-connotation are a part are: sensation—imagination—perception—perceptualization of the concept—verbalization—denotation—literal connotation—symbolic connotation. All processes preceding verbalization do not require representation by word symbols. They are not considered in this study.

Citing numerous other authors, as well as his own observations, Arieti indicated that the paleologician's world is closer to the phenomenological, i.e., to immediate perception, than to the world of the traditional logician. It coincides less with reality because of the extreme subjectivity of the paleologician. This subjectivity is evidenced through reduction in the connotative ability. Kurt Goldstein, as quoted by Arieti, observed that normal subjects with subsequent cerebral damage could not, following the damage, use metaphorical or figurative language. Arieti uses Benjamin's notion that the schizophrenic is unable to interpret proverbs correctly, since he always, more or less, gives a literal interpretation of them.

Arieti pinpoints three purposes served by loss of the ability to connote in the person diagnosed schizophrenic: (1) isolation from painful logical context; (2) increased emotional tone; and (3) acquisition of more subjective value, each of which brings the person using schizophrenic thought processes nearer the more comfortable perceptual level.

From Arieti's theory one would expect to find not only reduced use of connotation but also increased use of denotation by paleologicians. In verbalization even denotation is abandoned so that Y *is* why to the paleologician.

In summary, according to this second principle, paleological thought would be distinguished from the Aristotelian logic of "normal" individuals by a decreased connotation of terms, an increased denotation of words, and, in severe instances, by verbalization.

According to Arieti's principle of association, there are two normal ways by which ideas are associated:

1. According to the *law of contiguity:* If two mental processes occur simultaneously or in immediate succession, the recurrence of one tends to produce the recurrence of the other.
2. According to the *law of similarity:* If two mental representations have one or more characteristics in common, the occurrence of one of them tends to elicit the occurrence of the other.

In other words, two ideas associate by contiguity if they have a common predicate of time or space. If the associative link is a common essential predicate of quality or of function, the two ideas are said to be associated by similarity. When the ability to associate remains, but logical direction is diminished, as in severe anxiety, the ideas are connected but lack continuity.

According to Arieti, the person diagnosed schizophrenic will associate by similarity of verbalization rather than by similarity of connotation. The difference is most important, since associative similarity requires the ability to abstract and is the *absolute* prerequisite for Aristotelian logic. Paleologicians also associate by contiguity. Examples of association by contiguity are found in conversations heard in groups where ideas associated by commonality of temporal (or spatial) predicates guide the flow of communication, even in everyday experience.

## SUMMARY OF THE THEORY OF PALEOLOGIC THINKING

A review of Arieti's theory for this study led to the following general conclusions:

1. Thought processes used by persons diagnosed schizophrenic differ from those used by normal adult Western persons in the type of logic used, the nature of the associative link employed, the reduced use of connotation, the increased use of denotation, and the inability to shift from one mode of definition to the other.
2. The thinking process used by persons diagnosed schizophrenic is similar to that used by very young children and by members of primitive cultures.
3. Arieti concludes that the person diagnosed schizophrenic regresses along a continuum of reason away from Aristotelian logic toward lower,

more archaic forms of intellectual integration. This inference was made from the conclusion stated in 2; the assumption that paleologic is inferior to Aristotelian logic, within the Western societal conceptions of progress; recognition that cerebral damage and anxiety-provoking situations evoke the use of paleologic.

4. Paleologic is useful to the person diagnosed schizophrenic as a means of avoiding anxiety.

5. The use of paleologic tends to beget more paleologic.

6. The thinking process is a cultural, rather than a psychological, phenomenon.

7. Paleologic reasoning can be translated into Aristotelian thinking.

## REVIEW OF THE LITERATURE ON PALEOLOGIC THOUGHT BY AUTHORS OTHER THAN ARIETI

The review of the literature was so complete in 1956 and 1957, as the result of the work of Rabin and King,[10] that this author's task was appreciably limited. Various available reviews facilitated a comprehensive view of the literature. Arieti had made a comprehensive search of the literature prior to publication of his work in 1955.[11] Both sources cited investigated many disciplines and the works of writers from various countries. Arieti also utilized his own clinical experience.

The total review, including the works of the authors cited above, suggested that few empirical studies of formal aspects of thinking were done during the years reviewed.

The work of Bruner et al.[12] was based on empirical studies of concept formation and attainment. In their study a series of tests was administered to a normal population with a collegiate level of education. Arieti's assumption that thinking is formed by cultural rather than by psychological processes is supported by Bruner et al. Further, they state that category learning, which provides ready-made concepts, ". . . is one of the principal means by which a growing member of a society is socialized, for the categories that one is taught and comes to use habitually reflect the demands of the culture in which they arise." [13] If Arieti is correct in assuming that the process of socialization results in extreme or prolonged pain for people who then are diagnosed schizophrenic, then the conceptual

[10] Rabin, A. I., and King, G. F., op. cit., pp. 809–47.
[11] Arieti, S., op. cit., pp. 505–28.
[12] Bruner, J., Goodnow, J. J., and Austin, G. A., A Study of Thinking, pp. 330.
[13] Ibid., p. 232.

categories learned by them might tend to differ from those learned by people not so diagnosed.

Further, the Bruner study also supports Arieti's theory that thinking develops along a continuum from denotative to connotative interpretations of symbols. The work cited suggests that the development from concrete to abstract thinking is gradual. From "things I can drive a stake with" to the concept of "mechanical force" more freedom of definition from specific use is attained. If socialization is adequate for those persons diagnosed schizophrenic, the findings of Bruner would tend to support the hypotheses that posit decreased connotation and increased denotation in schizophrenia.

In the same study, it is postulated that "categorization is the means by which objects of the world about are identified. . . . when an event cannot be thus categorized and identified we experience terror in the face of the uncanny." [14] If the individual, later diagnosed schizophrenic, lacked adequate socializing persons or distrusted those in his environment, he would more often experience such terror than would the individual within an adequate socializing milieu. If, as Arieti postulates, this anxiety results in utilization of lower levels of integration, the categories used by persons diagnosed schizophrenic would tend to be more autistic. Both denotation and association by contiguity would be favored by the greater anxiety experienced from an inadequate system of categories.

Experiments by Wyatt and Campbell (1951) and Postman and Bruner (1948) [15] show that whenever completion of categorization is blocked, identification behavior that is abortive in the absence of adequate cues is manifested in future opportunities for categorization. The subject then perceives with inappropriate categorization which must be deconfirmed by subsequent stimulation before pragmatically adequate recognition can occur.[16] This supports Arieti's view that paleologic tends to beget paleologic.

Analysis of cue preference indicated that subjects more frequently utilized cues that had been "learned" as significant ones than was warranted by the ecological validity of those cues.[17] If this finding is extrapolated to the thought process seen in schizophrenia, cues "learned" to suggest painful results would be the more impressive ones which were used more often than other cues simultaneously present in a situation. If these impressive cues lacked validity for association by similarity or subject identification, predicate identification would be favored.

[14] *Ibid.*, p. 10.
[15] *Ibid.*, p. 40.
[16] *Ibid.*, pp. 15–16.
[17] *Ibid.*, p. 40.

One finding of the Bruner study implied that, in the absence of other information, people tend to fall back on cues that seemed to be useful in the past.[18] This again supports the view that persons diagnosed schizophrenic would tend to associate by contiguity or by similarity of verbalization and to identify by predicates.

Under stress, according to Bruner *et al.*, if a person must make identity of instances, he will come to place great reliance on cues that are immediately available for use. The person will tend to use the simpler, more easily ascertained cues rather than more complex ones of higher validity. This finding tends to confirm the hypothesis that in "normal nonstressful" situations individuals diagnosed schizophrenic would tend to use a different set of cues than persons not so diagnosed. This grows out of their higher level of anxiety. This difference in conceptualization would result in differences in the thought processes.

One other significant finding was that the college students who were the subjects in the Bruner *et al.* study often were unable to tell coherently how they proceeded, although the sequence of behavior showed systematically features of highly regular skill and order.[19] This finding suggested that the difficulties encountered in ascertaining the factors that contribute to conclusions of subjects in this present study were not unique.

Inhelder and Piaget's study [20] tends to support Arieti's theory that the normal thought processes move along a developmental continuum from paleologic to Aristotelian logic. The young child (0 to 2 years) learns to abstract some part of a physical entity as signifying the object as a concrete embodiment. In other words, parts are coordinated into wholes at a biological level. One might assume that this stage is equivalent to Arieti's perceptual level preceding verbalization. From the formation of language until about the age of six years, the child attempts to classify objects according to the recognition of function or quality. The child also begins to note consciously similarities and differences between two objects. The concept of permanence tends to be at a denotative level. Between the seventh and eleventh years the child learns to rank-order objects and is able to classify according to more, less, and equal. This indicates abstraction and association of abstracted qualities, even at a concrete level. The child begins to note the objects as distinctive systems in space. He also notes causal relationships. The child, however, still tends to think concretely. He

[18] *Ibid.*, p. 232.
[19] *Ibid.*, p. 241.
[20] Inhelder, B., and Piaget, J., *The Growth of Logical Thinking from Childhood to Adolescence*, p. 356.

cannot generalize from the immediate experience to all physical properties, however. The final actions of this period correspond to literal connotation as defined by Arieti.

Between the twelfth and fifteenth years the child enters a period in which operations tend to correspond to Arieti's symbolic connotation with personal control of formal logic. The child transforms concrete data about the real world into mental operations that are internalized and reversible. From this point on, the child is able to develop more and more elaborate systems. The increased development of symbolic connotation and association by similarity is essential to this elaboration of systems by means of true symbolic logic.

The empirical work of Piaget, briefly presented in the foregoing, tends to substantiate Arieti's theory regarding a developmental continuum of thought processes. If anxiety or poor socialization resulted in retreat or arrest, in any stage, for a person diagnosed schizophrenic, the indicators of Aristotelian logic would occur with less frequency than those of paleologic.

The theories of physical maturation suggest that facilitation of different association tracts accompanies each developmental stage.[21] These theories tend to substantiate the assumption of various levels of integration. Physiological changes accompanying profound anxiety might play an important role in inhibition of various association tracts whose facilitation preceded or triggered the onset of high levels of anxiety.

Freud's concept of the primary and secondary processes tends to support the developmental theory of thought. In the primary process, thoughts are organized around drives. Connections between these thoughts are thus subjective. The associations would be made by contiguity and identification by predicates, in the terms of Arieti. In the secondary process, thoughts are structured in regard to reality and therefore would exhibit more common (normal) associative links. In a culture where abstract thought patterns were used, the associations would be made more often by similarity than by contiguity. Identification would tend toward subject identification in such a culture. The altered thought process of schizophrenia could be regarded as developmentally inferior (i.e., regarding level) in such a culture.

Schilder's conception [22] of a striving toward objectivity as a major determinant in thought development also suggests a continuum from less objective to more objective associations. In a culture using abstract think-

---

[21] Rapaport, D., *Organization and Pathology of Thought*, pp. 689–751.
[22] *Ibid.*, p. 503 (footnote 52).

ing, the movement away from paleologic would be advantaged and would be manifested in the adolescent and the adult as the common pattern.

Arieti gave credit to the work of Eugen Bleuler as essential in the development of his theory. Reading this work [23] made evident the roots of the conception of association by verbalization utilized by Arieti. Bleuler stated that the basic symptom of schizophrenia is "loosening of associations." Bleuler assumed this was based on an organic process. Arieti assumes minimum biological potentials, yet he tends to regard the sociocultural factors as basic to the altered thought process of the person diagnosed schizophrenic.

Freud [24] wrote: "We may attempt a characterization of the schizophrenic's mode of thought by saying that he treats concrete things as though they were abstract." This statement supports the prediction that schizophrenic thought would tend to be more denotative and less connotative than the thought of persons not diagnosed schizophrenic. Since connotation is fundamental to association by similarity and subject identification, these two mechanisms could not be utilized by a person employing schizophrenic thought processes. By extension, Freud's statement supports the prediction that the two forementioned mechanisms would be absent.

Rabin and King,[25] in their review of psychological studies, have indicated a need for controlled investigation of both Arieti's theory of paleologic and the Von Doramus principle. These authors indicate that any research in the area of thinking, in reference to schizophrenia, suffers from certain methodological deficiencies. The inadequately described and heterogeneous composition of the "schizophrenic group" is regarded by these authors as a major difficulty. They suggest the material (regarding the deficit in abstract thinking as related to schizophrenics categorized as "early" or "in remission") should be collected from which the relationship between the level of conceptual thinking and chronicity might be inferred.

In brief, controlled experimental studies of thought processes, as observed in college students and in age groups arranged developmentally, tend to support Arieti's theory of a thought continuum. The theories of other writers, based on observations of persons diagnosed schizophrenic, give support of the predication that schizophrenic thought differs from normal in the nature of definition of terms and association of linkages. A review of psychological studies suggests a need for study of formal mechanisms used in thinking by individuals diagnosed schizophrenic.

[23] Bleuler, E., "The Basic Symptom of Schizophrenia," in David Rapaport's *Organization and Pathology of Thought*, pp. 581–650.
[24] Freud, S., "The Unconscious," *Collected Papers*, Vol. IV, p. 159.
[25] Rabin, A. I., and King, G. F., *op. cit.*, pp. 216–79.

# BIBLIOGRAPHY

ARIETI, SILVANO, *Interpretation of Schizophrenia*, Robert Bruner, New York: 1955.

BRUNER, JEROME, GOODNOW, J. J., and AUSTIN, G. A., *A Study of Thinking*, John Wiley and Sons, New York: 1956.

BLEULER, EUGEN, "The Basic Symptom of Schizophrenia," *Organization and Pathology of Thought*, David Rapaport (ed.), Columbia University Press, New York: 1951.

FREUD, SIGMUND, "The Unconscious," *Collected Papers*, Vol. IV, Hobart, London: 1946.

INHELDER, B., and PIAGET, J., *The Growth of Logical Thinking from Childhood to Adolescence*, Basic Books, New York: 1958.

RABIN, ALBERT I., and KING, GERALD F., "Psychological Studies," *Schizophrenia: A Review of the Syndrome*, Leopold Bellack (ed.), Logos Press, New York: 1958.

## SUGGESTED ADDITIONAL REFERENCES

BARTLETT, SIR FREDERICK, *Thinking: An Experimental and Social Study*, Basic Books, New York: 1958.

BOURNE, LYLE E., "Effects of Delay of Information Feedback and Task Complexity on the Identification of Concepts," *J. Exper. Psychol.*, 54:201–7, 1957.

GOLDBERGER, EMANUAL, "The Id and the Ego: A Developmental Interpretation," *Psychoanal. Rev.*, 44:235–88, 1957.

HERTZKA, ALFRED F., and GUILFORD, G. P., "Logical Reasoning," *J. Consult. Psychol.*, 19:405, 1955.

HUMPHREY, GEORGE, *Thinking: An Introduction to its Experimental Psychology*, John Wiley and Sons, New York: 1951.

JOHNSON, DONALD M., *The Psychology of Thought and Judgment*, Harper and Bros., New York: 1955.

KREYCHE, ROBERT J., *Logic for Undergraduates*, The Dryden Press, New York: 1954.

MC GILL, V. J., *Emotions and Reason*, Charles C Thomas, Springfield, Ill.: 1954.

MC KELLAR, PETER, *Imagination and Thinking*, Basic Books, New York: 1957.

PRABHAVEANANDA, SWAMI, and ISHERWOOD, CHRISTOPHER, *The Song of God: Bhagavad-Gita*, The New American Library, New York: 1954.

PRICE, H. H., *Thinking and Experience*, Harvard University Press, Cambridge, Mass.: 1953.

RAPAPORT, DAVID (ed.), *Organization and Pathology of Thought*, Columbia University Press, New York: 1951. (Parts of "Fantasy-Thinking," "Pathology of Thinking," and "Conclusion.")

ROUBICZEK, PAUL, *Thinking in Opposites*, The Beacon Press, Boston, Mass.: 1952.

SILLER, JEROME, "Socioeconomic Status and Conceptual Thinking," *J. Abnormal Soc. Psychol.*, 55:365–71, 1957.

TALLAND, GEORGE, "Criteria in Conceptual Transposition," *Am. J. Psychol.*, 70:263–76, 1957.

UNIVERSITY OF COLORADO, *Contemporary Approaches to Cognition*, A Symposium, University of Colorado. J. Bruner, E. Brunswik, L. Festinger, F. Heider, K. Muenzinger, Charles E. Osgood, D. Rapaport, contributors. Harvard University Press, Cambridge, Mass.: 1957.

USHENKO, ANDREW P., *The Problem of Logic*, Princeton University Press, Princeton, New Jersey: 1941.

WERNER, H., and KAPLAN, B., "Developmental Approach to Cognition: Its Relevance to the Psychological Interpretation of Anthropological and Ethnolinguistic Data," *American Anthropology*, October, 1956.

WERTHEIMER, MAX, *Productive Thinking*. Harper and Bros., New York: 1945.

# GLOSSARY

## CONTRIBUTOR'S DEFINITIONS OF CONCEPTS

*Adaptation:* Adaptation is the process by which an individual reduces felt needs by using automatic behavior patterns without experiencing learning.
(E. W. Carter)

*Adaptive Maneuvers:* These are automatic behavior patterns which one adopts to reduce anxiety without experiencing learning through the use of effective thought.
(F. R. Kumler)

*Aggression:* Aggression is any verbal and/or nonverbal, actual or attempted forceful abuse of the self, another person, or thing. There are observable behaviors antecedent to aggression. These antecedents defined operationally in order of their emergence yield the following explanation of aggressive behavior:

1. The person holds expectations.
2. The expectations are not met.
3. The person experiences a higher level of anxiety.
4. Aggression occurs.
5. Justification of aggression. (J. Clack)

*Anger:* The dynamics of anger include the following steps:

1. A blocked goal, reduced self-respect, or unmet expectations.
2. An unpleasant, uncanny, powerless feeling which is part of the concept of anxiety.
3. A change in feelings, sometimes without recognition of the anxiety, into feelings or actions of power, directed against the blocking object, a substitute, or the self, and
4. The feeling of relief. (D. R. Hays)

*Alcoholism:* Operationally, the development of alcoholism as a repetitive pattern can be defined in the following way:

A person has—

1. A problem,
2. Anxiety in relation to the problem,
3. Conversion of the energy of anxiety to behavior—drinking,
4. Withdrawal from problem through drinking,
5. Anxiety relieved temporarily,
6. Unsolved problem,
7. Recall of problem,
8. Anxiety in retrospect. (S. Rouslin)

*Autistic Invention:* Autistic invention involves the use of highly personal meanings attached to words and events. (S. W. Armstrong)

*Autistic Thinking:* Autistic thinking is largely a childhood tool through which thoughts, feelings, and words have a magical power of fulfilling needs, wants, and wishes. (R. S. Isani)

*Avoidance:* Avoidance is an action, verbal or nonverbal, by which the patient (person) keeps away from a situation. (G. Oden)

*Change:* Change is a process consisting of the phases of need, formulation, and acceptance, utilizing a concept of anxiety and a process and concept of learning. (S. F. Burd)

*Compulsion:* The tendency to repeat a certain kind of behavior without being able to inhibit it.

A person—

1. Has a thought or feeling that provokes discomfort,
2. Is not aware of the discomfort,
3. Feels a need to act or acts in a way that previously produced relief, usually opposite the original feeling or thought,
4. Performs the action,
5. Feels no more discomfort. (S. Rouslin)

—357

*Concept:* A concept is a term defined operationally so as to explain observations of behavior, in part, and to provide a structure for collecting more data so as to secure a complete and valid explanation. (S. F. Burd)

*Dissociation:* Dissociation may be defined as the separation from awareness of certain aspects (thoughts, feelings, and/or actions) of the individual's behavior, due to an experience of severe anxiety. Operationally, these steps occur in sequence:

1. In early life, certain thoughts, feelings, and/or actions of an individual are disapproved by significant other persons.
2. These standards for disapproval are incorporated as the individual's own.
3. Later in life, the individual experiences one of the disapproved thoughts, feelings, or actions.
4. Anxiety level rises to severe level.
5. The aspect, frequently the feeling, is barred from awareness.
6. Anxiety level is lowered.
7. Dissociated aspect continues to appear in disguised form in thoughts, feelings, and actions of the individual. (J. De Augustinis)

*Frustration:* The steps in the concept of frustration which can be observed and/or elicited [from the individual] include:

1. The setting of a goal,
2. Movement toward this goal,
3. An intervening obstacle,
4. Anger. (D. R. Hays)

*Giving:* Giving is a symbolic act of communication; the act meets the needs of two persons. Operationally defined, giving involves these sequential steps:

1. An individual has a need.
2. Need tension is felt.
3. Giving is a way to meet this need.
4. The individual chooses another person as a recipient.
5. The individual offers this other person a gift.
6. The gift is received.
7. Need tension decreases or
7. The receiver performs the expected reciprocal action(s).
8. Need tension decreases.

   or

7. The receiver *does not* perform expected reciprocal action(s).
8. The giver experiences an increased level of anxiety. (J. Clack)

*Hallucination:* A hallucination is an inner experience, expressed as though it were an outer event. It arises out of the dissociated motivations of the self-system and is an uncanny, yet real, experience for the person.

(K. H. Gravenkemper)

*Learning:* Learning is an active process which utilizes the thinking and perceiving abilities and knowledge previously acquired for three major purposes:

1. To explain events,
2. To facilitate change,
3. To solve problems. (H. E. Peplau)

*Loneliness:* Loneliness is in essence the inability to love, combined with a negative of being; or, to describe it otherwise, the lonely person has the terrifying experience of being unable to conceptualize himself as real, i.e., having existence. This is both a cognitive and affective unconscious dynamism; it is out of the person's awareness. (C. G. Francel)

*Manipulation:* Manipulation is a process by which one individual influences another individual to function in accord with his needs without regard for the other's needs or goals. It is an interpersonal process which takes many forms and which occurs unconsciously to some extent in all interpersonal behavior.

Manipulation may be defined by the following interpersonal operations:
1. One person has needs that are not met by the other person.
2. The anxiety level of the person with unmet needs rises.
3. There is disregard, consciously or unconsciously, of the other's needs or goals.
4. Adaptive maneuver(s) is (are) tried.
5. If the adaptive maneuver(s) elicits (elicit) the desired response, the needs are met, anxiety is reduced and the automatic behavior pattern continues. (F. R. Kumler)

*Obsessive-Compulsive Neurosis:* The emerging operations of an obsessive-compulsive neurosis are as follows:
1. An individual has a wish or a desire to act.
2. This wish or desire is seen as unacceptable by significant other persons, usually because it is related to hostile or aggressive feelings.
3. The unacceptability of the wish becomes a barrier to the individual's carrying out his wish or desire.
4. The individual feels this barrier of unacceptability as a threat to personality.
5. The individual experiences an increase of anxiety which occurs because the personality is threatened.
6. The individual develops adaptations to reduce or avoid the anxiety. These adaptations are routine or stereotyped ways of thinking and acting (obsessions and compulsions).
7. The original wish or desire to act is dissociated; the individual has the illusion of security.
8. These routine or stereotyped ways of thinking and acting are repeatedly reinforced in the process of growing up and maintain the illusion of security.
9. Ultimately, these routine and stereotyped methods of thinking and acting represent a denial of self. (A. Hadley)

*Operational Definition:* An operational definition provides statements of all observed behaviors (or inferences that classify all possible variations of each behavior) that are associated with the term (concept) in the order in which such behaviors emerge in the observed. (S. F. Burd)

*Problem-Solving Process:* This process involves eight steps resulting in satisfaction.
1. Conscious awareness of the problem.
2. Intention to deal with the problem.
3. Pertinent evidence gathered to understand the problem.
4. Consideration of means of action for solution.
5. Implementation of one means of action.
6. Observation of the implementation results.
7. Evaluation of the implementation results.
8. Revision in the light of Steps 1 through 7. (S. Rouslin)

*Rational Authority:* This is authority based on knowledge and competence which is used to encourage and guide those subject to it in realizing their potentialities. These potentialities involve the growth of the awareness of the integrity of the self as a separate and independent entity. The role of rational authority is temporary and requires constant self-evaluation. When the functions assigned to it are completed, it is dissolved. (F. R. Kumler)

*Role:* A role is a learned and organized pattern of social interactions. These interactions are based upon reciprocal expectations of actions and attitudes.
(A. M. Werner)

*Support:* Support is an interpersonal lay concept which is utilized to reduce anxiety of the patient and/or of the nurse by adaptive maneuver(s). Support is defined operationally in this way:

1. A person perceives another person as having an unmet need. This unmet need may or may not have been perceived correctly.
2. There is an increase in the anxiety level of the one or both persons.
3. This increased anxiety is empathized by the other individual.
4. One of the two persons utilizes adaptive maneuver(s).
5a. If the adaptive maneuver(s) is (are) successful, both persons experience a decrease in levels of anxiety.
5b. If the adaptive maneuver(s) is (are) not successful, anxiety of both persons continues to increase toward the level of panic. (E. W. Carter)

*Theme:* A theme is a recurring relation, view, or opinion held with respect to some aspect of living. It is the central idea inherent in many verbal and nonverbal details, rather than the details of verbalized material. (S. F. Burd)

*Therapeutic Nurse-Patient Relationship:* This is a relationship based upon the nurse's role as a rational authority. It requires the nurse's respect for the patient's potential for growth and provides for the stimulation of this potential. In the therapeutic relationship there is mutual participation in the task of utilizing the relationship as a learning experience directing maturation. The therapeutic relationship is not an end but, rather, a means to an end.
(F. R. Kumler)

*Thinking:* Thinking, as a process, includes:

1. Free association
2. Autistic thinking
3. Creative imagination
4. Reasoning
   a. problem
   b. definition of problem, isolation of data
   c. possible solutions
   d. evaluation of solutions, hypothesis
   e. observational or experimental test of solution
   f. steps b–f until solution is found. (G. Oden)

## THOUGHT DISORDERS

*Automatic Knowing:* A common cultural expression that people use is "you know" at the end of a statement. The use of "you know" becomes pathological when a person really thinks the listener knows what is about to be said.
(S. W. Armstrong)

*Depersonalization:* The individual's self-concept as well as a thought disorder is involved in depersonalization, which means that the person does not see himself as a total person. (S. W. Armstrong)

*Extensive Use of Modifiers:* Some individuals are so unsure of what they are saying that they use many modifiers in order to avoid making direct statements. (S. W. Armstrong)

*Global Adjectives:* Use of such ambiguous words as good, nice, bad, beautiful—these words do convey somewhat different meanings to different people. Adjectives can also be used by people to cover up their feelings.

(S. W. Armstrong)

*Global Pronouns:* This type of thought disorder involves the use of many pronouns without their referents. When questioned, sometimes the person is able to supply the referent and sometimes he is unable to do so.

(S. W. Armstrong)

*Imputing Intention and/or Ideas to Other People:* Some persons will predict what the other person thinks or intends to do without sufficient evidence on which to base the prediction. (S. W. Armstrong)

*Lack of Differentiation among Feelings, Thoughts, and Actions:* This thought disorder is common to many people, psychotic and nonpsychotic. Often people say they feel something that is really a thought or an opinion.

(S. W. Armstrong)

*Scattering:* A common thought disorder is scattering, in which the patient moves from one topic to another with no apparent connection between the topics. (S. W. Armstrong)

*Speaking in the Negative:* This thought disorder focuses on negative feelings, thoughts, and actions in their communication. (S. W. Armstrong)

*Switching the Subject:* In this thought disorder, the person talks around and around a subject, and even though he switches the subject, he keeps coming back to the original subject. (S. W. Armstrong)

*Waiting:* The three most frequently encountered aspects of the concept of waiting are the acts of *waiting for, waiting on,* and *waiting with* a person (or persons).

The subconcept *waiting for* can be defined as staying or resting in expectation till the arrival of some person or event.

The subconcept *waiting with* is closely related to the preceding subdivision—two or more persons are staying in expectation till the arrival of some person or event. This person or event may concern one or both, part or all, of the waiting persons; it may even affect them in varying ways.

The definitions being in readiness to perform services for someone and calling upon or visiting apply to the subconcept *waiting on.* (D. R. Hays)

*Withdrawal:* A behavioral reaction to anxiety, conflict, and frustration. A person—

1. Experiences anxiety or conflict or frustration,
2. Acts, or wants to act, aggressively according to feelings,
3. Perceives that actions are unacceptable to significant other persons,
4. Experiences anxiety,
5. Wants to please significant other person to ensure security,
6. Withdraws, reducing anxiety. (S. Rouslin)

# GENERAL BIBLIOGRAPHY

## BOOKS

ACKERMAN, NATHAN W., *The Psychodynamics of Family Life*, Basic Books, Inc., New York: 1958.

ALEXANDER, FRANZ, *Fundamentals of Psychoanalysis*, W. W. Norton and Company, Inc., New York: 1948.

———— and ROSS, HELEN, *Dynamic Psychiatry*, University of Chicago Press, Chicago, Ill.: 1952.

ALLPORT, F. H., *Theories of Perception and the Concept of Structure*, John Riley and Sons, Inc., New York: 1955.

ARIETI, S., *Interpretation of Schizophrenia*, Robert Brunner, New York: 1955.

———— (ed.), *American Handbook of Psychiatry*, Basic Books, Inc., New York: 1959.

BALDWIN, ALFRED, *Behavior and Development in Childhood*, The Dryden Press, New York: 1955.

BARTLETT, SIR FREDERICK, *Thinking: An Experimental and Social Study*, Basic Books, Inc., New York: 1958.

BELLACK, L. (ed.), *Schizophrenia: A Review of the Syndrome*, Logos Press, New York: 1958.

BERELSON, BERNARD, *Content Analysis in Communication Research*, The Free Press, Glencoe, Ill.: 1952.

BEST, CHARLES H., and TAYLOR, NORMAN BURKE, *The Physiological Basis of Medical Practice*, The Williams & Wilkins Co., Baltimore: 1939.

BIBER, B., MURPHY, L., and BLACK, I., *Life and Ways of the Seven to Eight Year Old*, Basic Books, Inc., New York: 1952.

BROADY, SYLVIA, *Patterns of Mothering*, International Universities Press, Inc., New York: 1956.

BROUSSEAU, A., *Essai Sur La Peur Aux Armées, 1914–1918*, Alcan, Paris: 1920.

BRUNER, JEROME, GOODNOW, J., and AUSTIN, G. A., *A Study of Thinking*, John Wiley and Sons, Inc., New York: 1956.

—363

BURTON, ARTHUR (ed.), *Psychotherapy of the Psychoses*, Basic Books, Inc., New York: 1961.

BURTON, G., *Personal, Impersonal and Interpersonal Relationships*, Springer Publishing Company, Inc., New York: 1958.

BUTLER, J. DONALD, *Four Philosophies*, Harper and Brothers, New York: 1957.

CALDWELL, J. M., RANSON, S. W., and SACHS, J. G., "Group Panic and Other Mass Disruptive Reactions," *U. S. Armed Forces Medical Journal*, 1951.

CLAPP, CHARLES, *Drinking's Not the Problem*, Thomas Crowell Company, New York: 1949.

CRITCHLEY, MAC DONALD, *The Language of Gestures*, Edward Arnold and Company, London: 1939.

——— *A Psychology of Gesture*, Methuen and Company, Ltd., London: 1948.

CROW, L. D., and CROW, A. (eds.), *Readings in General Psychology*, Barnes and Noble, Inc., New York: 1952.

CRUZE, W. W., *Psychology in Nursing*, McGraw-Hill Book Company, Inc., New York: 1955.

——— *Psychology for College Students*, Prentice-Hall, Inc., New York: 1951.

DENT, JOHN Y., *Anxiety and Its Treatment with Special Reference to Alcoholism*, John Murray, London: 1941.

DEWEY, JOHN, *How We Think*, D. C. Heath and Company, New York: 1910.

DOLLARD, JOHN, and MILLER, NEAL E., *Personality and Psychotherapy*, McGraw-Hill Book Company, Inc., New York: 1950.

——— *et al., Frustration and Aggression*, Yale University Press, New Haven: 1939.

EDWARDS, ALLEN L., *Statistical Methods for the Behavioral Sciences*, Rinehart and Company, Inc., New York: 1955.

EISENSTEIN, VICTOR W. (ed.), *Neurotic Interaction in Marriage*, Basic Books, Inc., New York: 1956.

ENGLISH, HORACE B., and ENGLISH, AVA C., *A Comprehensive Dictionary of Psychological and Psychoanalytical Terms*, Longmans, Green and Company, New York: 1958.

ENGLISH, O. SPURGEON, and PEARSON, GERALD H. J., *Emotional Problems of Living*, W. W. Norton and Company, New York: 1945.

FELDMAN, SANDOR, *Mannerisms of Speech and Gestures*, International Universities Press, Inc., New York: 1959.

FREUD, SIGMUND, "The Unconscious," *Collected Papers, Vol. IV*, Hobart, London: 1946.

FRIEDMAN, RONALD, *et al., Principles of Sociology: A Text With Readings*, Henry Holt and Company, Inc., New York: 1956.

FROMM, ERICH, *Escape From Freedom*, Rinehart & Company, Inc., New York: 1941.

FROMM-REICHMANN, FRIEDA, *Principles of Intensive Psychotherapy*, University of Chicago Press, Chicago: 1950.

——— *Psychoanalysis and Psychotherapy*, The University of Chicago Press, Chicago, Ill.: 1959.

FULTON, JOHN F., *A Textbook of Physiology*, 17th ed. W. B. Saunders Co., Baltimore: 1955.

GESELL., A., *The First Five Years of Life*, Harper and Brothers, New York: 1940.

GREEN, ARNOLD, *Sociology*, McGraw-Hill Book Company, Inc., New York: 1952.

GREENBLATT, M., LEVINSON, D., and WILLIAMS, R., *The Patient and the Mental Hospital*, The Free Press, Glencoe, Ill.: 1957.

GREENWALD, HAROLD, *The Call Girl*, Ballantine Books, New York: 1958.

HABERSTEIN, R. W., and E. A. CHRIST, *Professionalizer, Traditionalizer and Utilizer*, University of Missouri, Columbia, Mo.: 1955.

HALL, CALVIN S., and LINDZEY, GARDNER, *Theories of Personality*, John Wiley and Sons, Inc., New York: 1957.

HAMILTON, GORDON, *Theory and Practice of Social Case Work*, Columbia University Press, New York: 1951.

HARMER, BERTHA, and HENDERSON, VIRGINIA, *Textbook of Principles and Practice of Nursing*, 5th ed., The Macmillan Company, New York: 1955.

HODNETT, EDWARD, *The Art of Problem Solving*, Harper Brothers, New York: 1955.

HOFLING, CHARLES, and LEININGER, MADELINE M., *Basic Psychiatric Concepts in Nursing*, J. B. Lippincott Company, Philadelphia: 1960.

HORNEY, KAREN, *Our Inner Conflicts*, W. W. Norton & Co., New York: 1945.

——— *New Ways in Psychoanalysis*, W. W. Norton & Co., New York: 1939.

HUGHES, E. C., H. M., and DEUTSCHER, I., *Twenty Thousand Nurses Tell Their Story*, J. B. Lippincott Co., Philadelphia: 1958.

HUMPHREY, GEORGE, *Thinking; An Introduction to its Experimental Psychology*, John Wiley and Sons, New York: 1951.

INGRAM, MADELENE E., *Principles and Techniques of Psychiatric Nursing*, W. B. Saunders, Philadelphia: 1955.

INHELDER, S., and PIAGET, J., *The Growth of Logical Thinking*, Basic Books, Inc., New York: 1958.

JACKSON, DON D. (ed.), *The Etiology of Schizophrenia*, Basic Books, Inc., New York: 1960.

JAHODA, MARIE, DEUTSCH, M., and COOK, S., *Research Methods in Social Relationships, Part I: Basic Processes*, The Dryden Press, New York: 1951.

JANET, PIERRE, *The Major Symptoms of Hysteria*, The Macmillan Co., New York: 1913.

JELLINEK, E. M., *The Disease Concept of Alcoholism*, Hillhouse Press, New Haven, Conn.: 1960.

JENKINS, RICHARD L., *Breaking Patterns of Defeat*, J. B. Lippincott Co., Philadelphia: 1954.

JOHNSON, DONALD M., *The Psychology of Thought and Judgment*, Harper Brothers, Publishers, New York: 1955.

KALKMAN, MARION E., *Introduction to Psychiatric Nursing*, McGraw-Hill Book Co., New York: 1958.

KANT, FRITZ, *The Treatment of the Alcoholic*, Charles C Thomas, Springfield, Ill.: 1954.

KARPMAN, BENJAMIN, *The Hangover*, Charles C Thomas, Springfield, Ill.: 1957.

KELLY, GEORGE A., *The Psychology of Personal Constructs*, W. W. Norton & Co., New York: 1955.

KLUCKHOHN, CLYDE, and MURRAY, H. (eds.), *Personality in Nature, Society and Culture*, Alfred A. Knopf, Inc., New York: 1953.

KREYCHE, ROBERT J., *Logic for Undergraduates*, The Dryden Press, New York: 1954.

KRUSE, H. D. (ed.), *Alcoholism as a Medical Problem*. Hoeber-Harper, New York: 1956.

LA PEIRE, R., *Collective Behavior*, McGraw-Hill Book Company, New York: 1938.

LEARY, T., *Multilevel Measurement of Interpersonal Behavior, A Manual*, Psychological Consultation Service, Berkeley, Calif.: 1956.

———— *Interpersonal Diagnosis of Personality*, The Ronald Press Co., New York: 1957.

LEWIS, M. M., *How Children Learn to Speak*, George C. Harrup and Co., London: 1957.

LINDESMITH, A. R., and STRAUSS, A. L., *Social Psychology*, Dryden Press, New York: 1956.

LINDZEY, G. (ed.), *Handbook of Social Psychology*, Vol. I, Addison-Wesley Publishing Company, Cambridge, Mass.: 1954.

MAIER, NORMAN, *Frustration*, McGraw-Hill Book Co., New York: 1949.

MANN, MARTY, *Primer on Alcoholism*, Rinehart and Company, New York: 1950.

MASLOW, A. H., *Motivation and Personality*, Harper and Brothers, New York: 1954.

MASSERMAN, JULES H., *The Practice of Dynamic Psychiatry*, W. B. Saunders Co., Philadelphia: 1955.

MASSERMAN, JULES H., and MORENO, J. L. (eds.), *Progress in Psychotherapy*, Vol. 5, Grune and Stratton, New York: 1960.

MATHENEY, RUTH, and TOPALIS, MARY, *Psychiatric Nursing*, C. V. Mosby Co., St. Louis: 1957.

MAY, ROLLO, *The Meaning of Anxiety*, The Ronald Press, New York: 1950.

MC GILL, V. J., *Emotions and Reason*, Charles C Thomas, Springfield, Ill.: 1954.

MC KELLAR, PETER, *Imagination and Thinking*, Basic Books, Inc., New York: 1957.

MEERLOO, JOOST, A. M., *Patterns of Panic*, International Universities Press, New York: 1950.

MENNINGER, KARL, *A Psychiatrist's World*, Bernard E. Hall (ed.), The Viking Press, New York: 1954.

———— *Man Against Himself*, Harcourt, Brace and Company, New York: 1938.

MERENESS, DOROTHY, and KARNOSH, LOUIS J., *Psychiatry for Nurses*, C. V. Mosby Co., St. Louis: 1958.

MULLAHY, PATRICK, *Oedipus: Myth and Complex*, Grove Press, Inc., New York: 1948.

MULLER, THERESA C., *The Foundations of Human Behavior*, G. P. Putnam's Sons, New York: 1956.

MUNSON, E., *The Management of Men*, Henry Holt and Co., New York: 1921.

NICHOLS, RALPH G., and STEVENS, LEONARD A., *Are You Listening*, McGraw-Hill Book Company, New York: 1957.

NIGHTINGALE, FLORENCE, *Notes On Nursing*, Harrison, London: 1860.

NOYES, ARTHUR P., *Modern Clinical Psychiatry*, W. B. Saunders Co., Philadelphia: 1953.

OGBURN, W. F., *Encyclopedia of the Social Sciences*, Vol. 3, The Macmillan Company, New York: 1931.

PARSONS, TALCOTT, *Towards a General Theory of Action*, Harvard University Press, Cambridge: 1951.

PARSONS, TALCOTT, and BALES, R., *Family—Socialization and Interaction Process*, The Free Press, Glencoe, Ill.: 1955.

PEI, MARIO, *All About Language*, J. B. Lippincott Co., New York: 1954.

PEPLAU, HILDEGARD E., *Interpersonal Relations in Nursing*, G. P. Putnam's Sons, New York: 1952.

———— "Therapeutic Concepts: Aspects of Psychiatric Nursing," *The League Exchange*, No. 26, The National League for Nursing, New York: 1957.

POWDERMAKER, F., and FRANK, J., *Group Psychotherapy*, Harvard University Press, Cambridge, Mass.: 1953.

PRABHAVEANANDA, SWAMI, and ISHERWOOD, CHRISTOPHER, *The Song of God: Bhagavad-Gita*, The New American Library, New York: 1954.

PRICE, H. H., *Thinking and Experience*, Harvard University Press, Cambridge, Mass.: 1953.

PUNER, HELEN WALKER, *Freud, His Life and his Mind*, Dell Publishing Co., New York: 1957.

RAPAPORT, D. (ed.), *Organization and Pathology of Thought*, Columbia University Press, New York: 1951.

REDL, FRITZ, and WINERMAN, DAVID, *The Aggressive Child*, The Free Press of Glencoe, Ill.: 1957.

REIK, T., *Listening With a Third Ear*, Grove Press, New York: 1948.

REISSMAN, L., and ROHER, J. H., *Change and Dilemma in the Nursing Profession*, G. P. Putnam's Sons, New York: 1957.

RENDER, HELENA, and WEISS, OLGA, *Nurse-Patient Relationships in Psychiatry*, McGraw-Hill Publishing Co., New York: 1959.

RICHARDSON, ROY F., *The Psychology and Pedagogy of Anger*, Warwick & York, Baltimore: 1918.

RILEY, MATILDA, and RILEY, JOHN W., JR., "The Dyad, or Subject-Object Pair," *Scale Analysis*, Rutgers University Press, New Brunswick, New Jersey: 1954.

ROSEN, JOHN, *Direct Analysis*, Grune & Stratton, New York: 1953.

ROUBICZEK, PAUL, *Thinking in Opposites*, The Beacon Press, Boston, Mass.: 1952.

RUESCH, JURGEN, and BATESON, GREGORY, *Communication: The Social Matrix of Psychiatry*, W. W. Norton & Co., New York: 1951.

———— *Disturbed Communication*, W. W. Norton & Co., New York: 1957.

———— and KEES, W., *Nonverbal Communication*, University of California Press, Berkeley & Los Angeles: 1956.

SCHACHTEL, ERNEST G., *Metamorphosis*, Basic Books, Inc., New York: 1959.

SCHWARTZ, MORRIS, and SHOCKLEY, EMMY LANNING, *The Nurse and the Mental Patient*, Russell Sage Foundation, New York: 1956.

SEARS, ROBERT R., MACOBY, ELEANOR E., and LEVIN, HARRY, *Patterns of Child Rearing*, Row, Peterson and Company, White Plains, New York: 1957.

SECHEHAYE, MARGUERITE, *Autobiography of a Schizophrenic Girl*, Grune and Stratton, New York: 1951.

SELTIZ, C. M., JAHODA, M., DEUTSCH, M., and COOK, S., *Research Methods in Social Relations*, Henry Holt and Co., New York: 1959.

SHAFER, K. N., SAWYER, J. R., MC CLUSKEY, A. M., and LIFGREN, E. A., *Medical-Surgical Nursing*, C. V. Mosby Co., St. Louis, Mo.: 1958.

SHERFEY, M. J., "Psychopathology and Character Structure in Chronic Alcoholism," *Etiology of Chronic Alcoholism*, O. Diethelm (ed.), Charles C Thomas, Springfield, Ill.: 1955.

SLAVSON, S. R. (ed.), *The Fields of Group Psychotherapy*. International Universities Press, New York: 1956.

SODDY, KENNETH (ed.), *Mental Health and Infant Development*, Basic Books, Inc., New York: 1956.

STANTON, ALFRED, and SCHWARTZ, MORRIS, *The Mental Hospital*, Basic Books, Inc., New York: 1954.

STEELE, KATHERINE, and MANFREDA, MARGUERITE, *Psychiatric Nursing*, F. A. Davis Co., Philadelphia: 1959.

STEINMANN, A., *The Psychiatric Interview*, W. W. Norton & Co., New York: 1954.

STRECHER, EDWARD A., and CHAMBERS, FRANCIS T., *Alcohol, One Man's Meat*, The Macmillan Co., New York: 1938.

SULLIVAN, HARRY STACK, *The Psychiatric Interview*, W. W. Norton & Co., New York: 1954.

—— *Clinical Studies in Psychiatry*, W. W. Norton & Co., New York: 1956.

—— *The Interpersonal Theory of Psychiatry*, W. W. Norton & Co., New York: 1953.

—— *Conceptions of Modern Psychiatry*, W. W. Norton & Co., New York: 1953.

SYMONDS, PERCIVAL M., *The Dynamics of Human Adjustment*, Appleton-Century-Crofts, Inc., New York: 1946.

—— *Dynamics of Psychotherapy*, Vol. II, Grune and Stratton, New York: 1957.

UNIVERSITY OF COLORADO, *Contemporary Approaches to Cognition, A Symposium*, Harvard University Press, Cambridge, Mass.: 1957.

USHENKO, ANDREW P., *The Problem of Logic*, Princeton University Press, Princeton: 1941.

WALLERSTEIN, ROBERT S., *Hospital Treatment of Alcoholism*, Basic Books, Inc., New York: 1957.

WERTHEIMER, MAX, *Productive Thinking*, Harper and Brothers, New York: 1945.

WHITE, ROBERT W., *The Abnormal Personality*, The Ronald Press, New York: 1950.

WHITEHEAD, A. N., *Symbolism*, Capricorn Books, New York: 1959.

WILLIAMS, LINCOLN, *Tomorrow Will be Sober*, Harper and Brothers, New York: 1960.

WOLBERG, LEWIS R., *The Technique of Psychotherapy*, Grune and Stratton, New York: 1954.

WOLFF, CHARLOTTE, *Psychology of Gesture*, Methuen and Company, Ltd., London: 1948.

# PERIODICALS

AGRIN, ALFRED, "The Georgian Clinic," *Quart. J. Stud. Alcohol*, 21:113, 1960.

ALLISON, S. C., "Nondirective Group Therapy of Alcoholics in a State Hospital," *Quart. J. Stud. Alcohol*, Vol. 13, December, 1952.

ARIETI, S., "What is Effective in the Therapeutic Process," *Am. J. Psychoanal.*, 17:30, 1957.

ARMSTRONG, JOHN J., and GIBBINS, ROBERT J., "A Psychotherapeutic Technique with Large Groups in the Treatment of Alcoholics," *Quart. J. Stud. Alcohol*, 17:471, 1956.

BALES, ROBERT R., "Cultural Differences in Rates of Alcoholism," *Quart. J. Stud. Alcohol*, 6:418, 1946.

BATTEGAY, R., "Group Psychotherapy with Alcoholics and Analgesic Addicts," *Internat. J. Group Psychotherapy*, 8:428, 1958.

BELL, GORDON R., "Alcohol and Loneliness," *J. Soc. Ther.*, 2:171, 1956.

BENNIS, WARREN, "A Critique of Group Therapy Research," *Internat. J. Group Psychotherapy*, 10:63, 1960.

BIRDWHISTELL, RAY L., "Listen to the Body Bird," *Time*, 70:68, 1957.

BOURNE, LYLE E., "Effects of Delay of Information Feedback and Task Complexity on the Identification of Concepts," *J. Exper. Psychol.*, Vol. 54, 1957.

BOWMAN, KARL, "The Treatment of Alcoholics," *Quart. J. Stud. Alcohol*, 17:318, 1956.

BRIM, ORVILLE G., JR., "Attitude and Content-Intensity and Probability Expectations," *Am. Soc. Rev.*, Vol. 20, February, 1955.

BROWN, JAMES I., "The Measurement of Listening Ability," *School and Society*, 79:69, 1950.

BRUNNER-ORNE, MARTHA, "The Utilization of Group Psychotherapy in Enforced Treatment Programs for Alcoholics and Addicts," *Internat. J. Group Psycho-Therapy*, 6:292, 1956.

——— "Ward Group Sessions with Hospitalized Alcoholics and Motivation for Psychotherapy," *Internat. J. Group Psychotherapy*, 9:219, 1959.

——— and ORNE, MARTIN T., "Directive Group Therapy in the Treatment of Alcoholics: Technique and Rationale," *Internat. J. Group Psychotherapy*, 4:295, 1954.

BUERKLE, J., and BADGLEY, R., "Couple Role-Taking: The Yale Marital Interaction Battery," *Marriage and Family Living*, Vol. 21, February, 1959.

BURD, SHIRLEY FARLEY, "The Change From Institutional Living to Community Living," *Nursing World*, Vol. 133, October, 1959.

BUTTON, ALAN D., "The Psychodynamics of Alcoholism: A Survey of Eighty-Seven Cases," *Quart. J. Stud. Alcohol*, 17:443, 1956.

CHAFETY, MORRIS E., "Practical and Theoretical Considerations in the Psychotherapy of Alcoholism," *Quart. J. Stud. Alcohol*, 20:281, 1959.

CHAMBERS, JUANITA, "Maternal Deprivation and the Concept of Time in Children," *Am. J. Orthopsych.*, Vol. 21, No. 3.

CHASSAN, J., "On the Unreliability of Reliability and Some Other Consequences of the Assumption of Probabilistic Patient States," *Psychiatry*, Vol. 20, May, 1957.

CHILD, IRVIN L., POTTER, E. H., LEVINE, E. M., "Children's Textbooks and Personality Development: An Exploration in the Social Psychology of Education," *Psychological Monographs*, Vol. 60, No. 3, 1946.

CLANCY, JOHN, "Procrastination: A Defense Against Sobriety," *Quart. J. Stud. Alcohol*, Vol. 22, June, 1961.

CLARK, RUTH, "An Experimental Study of Silent Thinking," *Arch. Psychol.*, Vol. 11, No. 48, April, 1922.

CLAUSEN, JOHN A., et al., "The Impact of Mental Illness: Research Formulation," *J. Soc. Issues*, Vol. 11, No. 4, 1955.

——— and YARROW, M., "Paths to the Mental Hospital," *J. Soc. Issues*, Vol. 11, No. 4, 1955.

CLIEDMAN, LESTER H., ROSENTHAL, DAVID, FRANK, JEROME D., et al., "Group Therapy of Alcoholics with Concurrent Group Meetings of Their Wives," *Quart. J. Stud. Alcohol*, 17:633, 1956.

CLIFTON, STANLEY C., "A Technique for the Initial Interview with Male Alcoholics," *Quart. J. Stud. Alcohol*, 17:89, 1956.

COLE, N., BRANCH, C., and SHAW, O., "Mental Illness," *A.M.A. Arch. Neurol. Psychiat.*, Vol. 77, April, 1957.

CONFER, CHARLES M., "Reasoning as an Associative Process: III. The Role of Verbal Responses in Problem Solving," *J. Gen. Psychol.*, 57:55, 1957.

COUCH, C., "The Use of the Concept 'Role' and Its Derivatives in a Study of Marriage," *Marriage and Family Living*, Vol. 20, November, 1958.

CRIST, J., "Marriage Counseling Involving a Passive Husband and an Aggressive Wife," *Marriage and Family Living*, Vol. 20, May, 1958.

DEASY, L., and QUINN, O., "The Wife of the Mental Patient and the Hospital Psychiatrist," *J. Soc. Issues.* Vol. 11, No. 4, 1955.

DELEHANTY, E., "State Hospital Care of Alcoholics in Colorado," *J. Dis. Nerv. Sys.*, 8:40–42, 1947.

DEUTSH, M., and SOLOMON, L., "Some Methodological Suggestions for Research in a Family Counseling Setting," *Marriage and Family Living*, Vol. 20, February, 1958.

DINITZ, S., MANGUS, A., and PASAMANICK, B., "Integration and Conflict in Self-Other Conceptions as Factors in Mental Illness," *Sociometry*, Vol. 22, March, 1959.

DUNCKER, KARL, "On Problem Solving," *Psychol. Monographs*, 58:113, 1945.

ELDRED, STANLEY H., *et al.*, "A Procedure for the Systematic Analysis of Psychotherapeutic Interviews," *Psychiatry*, 17:337, 1954.

ELONEN, ANNA S., "The Effect of Child Rearing or Behavior in Different Cultures," *Am. J. Orthopsychiat.*, Vol. 21, No. 3, 1951.

ENDS, EARL J., and PAGE, CURTIS W., "A Study of Three Types of Group Psychotherapy with Hospitalized Male Inebriates," *Quart. J. Stud. Alcohol*, 18:263, 1957.

FEDERIGHI, E., "The Use of Chi-Square in Small Samples," *Am. Sociol. Rev.*, 15:770, 1950.

FERNANDEZ, THERESA M., "How to Deal with Overt Aggression," *Am. J. Nursing*, 59:113, 1959.

FOREMAN, PAUL B., "Panic Theory," *J. Sociol. Soc. Res.*, 37:295–304, 1953.

FORIZA, LORANT, "Brief Intensive Group Psychotherapy for the Treatment of Alcoholics," *The Psychiat. Quart. Supp.*, 29:43, 1955.

——— "Motivation of the Alcoholic for Recovery," *Quart. J. Stud. Alcohol*, 19:133, 1958.

FREEDMAN, A. M., "Day Hospitals for Severely Disturbed Schizophrenic Children," *Am. J. Psychiat.*, 115:893, 1958.

FREEMAN, H., and SIMMONS, O., "Wives, Mothers, and the Post-Hospital Performance of Mental Patients," *Social Forces*, 38:153, 1958.

GARRET, W., VAN, "Do You Ever Stop To Listen?," *American Mercury*, Vol. 83, November, 1956.

GOLDBERGER, EMANUAL, "The Id and the Ego: A Developmental Interpretation," *Psychoanal. Rev.*, Vol. 44, July, 1957.

GOVACCHINI, P., "Mutual Adaptation in Various Objects Relationships," *Internat. J. Psychoanal.*, 39:547, 1958.

GRAVENKEMPER, KATHERINE HEPP, "Hallucinations," *Nursing World*, Vol. 132, July, 1958.

GREENHILL, MAURICE, "Interviewing With a Purpose," *Am. J. Nursing*, Vol. 56, October, 1956.

GREGORY, B. A. J. C., "The Menstrual Cycle and Its Disorders in Psychiatric Patients," *J. Psychosomat. Res.*, 2:61–79, 1957.

HANFMAN, EUGENIA, and DASANIN, JACOB, "A Method for the Study of Concept Formation," *J. Psychol.*, 3:521–42, 1937.

HART, BETTY L., and ROHWEDER, ANN W., "Support in Nursing," *Am. J. Nursing*, Vol. 59, No. 10, 1959.

HAYS, DOROTHEA R., "Teaching a Concept of Anxiety to Patients," *Nursing Research*, Vol. 10, No. 2, 1961.

HEATH, R. C., "Group Psychotherapy of Alcohol Addiction," *Quart. J. Stud. Alcohol*, 5:555, 1945.

HERN, WOODBURN, "The Pathology of Boredom," *Scientific American*, Vol. 196, January, 1957.

HERTZKA, ALFRED F., and GUILFORD, G. P., "Logical Reasoning," *J. Consulting Psychology*, 19:405, 1955.

HEWITT, LESTER, "Student Perceptions of Traits Desired in Themselves as Dating and Marriage Partners," *Marriage and Family Living*, Vol. 20, November, 1958.

HIGGINS, JOHN W., "Psychodynamics in Excessive Drinking of Alcohol," *A.M.A. Arch. Neurol. & Psychiatry*, 69:713, 1953.

HIGHLEY, B. L., and NORRIS, C., "When A Student Dislikes A Patient," *Am. J. Nursing*, Vol. 57, September, 1957.

HOBART, C., "Disillusionment in Marriage, and Romanticism," *Marriage and Family Living*, 20:156, 1958.

HORTON, DONALD, "The Functions of Alcohol in Primitive Societies: A Cross Cultural Study," *Quart. J. Stud. Alcohol*, 4:199, 1943.

HUNTINGTON, R., "II., The Personality-Interaction Approach to Study of the Marital Relationship," *Marriage and Family Living*, 20:43, 1958.

HURTEAU, PHYLLIS, "The Psychiatric Nurse and The Mute Patient," Am. J. Nursing, Vol. 62, June, 1962.

INGLES, T., "The Worst Patient on the Floor," *Nursing Outlook*, Vol. 6, February, 1958.

——— "Mr. Parker—A 'Bad' Patient," *Nursing Outlook*, Vol. 6, April, 1958.

——— "Margaret—An Uncooperative Patient," *Nursing Outlook*, Vol. 6, May, 1958.

JACKSON, JOAN K., "The Definition and Measurement of Alcoholism, H-Technique Scales of Preoccupation with Alcohol and Psychological Involvement," *Quart. J. Stud. Alcohol*, 18:240, 1957.

JELLINEK, E. M., "The Problems of Alcohol," *Alcohol, Science, and Society* (Lectures with Discussions as given at Yale Summer School of Alcoholic Studies), *Quart. J. Stud. Alcohol*, 15:13, 1954.

JOURARD, SIDNEY, "How Well Do You Know Your Patients?," *Am. J. Nursing*, Vol. 59, November, 1959.

KANNER, LEO, and EISENBERG, LEON, "Review of Psychiatric Progress, 1957; Child Psychiatry," *Am. J. Psychiat.*, 114:609, 1958.

——— "Review of Psychiatric Progress, 1958; Child Psychiatry and Mental Deficiency," *Am. J. Psychiat.*, 115:608, 1959.

KAPLAN, A., and WOLF, L., "The Role of the Family in Relation to the Institutionalized Mental Patient," *Mental Hygiene*, 28:634, 1954.

KELLAND, C., "How Men and Women Act Facing Terror," *American Magazine*, Vol. 109, March, 1930.

KELLER, MARK, "Definition of Alcoholism," *Quart. J. Stud. Alcohol*, 21:125, 1960.

KINGHAM, RICHARD J., "Alcoholism and the Reinforcement of Theory of Learning," *Quart. J. Stud. Alcohol*, 19:320, 1958.

KROUT, MAURICE, "Autistic Gestures," *Psychol. Monographs*, 46, No. 4, 1935.

LA FORGE, R., and SUCZEK, R., "The Interpersonal Dimensions of Personality: III. An Interpersonal Check List," *J. Personality*, 24:94, 1955.

LEARY, T., "The Theory and Measurement Methodology of Interpersonal Communications," *Psychiatry*, 18:147, 1955.

LERNER, ARTHUR, "An Exploratory Approach in Group Counseling with Male Alcoholic Inmates in a City Jail," *Quart. J. Stud. Alcohol*, 14:427, 1953.

LEVINE, N., "The Mental Patient in the Community from the Viewpoint of the Family Agency," *Mental Hygiene*, 31:278, 1947.

LEVINSON, S., and WITHAY, M., "Sessions with Relatives of Mental Hospital Patients," *Mental Hygiene*, 39:118, 1955.

LEVY, ROBERT, "The Psychodynamic Functions of Alcohol," *Quart. J. Stud. Alcohol*, 19:649, 1958.

MANGUS, A., "Family Impacts on Mental Health," *Marriage and Family Living*, 19:256, 1957.

MARCONI, JUAN T., "The Concept of Alcoholism," *Quart. J. Stud. Alcohol*, 20:216, 1959.

MARSHALL, MARGARET A., "Hopelessness," *Nursing World*, Vol. 133, August, 1959.

MAXWELL, MILTON, "Interpersonal Factors in the Genesis and Treatment of Alcohol Addiction," *Social Forces*, 29:443, 1951.

MC CARTHY, R. G., "Group Therapy in an Outpatient Clinic for the Treatment of Alcoholism," *Quart. J. Stud. Alcohol*, 7(2):98, 1946.

MC CORD, WILLIAM, MC CORD, JOAN, and GUDEMAN, JON, "Some Current Theories of Alcoholism: A Longitudinal Evaluation," *Quart. J. Stud. Alcohol*, 20:727, 1959.

MERSAND, JOSEPH, "Why Teach Listening," *English Journal*, 40:260, 1951.

MOORE, R. A., and ROMSEUR, FRIEDA, "A Study of the Background of 100 Hospitalized Veterans with Alcoholism," *Quart. J. Stud. Alcohol*, 21:51, 1960.

NAVRATI, L., "On the Etiology of Alcoholism," *Quart. J. Stud. Alcohol*, 20:236, 1959.

PEI, MARIO, "Gesture Language," *Life*, Vol. 28, January 9, 1950.

PEPLAU, HILDEGARD E., "Themes in Nursing Situations: Safety," *Am. J. Nursing*, Vol. 53, November, 1953.

———— "Themes in Nursing Situations: Power," *Am. J. Nursing*, Vol. 53, October, 1953.

———— "Experiential Teaching," *Am. J. Nursing*, Vol. 57, July, 1957.

———— "Themes in Nursing Situations," *Am. J. Nursing*, Vol. 53, October, 1953.

———— "Interpersonal Techniques: Crux of Psychiatric Nursing," *Am. J. Nursing*, Vol. 62, June, 1962.

———— "Loneliness," *Am. J. Nursing*, Vol. 55, November, 1955.

PETTIT, L., "Attitudes of Relatives of Long Hospitalized Mental Patients Regarding Convalescent Leave," *Mental Hygiene*, Vol. 40, April, 1956.

PFEFFER, A. Z., FRIEDLAND, P., and WORTIS, H., "Group Therapy with Alcoholics, Preliminary Report," *Quart. J. Stud. Alcohol*, 1:217, 1949.

POPE, BENJAMIN, "Attitudes Toward Group Therapy in a Psychiatric Clinic for Alcoholics," *Quart. J. Stud. Alcohol*, 17:233, 1956.

QUARANTELLI, ENRICO, "The Behavior of Panic Participants," *J. Appl. Sociol.*, Vol. 41, 1957.

———— "The Nature and Conditions of Panic," *J. Sociol.*, Vol. 60, 1954.

RILEY, JOHN W., "The Social Implications of Problem Drinking," *Social Forces*, 27:301, 1949.

RINKEL, MAX, and SOLOMON, HARRY C., "Chemical Theories of Psychosis," *J. Clin. Exper. Psychol.*, 18:323, 1957.

RITRO, SAMUEL, and SOLNIT, ALBERT, "Influences of Early Mother-Child Inter-action on Identification Processes," *The Psychoanalytic Study of the Child,* Vol. 13, 1958.

ROBINSON, ALICE M., "Communicating With Schizophrenic Patients," *Am. J. Nursing,* Vol. 60, August, 1960.

ROGERS, M., "Reference Group Influences on Student Drinking Behavior," *Quart. J. Stud. Alcohol,* 19:244, 1958.

SCHWARTZ, C. G., "Perspectives on Deviance—Wives' Definitions of their Hus-bands' Mental Illness," *Psychiatry,* Vol. 20, August, 1957.

SCHWARTZ, D., "Uncooperative Patients?," *Am. J. Nursing,* Vol. 58, January, 1958.

SCOTT, B., "My Psychotherapy Helped My Entire Family," *Marriage and Fam-ily Living,* 20:128, 1958.

SCOTT, EDWARD M., "A Special Type of Group Therapy and Its Application To Alcoholics," *Quart. J. Stud. Alcohol,* 17:288, 1956.

——— "The Technique of Psychotherapy with Alcoholics," *Quart. J. Stud. Alcohol,* 22:69, 1961.

SEARS, ROBERT R., "Non-Aggressive Reaction to Frustration," *Psychol. Rev.,* 48:343, 1941.

SILLER, JEROME, "Socioeconomic Status and Conceptual Thinking," *J. Ab-normal Soc. Psychol.,* Vol. 55, November, 1957.

STEINMANN, A., "Lack of Communication Between Men and Women," *Mar-riage and Family Living,* 20:350, 1958.

STEWART, DAVID A., "Empathy in the Group Therapy of Alcoholics," *Quart. J. Stud. Alcohol,* 15:74, 1954.

STOMER, W. F., "Listening: How?," *English Journal,* Vol. 41, June, 1952.

STRAUSS, ANSELM, "The Literature on Panic," *J. Abnormal Soc. Psychol.,* Vol. 39, 1944.

STRAYER, ROBER, "Social Integration of Alcoholics Through Prolonged Group Therapy," *Quart. J. Stud. Alcohol,* 22:471, 1961.

STRECKER, EDWARD A., "Psychotherapy in Pathological Drinking," *J.A.M.A.,* 147(9):74, 1951.

TALLAND, GEORGE, "Criteria in Conceptual Transposition," *Am. J. Psychol.,* Vol. 70, 1957.

THOMPSON, CHARLES E., and KOLB, WILLIAM P., "Group Psychotherapy in As-sociation with Alcoholics Anonymous," *Am. J. Psychiat.,* 110:29, 1953.

TRAEGER, HARVEY, "How You Can Help the Alcoholic Offender," *Federal Probation,* 22:25, 1958.

TUDOR, GWEN E., "A Sociopsychiatric Nursing Approach to Intervention in a Problem of Mutual Withdrawal on a Mental Hospital Ward," *Psychiatry,* Vol. 15, May, 1952.

VARLEY, BARBARA K., "Reaching Out, Therapy With Schizophrenic Patients," *Am. J. Orthopsychiat.,* 29:407, 1959.

VOGEL, SIDNEY, "Some Aspects of Group Psychotherapy with Alcoholics," *Internat. J. Group Psychotherapy,* 7:302, 1957.

WARD, A., and JONES, G., "Helping the Families of Our Mentally Sick," *Mental Hygiene,* 38:576, 1954.

WASHBURNE, CHANDLER, "Alcohol, Self, and the Group," *Quart. J. Stud. Alco-hol,* 17:108, 1956.

WEISMAN, G., "Silence and Psychotherapy," *Psychiatry, J. Study Interpersonal Processes,* 18:241, 1955.

WERNER, H., and KAPLAN, B., "Developmental Approach to Cognition: Its

Relevance to the Psychological Interpretation of Anthropological and Ethnolinguistic Data," *Am. Anthrop.*, October, 1956.

WYNN, D. R., "Good Listener," *J. Nat. Educ.*, 44:502, 1953.

YARROW, M., *et al.*, "The Psychological Meaning of Mental Illness in the Family," *J. Social Issues.* 11(4):12, 1955.

YARROW, M. R., CLAUSEN, J., and ROBBINS, P., "The Social Meaning of Mental Illness," *J. Social Issues*, 11(4):33, 1955.

ZELKO, H. P., "Art of Listening," *Rotarian*, 87(6):127, 1955.

ZILBOORG, GREGORY, "Loneliness," *Atlantic Monthly*, 161(1):45, 1938.

## UNPUBLISHED REPORTS AND PAPERS

BREGG, ELIZABETH A., LEDDY, MARY C., and MAC KENZIE, LILLIAN G., *A Study on the Nurse's Concept of Death*, master's thesis, Columbia University, New York: 1953.

COX, JOYCE E., DAVIS, M. E., FERNANDEZ, T. M., JOHANNESON, L., and TOSIELLO, F. C., *Trends and Directions*, master's thesis, Columbia University, New York: 1953.

FARLEY, SHIRLEY, *Family Views on Mental Illness*, master's thesis, Graduate School, Rutgers, The State University of New Jersey, New Brunswick: 1957.

HEPP, KATHERINE, *Two Instruments to Inventory and Classify Problems*, master's thesis, Graduate School, Rutgers, The State University of New Jersey, New Brunswick: 1957.

RICHTER, BETTIJEAN, *Exploratory Empirical Testing of Arieti's Theory of Paleologic*, master's thesis, Graduate School, Rutgers, The State University of New Jersey, New Brunswick: 1960.

RICHTER, DOROTHEA, *Teaching a Concept of Anxiety to Patients*, master's thesis, Graduate School, Rutgers, The State University of New Jersey, New Brunswick: 1957.

SETTLAGE, CALVIN, F., "The Values of Limits in Child Rearing," unpublished paper, Family Service of Philadelphia, February, 1958.

SMOYAK, SHIRLEY A., *Marriage and Mental Illness*, master's thesis, Graduate School, Rutgers, The State University of New Jersey, New Brunswick: 1959.

WERNER, ANITA M., *An Exploratory Investigation of Teaching a Problem Solving Process in Group Therapy to Patients Diagnosed Chronic Alcoholism*, master's thesis, Graduate School, Rutgers, The State University of New Jersey, New Brunswick: 1962.

# INDEX

—375

Trust, 73–76
  development, 73–74
  nursing intervention, 74–76
Tudor, Gwen E., 106

Umland, Theo J., 87–89

Value judgments, 63, 79, 128–29, 181,
    203, 252–70
"Veil" phenomenon, 189–94
  nursing intervention, 191–94
  roots and purpose, 194
  theoretical framework, 189–90

Verbal communication, 18–26, 77. *See also*
    Nursing intervention technique
  nursing intervention, 19–24

Waiting, 67–72
  distortions, 70–72
  expectations, 68
  personality development, 69–70
  power, 69
  readiness, 69
  time, 68
Weiss, Olga, 278
Werner, Anita M., 59–62, 73–76, 239–47,
    360